D1527733

NIGHT EATING SYNDROME

Also from Albert J. Stunkard

Handbook of Obesity Treatment
Thomas A. Wadden and Albert J. Stunkard, Editors

Night Eating Syndrome

Research, Assessment,
and Treatment

Edited by

Jennifer D. Lundgren
Kelly C. Allison
Albert J. Stunkard

Foreword by James E. Mitchell

THE GUILFORD PRESS
New York   London

© 2012 The Guilford Press
A Division of Guilford Publications, Inc.
72 Spring Street, New York, NY 10012
www.guilford.com

Printed in the United States of America

This book is printed on acid-free paper.

Last digit is print number: 9 8 7 6 5 4 3 2 1

The authors have checked with sources believed to be reliable in their efforts to provide information
that is complete and generally in accord with the standards of practice that are accepted at the
time of publication. However, in view of the possibility of human error or changes in behavioral,
mental health, or medical sciences, neither the authors, nor the editors and publisher, nor any
other party who has been involved in the preparation or publication of this work warrants
that the information contained herein is in every respect accurate or complete, and they are not
responsible for any errors or omissions or the results obtained from the use of such information.
Readers are encouraged to confirm the information contained in this book with other sources.

Library of Congress Cataloging-in-Publication Data is available from the publisher

ISBN 978-1-4625-0630-9

For Justin and Sam, who remind me
of the important things in life
—J. D. L.

For my husband, Jim, and my sons, Tyler and Xavier,
who provide me with the smiles and support
that keep my perspective balanced
—K. C. A.

For my wife, Margaret,
my daughter and son-in-law, Alana and Keith,
and my wonderful grandchildren, Maya and Luca,
whom I treasure beyond words
—A. J. S.

About the Editors

Jennifer D. Lundgren, PhD, is Associate Professor and Chair of the Department of Psychology at the University of Missouri–Kansas City. Her research focuses on eating disorders and obesity.

Kelly C. Allison, PhD, is Assistant Professor of Psychology in the Department of Psychiatry at the Perelman School of Medicine at the University of Pennsylvania, where she is also Director of Education at the Center for Weight and Eating Disorders.

Albert J. Stunkard, MD, is Emeritus Professor of Psychiatry at the Perelman School of Medicine at the University of Pennsylvania. He is the founder of the Center for Weight and Eating Disorders, where an endowed professorship has been named for him, and is a member of the Institute of Medicine and the National Academy of Sciences.

Contributors

Kelly C. Allison, PhD (*see* "About the Editors").

Drew A. Anderson, PhD, is Associate Professor and Director of Clinical Training at the University at Albany, State University of New York.

Raymond Boston, PhD, is Professor of Applied Biomathematics in the Department of Clinical Studies, School of Veterinary Medicine, and Professor of Biostatistics in the Department of Biostatistics and Epidemiology at the Perelman School of Medicine at the University of Pennsylvania. He is also a Senior Scholar in the Center for Clinical Epidemiology and Biostatistics.

Cynthia M. Bulik, PhD, is the Jordan Distinguished Professor of Eating Disorders in the Department of Psychiatry at the University of North Carolina at Chapel Hill, where she is also Professor of Nutrition in the Gillings School of Global Public Health and Director of the University of North Carolina Eating Disorders Program.

Susan L. Colles, PhD, is a researcher and lecturer in the Master of Dietetics program at the University of South Australia. She is a clinical dietitian with expertise in the nutritional and behavioral management of bariatric surgery recipients. Her research focuses primarily on associations among eating-related cognitions, behavioral patterns, and body weight.

Mario A. Cristancho, MD, is a member of the Clinical Research Scholars Program of the Department of Psychiatry at the Perelman School of Medicine at the University of Pennsylvania.

Ross D. Crosby, PhD, is Director of Biomedical Statistics at the Neuropsychiatric Research Institute and Professor of Clinical Neuroscience at the University of North Dakota School of Medicine and Health Sciences.

Scott J. Crow, MD, is Professor in the Department of Psychiatry at the University of Minnesota, Past President of the Academy for Eating Disorders, and Director of the Clinical Populations–Disordered Eating Assessment Core of the Minnesota Obesity Center. His clinical and research focus is on the clinical course and management of anorexia nervosa, bulimia nervosa, and binge-eating disorder.

John B. Dixon, PhD, is National Health and Medical Research Council Senior Research Fellow, combining positions in vascular and hypertension–obesity research at Baker IDI Heart and Diabetes Institute and the Department of General Practice, Monash University, Melbourne, Australia.

Scott G. Engel, PhD, is Research Scientist at the Neuropsychiatric Research Institute and Assistant Professor of Clinical Neuroscience at the University of North Dakota School of Medicine and Health Sciences.

Allan Geliebter, PhD, is Senior Research Scientist in the Department of Psychiatry at Columbia University College of Physicians and Surgeons and Professor of Psychology at Touro Graduate School in New York.

Marci E. Gluck, PhD, is Research Clinical Psychologist in the Obesity and Diabetes Clinical Research Section of the National Institute of Diabetes and Digestive and Kidney Diseases in Phoenix, Arizona.

Michael J. Howell, MD, is Assistant Professor in the Department of Neurology at the University of Minnesota, where he is Director of the Parasomnia Program. His clinical and research focus is on abnormal nocturnal behaviors arising from sleep (parasomnias).

Yael Latzer, DSc, is Associate Professor in the Faculty of Social Welfare and Health Sciences at the University of Haifa and the founder and director of the Institute for the Treatment and Study of Eating Disorders in the Division of Psychiatry at Rambam Health Care Campus, Haifa, Israel.

Jennifer D. Lundgren, PhD (*see* "About the Editors").

James E. Mitchell, MD, is the NRI/Lee A. Christoferson M.D. Professor and Chairman of the Department of Clinical Neuroscience at the University of North Dakota School of Medicine and Health Sciences. He is also the Chester Fritz Distinguished University Professor at the University of North Dakota and President and Scientific Director of the Neuropsychiatric Research Institute. Dr. Mitchell's research has focused on eating disorders, obesity, and bariatric surgery.

Meghan E. Murphy, MA, is a doctoral student in clinical psychology at the University of Missouri–Kansas City. She is currently a clinical psychology intern at the VA Western New York Health Care System in Buffalo, New York.

Glenys K. Noble, PhD, is Lecturer of Equine Science in the School of Animal and Veterinary Sciences at Charles Sturt University, New South Wales, Australia.

John P. O'Reardon, MD, is Associate Professor of Psychiatry at the Perelman School of Medicine at the University of Pennsylvania. His clinical and research interests include treatment-resistant mood disorders; the development of novel neuromodulation therapies in psychiatry such as transcranial magnetic stimulation, vagus nerve stimulation, and deep brain stimulation; cognitive therapy; and night eating syndrome.

Kajal R. Patel, MD, is Fellow in Psychosomatic Medicine in the Department of Psychiatry at the Perelman School of Medicine at the University of Pennsylvania.

Laura Pawlow, PhD, is Associate Professor in the Department of Psychology at Southern Illinois University Edwardsville. Her research and clinical interests include weight management.

Melisa V. Rempfer, PhD, is Associate Professor in the Department of Psychology at the University of Missouri–Kansas City, where her research focuses on serious mental illness.

Tammy L. Root, PhD, is Assistant Professor in the Department of Psychiatry at the University of North Carolina at Chapel Hill. She also serves as faculty at Walden University.

Cristin D. Runfola, MS, is a clinical psychology doctoral candidate at Palo Alto University and an eating disorders predoctoral psychology intern in the Department of Psychiatry at the University of North Carolina at Chapel Hill.

Albert J. Stunkard, MD (*see* "About the Editors").

Orna Tzischinsky, DSc, is Associate Professor in the Psychology Department at Emek Yezreel Academic College, Emek Yezreel, Israel, and a senior researcher in the Sleep Laboratory at the Technion, Israel Institute of Technology, Haifa, Israel.

Tatiana Ungredda, MA, MEd, is a clinical psychology doctoral candidate at Texas A&M University in College Station, Texas.

Piergiuseppe Vinai, MD, is a psychologist, psychotherapist, and teacher at the Italian Society of Behavioral and Cognitive Therapy (SITCC) and at the Post Graduate Psychotherapy Cognitive School in Milan. He is also the cofounder of the nonprofit research group GNOSIS in Cuneo, Italy.

Foreword

Albert J. (Mickey to everyone who knows him) Stunkard, along with his colleagues William J. Grace and Harold G. Wolff, wrote a seminal paper in 1955 describing night eating syndrome (NES) for the first time. Mickey, always the astute clinician and careful observer, described an interesting and important problem that hadn't been noted previously. What was also particularly interesting was that the paper failed to stimulate much interest in, or research on, the disorder until the last two decades, when the concept was revitalized by Mickey and others. Now we have a much better clinical and scientific understanding of NES, thanks in large part to the editors and chapter authors of this volume, including Jennifer D. Lundgren, Kelly C. Allison, and Mickey himself.

The book is laid out in a way that is both comprehensive and user friendly. First, the editors offer an introduction to NES. Then, Mickey reviews the history of NES, which is only appropriate given his pivotal role in our understanding of patients with this disorder. This is followed by three thoughtful chapters on the psychobiology of NES. The chapters offer interesting overviews on topics such as circadian rhythms and neuroendocrine aspects of NES. The contributors of these chapters represent the group of individuals who have done much of the pioneering work in the psychobiology of NES.

The next section provides a detailed examination of the relationship between NES and other disorders and procedures, including obesity, bariatric surgery, eating disorders, other psychiatric disorders, and sleep/movement disorders. This again provides a comprehensive, well-written overview of the research data in this area, the clinical implications of these data, and the controversies in this area. Further work is needed to address how NES should fit into the nomenclature and what overlap NES has with other conditions.

Next come two chapters addressing conceptual issues concerning assessment of NES and the assessment instruments that have been developed for this purpose, including the Night Eating Syndrome History and Inventory. The latest version of this instrument grew out of a meeting of individuals interested in NES that was held in Minneapolis (which I had the pleasure of attending) and has provided for better standardization for data collection in clinical practice.

This is followed by a section on treatment approaches for NES. Although the controlled treatment literature on NES is still modest, certain psychopharmacological agents and psychotherapeutic techniques do appear to affect NES. Chapter 14 offers a detailed presentation of the cognitive-behavioral treatment manual that Kelly Allison and Mickey developed. The book concludes with a thoughtful epilogue by the editors.

Overall, this volume provides a very useful overview and thorough introduction to NES. It will be of great value to both clinicians and researchers and highlights not only what has been learned but what remains controversial. Jennifer, Kelly, and Mickey are to be congratulated for pulling together the best people working in this area, offering an up-to-date, comprehensive, yet accessible compilation of the status of NES. One has the sense that this volume is not only very timely, but will also focus increased clinical interest and research on this important topic.

JAMES A. MITCHELL, MD

Acknowledgments

This edited volume is the culmination of many years of research that have advanced our understanding of night eating syndrome (NES). We are pleased to have so many wonderful colleagues who are now actively engaged in investigating this disorder and who have contributed to this book. It has truly been an international effort.

We would also like to thank the many patients and participants we have seen who have shared their personal stories and participated in our studies in the service of advancing our knowledge of the underpinnings and possible treatments for NES.

It is sometimes difficult to work on an issue that is not well recognized. Therefore, the unwavering support of our colleagues at our universities has been greatly appreciated. This includes the faculty and staff of the Center for Weight and Eating Disorders in the Department of Psychiatry at the Perelman School of Medicine at the University of Pennsylvania, and of the Department of Psychology at the University of Missouri–Kansas City. Drs. Thomas Wadden, David Sarwer, Robert Berkowitz, Reneé Moore, Lucy Faulconbridge, Tanja Kral, and Melisa Rempfer have offered their expertise, insights, and friendship throughout this process.

Thanks to The Guilford Press and our editorial team, Jim Nageotte, Jane Keislar, and Jeannie Tang, for their help in assembling and presenting the material from start to finish. They have been a pleasure to work with and we are grateful for their commitment to disseminating this work on NES. We would also like to thank Dr. Jim Mitchell for his encouragement and contribution to this volume.

Finally, we would like to thank our families and friends, who may not have always understood our passion for this work but who were always there to support it.

Contents

PART III. RELATION TO OTHER CLINICAL SYNDROMES

PART IV. ASSESSMENT

PART V. TREATMENT

PART I

INTRODUCTION AND HISTORY

Chapter 1

Introduction to Night Eating Syndrome

Past, Present, and Future

Jennifer D. Lundgren
Kelly C. Allison
Albert J. Stunkard

More than five decades have passed since the eating pattern now known as night eating syndrome (NES) was first recognized in the medical literature. Inarguably, NES is better understood now than it was in the 1950s, but in many ways our conceptualization, assessment, and treatment of NES is still in its infancy. We thought it was both timely and appropriate to provide the research and clinical communities with a comprehensive resource to help understand and treat NES better.

In preparing this book, our aim has been to help those who suffer from NES by providing the professional reader with the scientific knowledge base and clinical tools necessary to study and treat NES. As such, this book is written for the scientific and clinical communities, but most important, it is written to help those who suffer from NES.

Case Examples

Each of us has worked closely with individuals who have struggled to overcome their night eating. We are grateful to those whose personal experiences with NES have informed our research and led to better assessment and treatment for this condition. Although everyone's story is different, those with NES often share similar core experiences. These case examples illustrate the impact that NES can have on people who suffer from it.

Lisa

Lisa presented self-referred for treatment of her NES. She also reported struggling with panic disorder. She is a 19-year-old single, Caucasian female who is currently a sophomore in college. Her parents are married, and she has one sister. All of her family members also struggle with some form of anxiety, including her sister, who has obsessive–compulsive disorder. Lisa reports a history of panic disorder since her sophomore year of high school. Last year, she "broke down" and finished the spring semester from home. She began taking a selective serotonin reuptake inhibitor (SSRI) to treat her anxiety, but she began waking up during the night with a "gnawing" feeling in her stomach, compelling her to eat. These nocturnal ingestions began once per night within the first 2 weeks of taking the SSRI, but increased to its current intensity of three to five each night as her dose increased. She discontinued the SSRI in September, but her night eating has continued.

Lisa returned to school this semester. She currently lives in a house with five female roommates. She has a single bedroom, which is next to the kitchen. She reports that she enjoys her current living situation.

Lisa reports that she reached her highest weight of 135 pounds at the age of 15. After that, she dropped down to 110 pounds. She did not receive treatment for anorexia, and she reports that she continued menstruating regularly. She does report having a history of "control issues" with eating. Her current weight at evaluation was 118.6 pounds. She stated that she is comfortable with her current weight, but is very worried that her night eating will increase her weight.

To deal with the anxiety about weight gain linked to her nocturnal ingestions, Lisa compensates with exercise. She works out for approximately 90 minutes per day, 7 days per week. These workouts include a variety of activities, including spin class, running on the treadmill, and other activities at the gym. She was up to running 13 miles, but she hurt her knee and was forced to modify her routine. She did not cut back on her overall time spent engaging in physical activity, despite this injury.

Lisa wakes most days at about 9:00 A.M. Her classes begin at about 10:30 A.M. When she wakes up, she is not hungry. She has a small breakfast, typically a yogurt or oatmeal, sometime before noon. She next eats at about 3:00 P.M., when she eats a soup or salad or oatmeal or cereal. She often fits in her workout after classes. Dinner consists of sushi or a salad. She does not eat much meat, but prefers nuts, tofu, fish, and meal-replacement bars as her sources of protein. At night, she usually snacks just before going to bed to make sure she is full. She typically has some combination of peanut butter, popcorn, frozen yogurt, and whipped topping.

She goes to bed between 1:00 and 2:00 A.M. and it usually takes her about 30 minutes to fall asleep. Initial insomnia is a long-standing issue, and she has been taking an over-the-counter antihistamine to help her fall asleep. She wakes up about 1 hour after falling asleep and eats each time she is up, ranging from three to five times per night. She snacks on pretzels, peanut butter, cereal, and other foods that she has eaten during the day. Sometimes her portion is controlled, but if there is a specific food, such as birthday cake, in the house, she will eat through the majority of the cake in one night. When she is drinking alcohol, she wakes to eat more often and consumes much more food, such as a box of cereal. She typically drinks two to three times per week and has two to five drinks each time. She claims that the urge to eat during the night is overwhelming. Despite keeping flavored water in her bedroom, she is overcome by what she describes as a physical sensation of needing to eat and feels unable to stay in her room and resume sleep without eating. Overall, she meets criteria for NES, which is also supported by a score of 39 on the Night Eating Questionnaire (NEQ).

As stated above, Lisa has had a history of panic disorder since she was a sophomore in high school. Her first attempt at medication treatment was with an SSRI, but taking this medication coincided with her onset of NES, even though SSRIs have shown efficacy in treating NES in research studies. Lisa reports that she feels as though she is going to have a panic attack every day, but most days she can control them. She states that they come on out of the blue. She is curious about taking another medication to control them, but is wary of anti-anxiety medications, given her last experience.

Lisa has strong friendships and is involved in campus life. She does not have a boyfriend currently, but is dating. Her roommates are aware of her struggles with night eating and try to be supportive. She is wary of having a bed partner at this point because of her night eating. She drinks alcohol two to three times per week and engages in binge drinking on some of those occasions. She is aware that this exacerbates her nocturnal ingestions.

Lisa reports problems with acid reflux, for which she takes Prevacid.

She is also on an oral contraceptive. Finally, she is taking a 5-hydroxy-tryptophan supplement and an antihistamine to help with her mood and sleep. She is considering trying another SSRI to help with her panic and night eating symptoms.

Bridget

Bridget was referred for problems with NES as she prepared for bariatric surgery. She is twice divorced and is now living with her husband and stepson, who is a senior in high school. Her husband is supportive of her efforts, but she has had trouble controlling the type and amount of food in the house during their 3 years of marriage. Since then, she has gained almost 100 pounds.

Bridget reports a history of eating during the evening and night since childhood. She remembers that her mother and sister also had NES. Her father and brother did not. She reports that she has always functioned best at night, particularly from 10:00 P.M. to 1:00 A.M. She wakes to eat almost every night, usually between 1:30 and 2:00 A.M. Her initial thought is, "What's in the fridge?" She will go eat the particular food she is craving and subsequently is able to return to sleep quickly. Typical foods consumed during nocturnal ingestions include bread, cereal (one or two bowls), and ice cream.

Bridget believed she was overweight as a child, but looking at pictures, she realizes that she was not particularly overweight. She is active and has enjoyed exercise throughout her life. In her early to mid-30s, she was running marathons and was at a healthy weight. Her weight slowly increased after her activity was curtailed. She is currently at her highest weight, with a body mass index of 42 kg/m^2.

She has not exercised much recently. She complains that her weight interferes with her activity and contributes to her fatigue. After work she may drive to the gym, but then take a nap in her car instead of going in and exercising. She typically has difficulties with seasonal affective disorder (SAD), and she believes her fatigue in the late afternoon during the winter is worsened by this disorder.

Bridget wakes between 7:30 and 7:45 A.M. and is not at all hungry. She first eats between 11:00 A.M. and 1:00 P.M., when she will have a lunch of soup, bread, and coffee. She occasionally has an afternoon snack, for example a snack pack of Oreo cookies. After work she eats dinner at 7:30 P.M. A cook prepares her meals, which are nutritionally balanced. However, she reports eating very large portions. After dinners she continues eating leftovers, chips, and other available snacks. She describes herself as restless, and part of her grazing behavior is spurred by this restlessness, as well as boredom in the evening. She eats just before going to bed, typically between 11:30 and midnight, to try to prevent nocturnal ingestions. She only occasionally experiences initial insomnia.

Between 1:30 and 2:00 A.M. she wakes with the urge to eat. Although she may use the bathroom at this time, the main reason for arousal is to seek food. Within 5 minutes of eating her preferred snack, she falls back to sleep. She is awake and aware during these nocturnal eating episodes. She repeats this behavior every night, once per night. Bridget has controlled this behavior in the past by keeping most foods out of the house. She believes that surgery will help her control her intake. Her stepson will be leaving for college in the fall, which will also help her limit foods that are brought into the house.

Bridget has a history of major depressive disorder (MDD), with her first episode in the early 1990s. She received psychotherapy and fluoxetine with some success. Her second episode of MDD occurred in the late 1990s, when she was diagnosed with melanoma. She was switched to escitalopram and has stayed on this medication at 10 mg per day. Her score of 7 on the Beck Depression Inventory–II indicates mild levels of depressed mood currently. Her medical practice with children with serious illnesses certainly contributes to her struggles with depression. She also reports symptoms consistent with SAD. She uses bright light therapy inconsistently to help these symptoms.

Bridget did not report significant anxiety symptoms, with a Beck Anxiety Inventory score of 4 and no previous anxiety diagnosis. However, she seemed anxious in the interview, with some pressured speech, stuttering, and perspiration. In addition, she describes feeling restless in the evenings when she is trying to relax with her husband. She is unable to sit still to watch her favorite television shows, which contributes to her evening grazing. Bridget has an extensive family history of mental illness. Her mother has bipolar disorder, and her sister has borderline personality disorder and MDD. Her sister is deceased, and Bridget suspects she committed suicide.

Bridget experiences cluster headaches. She takes Imitrex to help control these. She believes they are seasonal and coincide with her SAD. She also has high cholesterol, hypertension, and gastroesophageal reflux disease (GERD). These are also controlled by medications, and she hopes that the gastric bypass procedure will help reduce the signs and symptoms related to these diseases. She is also a cancer survivor of melanoma, which she suffered in the late 1990s.

Paul

Paul presented for treatment of his NES and for weight loss. He was referred by a sleep center. He is on many medications to manage his chronic neck pain, which have likely contributed to his weight gain and possibly influence his night eating symptoms.

Paul was a computer specialist when he developed serious and chronic neck pain more than a decade ago. He stopped working several years ago and has only been able to work part-time since then. Paul lives with his domestic partner, an adopted teenage son, a foster daughter, a dog, and a cat. His children present multiple challenges. These family issues, along with his pain, have created and maintain the high levels of chronic stress in his life.

Paul's pain has caused insomnia. About 3 years ago, he remembers starting to eat ice cream during the night to help ease the pain and likely to help soothe his stomach due to discomfort from his numerous medications. Since then, his nocturnal ingestions have steadily increased. He currently wakes to eat one to three times each night.

Paul reports maintaining a normal weight as a child and into early adulthood. He exercised frequently until his chronic neck pain began. He is now at his heaviest weight. Over the last 10 years he has been treated with several medications that are known to cause weight gain, which have interfered with his efforts to lose weight.

Currently, Paul wakes at about 7:30 each morning. He has a 40- to 60-minute commute to work. If he eats breakfast before driving, he has a yogurt, cereal, and juice. His morning snack typically consists of pretzels. Lunchtime is variable and can often be delayed until 2:00 P.M.. He has leftovers or purchases his lunch, such as sushi or a chicken sandwich. In the afternoon he has one to two cups of tapioca pudding or a cookie and milk. He typically walks the dog for 1 mile either before or after dinner. Dinner is usually between 7:00 and 8:00 P.M.. He and his partner cook nutritious meals. Paul avoids processed foods and attempts to eat fresh foods.

After dinner he reads, surfs the Internet, or takes care of household duties. He has between one to three snacks in the evening, which he usually feels compelled to eat. He consumes a snack just before going to bed in order to stave off the gnawing feeling he describes in his stomach, which he attributes to his nighttime medications, including Niaspan, Lexapro, oxycodone, Rozerem, and Benadryl. He goes to bed at 10:00 P.M., using a continuous positive airway pressure (CPAP) machine to treat his sleep apnea. About once per week he sleeps through the night, but typically he wakes between 1 to 2 hours after falling asleep. He feels hunger and believes that he cannot fall back to sleep unless he eats. He describes it as an overwhelming, consuming feeling, as if it is "chemically driven." He consumes snacks such as tapioca, cookies, pie, ice cream, popcorn, and sometimes he cooks. He may eat in the kitchen or bring food up to the office while using the Internet. He repeats this up to three times each night. Paul's score of 34 on the NEQ meets the clinical cut score for NES, and he meets the diagnostic criteria for NES.

Paul has a long history of clinical depression. He has a therapist whom he sees with his partner to deal with his depression, cope with his pain, and to keep their relationship strong amid their many life stressors. He takes Lexapro (10 mg) and Cymbalta (60 mg, twice per day), as prescribed by his psychiatrist, to alleviate his depression. His score of 22 on the Beck Depression Inventory suggests a moderate level of depressive symptoms, consistent with his self-description. He has passive suicidal ideation, but no plan. His score of 2 on the Beck Anxiety Inventory suggests minimal anxiety symptoms currently. Paul works to keep his relationship strong. He leads a busy life despite his pain, although his level of activity exhausts him by the end of each day.

As these case examples illustrate, the core feature of NES, since its original description in 1955 (Stunkard, Grace, & Wolf, 1955), has been a circadian-delayed pattern of food intake, which manifests behaviorally as excessive food consumption in the evening relative to total daily food intake (i.e., evening hyperphagia) and/or waking at night and eating (i.e., nocturnal ingestion). As more people with nighttime eating problems have been studied, the definition of NES has developed. In March 2008, several eating and sleep researchers convened for the first International Symposium on NES. From this meeting came a comprehensive set of research diagnostic criteria for NES, which have been published in the *International Journal of Eating Disorders* (Allison et al., 2010) and are outlined in Table 1.1.

These criteria are a step in the right direction toward a comprehensive, evidence-based conceptualization of NES, but as several of the chapters in this book illustrate, much more research is necessary to validate these diagnostic criteria and to establish their clinical utility.

TABLE 1.1. Research Diagnostic Criteria for NES

A. The daily pattern of eating demonstrates a significantly increased intake in the evening and/or nighttime, as manifested by one or both of the following:

  1. At least 25% of food intake is consumed after the evening meal
  2. At least two episodes of nocturnal eating per week

B. Awareness and recall of evening and nocturnal eating episodes are present.

(continued)

TABLE 1.1. *(continued)*

C. The clinical picture is characterized by at least three of the following features:

1. Lack of desire to eat in the morning and/or breakfast is omitted on four or more mornings per week
2. Presence of a strong urge to eat between dinner and sleep onset and/or during the night
3. Sleep onset and/or sleep maintenance insomnia are present four or more nights per week
4. Presence of a belief that one must eat in order to initiate or return to sleep
5. Mood is frequently depressed and/or mood worsens in the evening

D. The disorder is associated with significant distress and/or impairment in functioning.

E. The disordered pattern of eating has been maintained for at least 3 months.

F. The disorder is not secondary to substance abuse or dependence, medical disorder, medication, or another psychiatric disorder.

Note. From Allison et al. (2010). Copyright 2010 by John Wiley & Sons, Inc. Reprinted by permission.

A Guide to This Book

This book is designed to be a resource for both scientists and practitioners. In that regard, it both reviews the scientific knowledge base of NES and functions as a clinical tool box for treatment providers. The book is presented in six parts.

Part I. Introduction and History

- *History of NES.* Chapter 2 (Stunkard) reviews the original conceptualization of NES and chronicles its development through the recently introduced research diagnostic criteria (Allison et al., 2010) and proposal for inclusion in the forthcoming edition of the *Diagnostic and Statistical Manual of Mental Disorders* (DSM-5) as an eating disorder not otherwise specified (EDNOS; *www.dsm5.org*). In this chapter, Stunkard provides an account of his first clinical patients whom he diagnosed with NES.

Part II. Biology

- *Pathophysiological and neuroendocrine aspects of NES.* Recent advances in brain imaging techniques have contributed to a better understanding of neurotransmitter systems and brain areas associated with eating, sleep, and mood disturbance. Similarly, at least three neuroendocrine systems may be involved in NES: (1) the glucocorticoid system, because it is responsive to stress, (2) the melanocortin system because of its involvement in circadian rhythms, and (3) the serotonergic system, for which there is the most evidence. Chapter 3 (Ungredda, Gluck, & Geliebter) reviews the literature implicating these systems, and suggestions for future neuroendocrine and pathophysiological research are discussed.

• *Circadian rhythms associated with NES.* The most central feature of NES is the circadian-delayed food intake. As such, animal models of circadian-altered food intake and sleep–wake patterns may be useful in understanding the etiology of NES. Chapter 4 (Lundgren, Boston, & Noble) reviews the human and animal literature on circadian eating and sleeping patterns, including circadian neuroendocrine and eating patterns in persons with NES. New models for quantifying circadian eating patterns are presented.

• *Behavioral and molecular genetics of NES.* Genetic factors likely contribute to the development and maintenance of NES. Chapter 5 (Runfola, Root, & Bulik) reviews both the behavioral (family and twin studies) and molecular genetics literature on NES and other eating disorders and provides future directions for studies in this area.

Part III. Relation to Other Clinical Syndromes

• *Relationship of NES with obesity, bariatric surgery, and physical health.* Although NES was first described as a syndrome affecting obese individuals, the relationship of NES to obesity remains inconclusive. Chapter 6 (Colles & Dixon) reviews the sometimes contradictory literature on night eating and obesity. In addition, as more obese individuals seek bariatric surgery, the effect of night eating on treatment outcome and prognosis is an important clinical question. This chapter also reviews studies of NES in bariatric surgery populations and offers suggestions for health care providers who encounter patients with NES in bariatric surgery clinics. Finally, over the past decade researchers have begun to study the effect of NES on physical health, including metabolic syndrome, diabetes, and oral health. These findings are reviewed and suggestions for improving research on the health implications of NES are presented.

• *NES and other eating disorders.* Recent research in both the United States and abroad has found high rates of night eating behavior among patients with other eating disorders (anorexia nervosa, bulimia nervosa, and binge-eating disorder). The relationship of NES to other eating disorders, especially within the context of proposed changes in DSM-5, are reviewed in Chapter 7 (Latzer & Tzischinsky).

• *NES and other psychiatric disorders.* Night eating has long been associated with psychiatric comorbidity. Chapter 8 (Rempfer & Murphy) reviews the literature, finding high rates of NES among psychiatric samples and high rates of psychiatric disorders among persons with NES. Potential reasons for the high rates of comorbidity are discussed.

• *Nocturnal eating and sleep disorders.* In characterizing, assessing, and treating NES, it is crucial to understand its relationship to sleep and movement disorders such as the parasomnia, sleep-related eating disorder. Chapter 9 (Howell & Crow) describes the differences and similarities between NES and other sleep and movement disorders, and suggestions are made made for future research to understand better the relationships among these disorders.

Part IV. Assessment

• *Conceptual issues in the assessment of eating behavior, mood, and sleep in NES.* The primary behavioral feature of NES is a delay in the circadian intake of food. Sleep and mood disturbance are other key features of NES. As the field moves forward, it is essential that the assessment of food, sleep, and mood be valid and reliable. Chapter 10 (Anderson, Engel, & Crosby) introduces the reader to common challenges in the assessment of eating, sleep, and mood in the context of NES and offers strategies for effective assessment practices in both research and clinical settings.

• *Assessment instruments for NES.* Several assessment tools have been developed specifically to assess the symptoms of and to make a diagnosis of NES. These include the NEQ, the Night Eating Syndrome History and Inventory (NESHI), and the Night Eating Diagnostic Questionnaire (NEDQ), and portions of the Eating Disorder Examination (EDE). Chapter 11 (Lundgren, Allison, Vinai, & Gluck) describes the currently available NES assessment instruments, with particular emphasis on the NESHI, a semistructured interview that assesses the history of and current eating, sleep, and mood patterns in the context of NES.

Part V. Treatment

• *Pharmacological treatment of NES.* Pharmacotherapy is the most commonly reported treatment for NES in the literature. The most promising agents are SSRIs, but other agents (e.g., topiramate) can be used successfully, as reported in case studies. Chapter 12 (Patel, O'Reardon, & Cristancho) critically reviews the evidence base for pharmacological interventions, offering researchers suggestions for further study and offering clinicians an evidence-based starting place for treating NES.

• *Psychotherapy/cognitive-behavioral therapy for NES.* Pharmacotherapy is not the only treatment option for NES, and psychotherapy (as it is for other eating and sleep disorders) is an important part of a comprehensive approach to the treatment of NES. Chapter 13 (Allison) reviews the conceptual background for the use of cognitive-behavioral therapy (CBT) in the treatment of NES, as well as empirical evidence for its efficacy.

• *Cognitive-behavioral treatment manual for NES.* Chapter 14 (Allison) presents a detailed CBT treatment manual for NES, developed by the author and her colleagues at the University of Pennsylvania.

• *Other approaches in treatment of NES.* Chapter 15 (Pawlow) reviews the evidence for alternative approaches to the treatment of NES, including relaxation and stress management, phototherapy, and behavioral weight loss.

In summary, we hope that readers of this book find the material informative and use it to advance future research and clinical efforts, with the ultimate goal of helping those who suffer from NES and related conditions.

References

Allison, K. C., Lundgren, J. D., O'Reardon, J. P., Geliebter, A., Gluck, M., Vinai, P., et al. (2010). Proposed diagnostic criteria for night eating syndrome. *International Journal of Eating Disorders, 43,* 241–247.

Stunkard, A. J., Grace, W. J., & Wolff, H. G. (1955). The night-eating syndrome: A pattern of food intake among certain obese patients. *American Journal of Medicine, 19,* 78–86.

Chapter 2

A History of Night Eating Syndrome

The First Patient

Albert J. Stunkard

The First Patient

In 1953, soon after I began training in psychiatry, I was assigned to the topic of obesity. Very shortly, I encountered a new obese patient whose story led to recognition of what is now called night eating syndrome (NES). Prior to that time, none of the many studies on obesity had considered the eating patterns of obese persons in more than a cursory manner.

I had become fully involved in the study of obesity when I was invited to give a talk at the weekly meeting of the Psychosomatic Research Group at the New York Hospital. This invitation led me to look for a topic that might interest members of the group. At the time there were no burning questions about human obesity. Obesity was dismissed as an unfortunate disorder, manifested by a disturbance in the psychoanalytic "oral" phase of personality development. No questions about this issue had been proposed, and it was a problem to decide how to formulate testable hypotheses.

A measure of the satisfaction with which the origins of human obesity was viewed was that the meeting produced almost no questions about the etiology of obesity. It was as if everything that could be known about human obesity was already known. There was no great satisfaction with the results of treatment for obesity; it was generally agreed that obese patients rarely lost much weight in treatment. But psychoanalytic theory provided an explanation, as one of my professors expressed it, "Obesity is due to fixation of the libido at a very early stage of personality development. These early oral fixations are the most difficult to handle, but it is a good topic to work on if you can stand the intense orality of the obese. You can learn a lot about primitive character structures and a great deal about yourself." Such views were not uncommon at the time and were not accompanied by advice on how to cope with the problems presented by these patients.

In preparing the talk for our weekly research meeting, I decided to present an obese patient as a stimulus for ideas about obesity. At the time, I was treating an obese adolescent girl and thought that her story would be a suitable stimulus for discussion.

"Ms. M.[1]" was a 15-year-old girl who weighed 210 pounds and was gaining weight. She was 5 feet 3 inches tall and appeared matronly. Her brown dress and chubby, expressionless face gave her the appearance of a little old woman. Although I started treating Ms. M. as part of a research program on obesity, at first she said nothing about her weight. In fact, she had been brought to the hospital by her mother for an entirely different problem. She had been experiencing episodes of abdominal pain that her mother ascribed to "nerves." The note from the referring physician, however, did not mention Ms. M.'s "nerves" or her obesity, and, ironically, reported that, "Ms. M. is always happy, sociable, good in school, and has plenty of dates. Her family relationships are excellent."

In the course of learning about her abdominal pain, I asked Ms. M. what sort of things made her nervous and whether she thought that "nerves" might cause her pain. With a sweet smile, she told me that "the other doctor" had said that she had to come to the psychiatric clinic because she was nervous.

She continued, "I actually hardly ever feel nervous and do not think that nervousness could have anything to do with my pain."

Smiling again, Ms. M. repeated the content of the referring physician's note: things were going very well in her life; she enjoyed her school work, and regretted only that her pains kept her from attending school as much as she would have liked. She then described a happy home life with her mother and father, and described with enthusiasm how they sang and played games together in the evenings.

---

[1] All patient characteristics have been modified for anonymity.

This account made me, as a beginning psychiatric resident, concerned that there were no psychological problems which we could address. I need not have been concerned.

At Ms. M.'s next visit, she began, "I must start off by confessing that I didn't tell the truth about all the questions you asked me. One of the things you asked me about was about girl friends and things like that and I said that I had them, but I don't. And I never had a date with a boy."

Ms. M. then turned to the family's financial status. On the brink of poverty, she and her mother used to spend Friday mornings visiting those neighbors from whom they believed that they had the best chance of borrowing money. Then they would return home to give whatever they had collected to her father to help him restore funds that he had appropriated from his office.

I began my presentation to the research group with a description of Ms. M.'s background, including a brief account of her eating pattern. Then we began to listen to a recording of a treatment session.

Suddenly, one of the research group members, a young woman physician, became upset. Gasping for breath, she rose from her chair and began to stagger out of the room. Puzzled, I followed her, not realizing until I reached her that she was obese. When I saw her face, it mirrored anguish bordering on panic. Only reluctantly could she be persuaded to return to the conference room. She then tried to explain to a baffled group what had happened to precipitate her attack of acute anxiety.

"It wasn't anything about the family. That was nothing. It was how that girl talked about the way she eats: nothing for breakfast. She is never hungry at all in the morning. Then, at night, she can't stop eating. Supper doesn't satisfy her and she just eats on and on. She even gets up out of bed to eat . . . that's how I eat and I never heard about it from anyone else in my whole life!"

I have never forgotten that shock of recognition by the woman physician. It made me realize that an eating pattern could mean so much more to an obese woman than even the troubling story of the family to which she had been listening.

This experience was so intriguing that I decided to investigate the curious eating pattern that the patients had described. I quickly learned that skipping breakfast, as Ms. M. and the obese woman physician did, was not uncommon among obese persons. This is particularly true of those who do not snack in the morning and have little or no appetite for lunch. Then, during the late afternoon and evening they began to eat more and more heavily. Sometimes they wake up, agitated and in turmoil, and get out of bed to eat.

Next Steps

In the following months, I tried to learn more about this distinctive eating pattern. I began by reviewing the literature to see what had been reported about eating patterns of obese persons. To my surprise, none of the many papers on obesity had dealt with eating patterns of obese persons in much detail. The rare papers on the topic reported that obese persons eat more frequently than non-obese persons (Freed, 1947), less frequently (Richardson, 1952), or even that decreased activity, rather than increased food intake, led to obesity (Greene, 1939). I began to think that I might have stumbled upon a unique eating pattern—morning anorexia and evening hyperphagia. Searching for examples of this eating pattern continued to the discovery of non-obese night eaters and raised the question of whether they were on the path to obesity.

This eating pattern intrigued me sufficiently to study it further. An opportunity arose by the application of "Mrs. R." for treatment at our clinic. She was a 28-year-old housewife, referred for treatment of obesity, which was accompanied by attacks of phlebitis of her right leg. The seventh of 10 living children, Mrs. R. remembered her mother with great bitterness, and complained that she had been exploited by her mother. Her childhood had been a time of hardship and deprivation, and her father's sporadic employment never permitted the family more than a marginal existence. At 19, Mrs. R. married the neighborhood alcoholic in an attempt to escape her home environment. She escaped into even more unfortunate circumstances and soon bitterly regretted it. But children followed and she found herself enmeshed in inescapable obligations. This led to overeating. Within 6 years of her marriage, Mrs. R. had added 110 pounds to her 5-foot-5-inch frame, reaching a weight of 290 pounds. Her weight had stayed at this level for 3 years when she came to the clinic.

Mrs. R.'s manner was pleasant and friendly, but her communication had an oddly impersonal quality. She was usually late for appointments and her attendance was irregular.

Mrs. R. manifested a classic night-eating pattern. She awoke in the morning with no appetite and ate no breakfast and little for lunch. Supper, in the early evening, was large, but only temporarily satisfying. During the rest of the evening and often until early morning, she nibbled at various foods distinguished mainly by their sweetness. She said that this eating helped reduce her anxiety.

Mrs. R.'s anxiety was most severe when she was alone, when she would worry about someone breaking into her house and harming her.

She attempted to control this anxiety, usually unsuccessfully, by keeping the radio and lights on. Sometimes, the presence of Mrs. R.'s husband reassured her. More often, they would quarrel, which also increased her anxiety. She usually stayed up eating until midnight and sometimes even later.

Soon after Mrs. R. had described her night-eating pattern, she developed a severe recurrence of her phlebitis, for which she was hospitalized. To my surprise, Mrs. R. greeted this development with relief and did not overeat the next evening. The morning after she entered the hospital, she awoke with an appetite for breakfast for the first time in months. She went on to eat an average-size lunch and a small supper and had no desire to eat during the evening or night. This absence of night eating was the more remarkable in that Mrs. R.'s phlebitis kept her awake much of the night during her first week in the hospital. Thereafter, she slept well, adhered with no difficulty to an 800-calorie diet, and lost 28 pounds in a month. This marked change in Mrs. R.'s eating pattern was paralleled by a great decrease in her anxiety.

At the time, I believed that this eating pattern was confined to obese persons. Accordingly, I tried to assess its extent in a group of 25 obese persons, who had been referred to the obesity clinic for treatment of their obesity, because of its severity or problems in its management (Stunkard, Grace, & Wolff, 1955). This effort was by no means a controlled study, but simply a first approach to the problem of night eating. I had made no attempt to select subjects by any particular criterion, and to my surprise, the sample of 25 persons included only two men. This disparity has occurred in subsequent treatment-seeking samples, but the proportions have varied in community samples over the years.

The median age of the night eating patients in our sample was 35 years, with a range from 18 to 56. The patients' average percentage of overweight was 68%, varying from 22% to 137%. A control group of 38 patients was selected, matched for age and body weight, none of whom reported night eating.

My first step was to propose provisional criteria for NES. These criteria were: (1) consumption of large amounts of the total caloric intake, and a major part of the excess intake, during the evening and night, (2) sleeplessness until midnight more than half the time, and (3) negligible food intake in the morning.

This pattern was reported by 16 of the 25 obese patients whom I had been treating in the clinic, and four manifested the pattern with slight variations. Most of the 16 patients with NES reported that they ate at night during two closely related situations: periods of wakefulness and periods of life stress.

I began to look for characteristics that differentiated these night eaters from obese control subjects. The first difference was in their efforts at weight reduction. Of the 16 patients who reported the full NES, only two had ever succeeded in losing more than one-third of their excess weight. Five patients with NES lost from 10 to 30 pounds and then promptly regained them. By contrast, nine patients who had not reported the syndrome lost an average of 67% of their excess weight. It began to appear that the NES might serve as an index of refractoriness to efforts at weight reduction. Thus the weight loss of four of the five patients who had lost weight occurred during temporary remissions of their NES.

In eight of the 16 patients with NES, weight loss was accompanied by emotional disturbance. Four of these patients presented a picture of what was then termed "neurasthenia," characterized by feelings of futility and inordinate fatigue (Mitchell, 1889). These patients were confined to bed, in one case for as long as 4 months. Three patients stopped weight-reducing efforts because of depressive reactions and in one case following the onset of severe anxiety. Thus, of the 11 patients with a past history of significant weight loss, only three achieved this goal without emotional illness.

This large incidence of disability during attempts at weight reduction by patients with NES differed sharply from the apparent infrequency of such complications in a control group of 38 obese women who did not manifest NES (Stunkard et al., 1955).

It had long been recognized that some patients cannot maintain a reducing diet long enough to make it worthwhile. It has also been pointed out that some patients cannot lose weight without emotional disturbance and should probably not even try (Stunkard, 1957). There had been no criteria to select patients who might undertake dieting with safety and reasonable hope of success. The delineation of NES appeared to identify such persons.

The Next Chapter in NES History

After I left my residency I pursued the study of weight and eating disorders. The experience with the NES encouraged me to look for other unusual eating patterns. The NES appeared to represent a *failure of satiety*. Could overeating result also from an *increased hunger drive*? The question kept coming back and was answered by the discovery of binge-eating disorder (BED). The defining feature of BED is "eating, during a discrete period of time (within a 2-hour period) an amount of food that is definitely larger than most people would eat during a similar period of time under similar circumstances" (American Psychiatric Association, 2000).

My colleagues and I at the University of Pennsylvania were studying the characteristics and treatment of BED in the 1990s when my curiosity regarding NES returned. At the European Congress on Obesity in Copenhagen in the spring of 1995, I posed questions to international experts in the field regarding their ideas of night eating to help start an intellectual discussion on its diagnostic features and the best way to assess them. Responses poured in from colleagues in North America, Europe, Asia, and South America. This coincided with an increased interest in addressing the rising prevalence of obesity and a desire to find patterns of eating that could be addressed to reduce distress and control weight. Thus the 1990s proved to be a time of renewed interest in NES, as several studies described its prevalence and clinical features (e.g., Adami, Meneghelli, & Scopinaro, 1999; Birketvedt et al., 1999; Greeno, Wing, & Marcus, 1995; Rand, Macgregor, & Stunkard, 1997; Spaggiari, Granella, Parrino, Marchesi, Melli, et al., 1994; Stunkard et al., 1996).

The first intensive outpatient and inpatient studies of NES were performed during this time (Birketvedt et al., 1999). We identified the occurrence of nocturnal ingestions in this study with the help of the technology of actigraphy. We also noted abnormalities in neuroendocrine markers such as leptin, cortisol, and melatonin (Birketvedt et al., 1999). This was the first report to suggest that NES interfered with the optimal expression of these eating-, stress-, and sleep-related hormones. This suggested that the behaviors associated with NES have measurable biological correlates. These studies served as the impetus for the next phase of research concerning the definition and development of new treatment approaches for NES in the 2000s.

The Present

The nature of the NES has been studied further over the last decade. The provisional criteria from the initial study of night eating (Stunkard et al., 1955) were refined and applied in a series of clinical trials. These trials indicated that the selection of preliminary criteria had been prescient. All three of the preliminary criteria were replicated in more systematic studies and have been proposed as research diagnostic criteria (Allison et al., 2010).

In recent years, the various findings about the NES have been organized into a biobehavioral model designed to predict effective treatment (Stunkard, Allison, Lundgren, & O'Reardon, 2009). Figure 2.1 depicts the very different eating behaviors of night eaters and control subjects in both the first and third hours of the day (O'Reardon et al., 2004).

The originally proposed core behaviors of the NES, evening and nighttime hyperphagia and morning anorexia, suggested that the disorder represented a delay in the circadian rhythm of food intake. This suggestion was assessed by Boston, Moate, Allison, Lundren, and Stunkard (2008), who modeled circadian rhythms of food intake among night eaters and control subjects by means of parametric deconvolution. These findings are well illustrated in Chapter 4 (Lundgren, Boston, & Noble), which includes a novel equation that describes the 24-hour temporal eating patterns of subjects with NES. The model accurately described and quantified the temporal eating patterns of both night eaters and control subjects. Both normal weight and overweight subjects with NES manifested differences between the timing of eating patterns and the caloric intake in a control group of non-night eaters.

Circadian eating patterns of night eaters were found also by Goel, Stunkard, Rogers, Van Dongen, Allison, et al. (2009), as described in Chapter 4. They showed that the phase and amplitude of behavioral and neuroendocrine circadian rhythms of patients with NES differed strikingly from those of control subjects. The night eaters showed a delay in the circadian pattern of food intake and Goel et al. (2009) reported phase and amplitude of behavioral and neuroendocrine circadian rhythms of 15 night eaters. These patterns were compared to those of 14 control subjects, who displayed normal phase and amplitude for all circadian rhythms. The patients with NES showed a phase delay in the timing of meals, and total caloric, fat, and carbohydrate intake.

An examination of these findings, which are described in more detail in Chapter 4 (Lundgren, Boston, & Noble), have led to the conceptualization that NES may result from a dissociation between central (suprachiasmatic nucleus) timing mechanisms and oscillators elsewhere in the central nervous system or periphery (such as the stomach or liver). These results suggest that chronobiological treatments of NES may be useful, and this possibility has been explored. For example, bright light therapy has reduced night eating in individual cases (Friedman, Even, Dardennes, & Guelfi, 2002, 2004) and should be evaluated in controlled clinical trials (see Pawlow, Chapter 15, for a review).

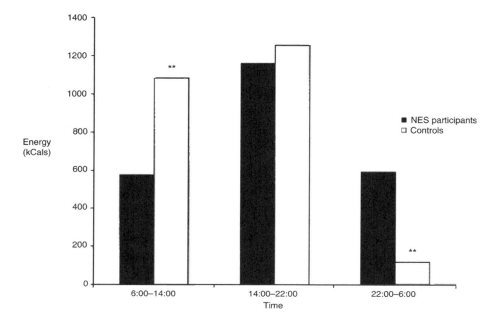

FIGURE 2.1. Caloric intake in 8-hour increments for NES and control groups. Food intake is lower in the first part of the day and higher in the latter third of the day in the NES group. $**p < .01$. From O'Reardon et al. (2004). Reprinted by permission of Nature Publishing Group.

Discussion

The nature of NES has been studied further over the course of the last 50 years. The provisional criteria from the initial study of night eating (Stunkard et al., 1955) were refined and applied in a series of clinical trials. These clinical trials indicated that the selection of preliminary criteria had been prescient. All three of these preliminary criteria were replicated in more systematic studies and have been proposed as research diagnostic criteria (Allison et al., 2010).

The past half-century has proven to be a period of discovery and intense study of both normative and disordered eating patterns, the scope of which was unfathomable when I wrote my first paper on NES in 1955. The core features of evening hyperphagia and waking to eat have stood the test of time, and progress has been made in understanding the circadian nature of this disorder. I hope that the next half-century holds more discoveries in diagnostics and treatments for those who suffer with NES.

References

Adami, G. F., Meneghelli, A., & Scopinaro, N. (1999). Night eating and binge eating disorder in obese patients. *International Journal of Eating Disorders, 25*, 335–338.

Allison, K. C., Lundgren, J. D., O'Reardon, J. P., Geliebter, A., Gluck, M. E., Vinai, P., et al. (2010). Proposed diagnostic criteria for night eating syndrome. *International Journal of Eating Disorders, 43*, 241–247.

American Psychiatric Association. (2000). *Diagnostic and statistical manual of mental disorders* (4th ed., text rev.). Washington, DC: Author.

Birketvedt, G. S., Florholmen, J., Sundsfjord J., Osterud, B., Dinges, D., Bilker, W., et al. (1999). Behavioral and neuroendocrine characteristics of the night eating syndrome. *Journal of the American Medical Association, 282*, 657–663.

Boston, R. C., Moate, P. J., Allison, K. C., Lundgren, J. D., & Stunkard, A. J. (2008). Modeling circadian rhythms of food intake by means of parametric deconvolution: Results from studies of the night eating syndrome. *American Journal of Clinical Nutrition, 87*, 1672–1677.

Bruch, H. (1952). Psychological aspects of reducing. *Psychosomatic Medicine, 14*, 337.

Freed, S. C. (1947). Psychic factors in the development and treatment of obesity. *Journal of the American Medical Association, 133*, 369.

Friedman S., Even C., Dardennes R., & Guelfi J. D. (2002). Light therapy, obesity, and night eating syndrome. *American Journal of Psychiatry, 159*, 875–876.

Friedman S., Even C., Dardennes R., & Guelfi J. D. (2004). Light therapy, non-seasonal depression, and night eating syndrome. *Canadian Journal of Psychiatry, 49*, 790.

Goel, N., Stunkard, A. J., Rogers, N. L., Van Dongen, H. P., Allison, K. C., O'Reardon, J. P., et al. (2009). Circadian rhythm profiles in women with night eating syndrome. *Journal of Biological Rhythms, 24*(1), 85–94.

Greene, J. A. (1939). Clinical study of the etiology of obesity. *Annals of Internal Medicine, 12*, 1797.

Greeno, C. G., Wing, R. R., & Marcus, M. D. (1995). Nocturnal eating in beinge eating disorder and matched-weight controls. *International Journal of Eating Disorders, 18*, 343–349.

Hamburger, W. W. (1951). Emotional aspects of obesity. *Medical Clinics of North America, 35*, 483.

Keys, A., & Brozek, J. (1953). Body fat in adult man. *Physiological Review, 33*, 245.

Mitchell, S. W. (1889). The poison of serpents. *The Century Magazine, 38*, 503–515.

O'Reardon, J. P., Ringel, B. L., Dinges, D. F., Allison, K. C., Rogers, N. S., Martino, N. S., et al. (2004). Circadian eating and sleeping patterns in the night eating syndrome. *Obesity Research, 12*, 1789–1796.

Rand, C. S., Macgregor, A. M., & Stunkard, A. J. (1997). The night eating syndrome in the general population and among postoperative obesity surgery patients. *International Journal of Eating Disorders, 22,* 65–69.

Richardson, J. S. (1952). The treatment of maternal obesity. *Lancet, 1,* 525.

Spaggiari, M. C., Granella, F., Parrino, L., Marchesi, C., Melli, I., & Terzano, M. G. (1994). Nocturnal eating syndrome in adults. *Sleep, 17*(4), 339–344.

Stunkard, A. J. (1957). The "dieting depression." Incidence and clinical characteristics of untoward responses to weight reduction regimes. *American Journal of Medince, 23,* 77–86.

Stunkard, A. J., Allison, K. C., Lundgren, J. D., & O'Reardon, J. P. (2009). A biobehavioural model of the night eating syndrome. *Obesity Reviews, 10*(Suppl. 2), 69–77.

Stunkard, A. J., Berkowitz, R., Wadden, T., Tanrikut, C., Reiss E., & Young, L. (1996). Binge eating disorder and the night eating syndrome. *International Journal of Obesity and Related Metabolic Disorders, 20,* 1–6.

Stunkard, A. J., Grace, W. J., & Wolff, H. G. (1955). The night eating syndrome. A pattern of food intake among certain obese patients. *American Journal of Medicine, 19,* 78–86.

PART II

BIOLOGY

Chapter 3

Pathophysiological and Neuroendocrine Aspects of Night Eating Syndrome

Tatiana Ungredda
Marci E. Gluck
Allan Geliebter

Night eating syndrome (NES) is an eating disorder characterized most recently by 25% or more of one's daily energy intake after the evening meal and/or waking up during sleep (with some awareness, rather than in a state of sleep) to eat at least two times per week (Allison et al., 2010). NES is usually accompanied by trouble sleeping. The causes of night eating remain largely unknown, although recent research suggests that biological factors contribute to the development and maintenance of the disorder. Some studies have begun exploring potential treatments based on these biological aspects (Friedman, Even, Dardennes, & Guelfi, 2002; O'Reardon et al., 2006; O'Reardon, Stunkard, & Allison, 2004; Rosenhagen, Uhr, Schüssler, & Steiger, 2005; Spaggiari, Granella, Parrino, Marchesi, Melli, et al., 1994). NES, therefore, appears to involve desynchronization between the circadian rhythms of eating and sleep, resulting in a delayed pattern of eating (O'Reardon, Ringel, et al., 2004).

The suprachiasmatic nucleus (SCN) of the hypothalamus helps orchestrate the schedule for sleep, eating, and endocrine activity, based on the circadian day–night cycle. It receives information through the optic chiasm about light signals to the eye and then transmits them to peripheral oscillators located in various organs to synchronize central and peripheral hormone action related to sleep and eating. A number of articles on NES have explored these circadian rhythms and the neuroendocrine system. Although there is significant overlap in the circadian and neuroendocrine systems, circadian rhythm will be reviewed in Chapter 4 (Lundgren, Boston, & Noble), and neuroendocrine features of NES will be reviewed in this chapter.

Peripheral Nervous System

Stress Hormones

There is evidence that major life stressors can trigger night eating (Stunkard, Grace, & Wolff, 1955), leading some investigators to focus on the role of cortisol in NES. Cortisol, a hormone released by the adrenal cortex in response to stress, has been associated with weight gain (Bjorntorp & Rosmond, 2000) and overeating (Epel, Lapidus, McEwen, & Brownell, 2001). In the first study to examine cortisol in NES, Birketvedt et al. (1999) compared 12 night eaters (7 lean, 5 obese) and 21 nonnight eaters (14 lean, 11 obese). They were fed fixed meals at 8:00 A.M., 12:00 P.M., 4:00 P.M., and 8:00 P.M., each meal providing 1,255 kJ (300 kcal), with no additional food past 8:00 P.M., hence, a calorically restrictive diet. Blood was drawn every 2 hours for 24 hours, which showed that cortisol levels were significantly higher from 8:00 A.M. to 2:00 A.M. in the night eaters (combined weight groups) than those of the controls ($p < .002$). The authors hypothesized that, in NES, there are disturbances in the hypothalamic–pituitary–adrenal (HPA) axis, which regulate the cortisol stress response.

Birketvedt, Sundsfjord, and Florholmen (2002) studied five night eaters and five weight-matched controls from the previous study and administered 100 µg of corticotropin-releasing hormone (CRH) at 8:00 A.M. to elicit adrenocorticotropic hormone (ACTH) response in order to stimulate cortisol secretion. Blood was drawn every 10 minutes for 2 hours and at 30 minutes for the next hour, and analyzed to measure plasma ACTH levels. CRH induced a gradual elevation of ACTH, which rose less in the NES group ($p = .04$) at 10, 20, 30, 40, 50, and 60 minutes following the infusion. Plasma cortisol followed a similar pattern and was significantly less elevated in the night eaters than the controls at 20, 30, 40, 50, 60, 90, and 120 minutes ($p = .001$).

The authors suggested that night eaters have an attenuated pituitary and adrenal secretory capacity due to chronic stress exposure. These results may correspond to the greater elevation of cortisol in the night eaters from the previous study (Birketvedt et al., 2002) as an overactive HPA axis in NES, resulting in higher cortisol levels, may eventually become less sensitive to further CRH stimulation.

In another study, Allison et al. (2005) recruited 15 female participants with NES (more than 50% of calories after the evening meal) and 14 controls. Plasma levels of cortisol and prolactin, also increased by stress, were collected for 24 hours (every 2 hours from 8:00 A.M. to 8:00 P.M., and every hour from 9:00 P.M. to 9:00 A.M.). Participants received three large meals and ad libitum snacks, averaging a total of 2,900 kcal per day. The results did not show a difference in cortisol (Figure 3.1, panel C) or prolactin concentrations between groups. The results that contradict the Birketvedt et al. (2002) study may be related to the differing feeding protocols. The relative caloric deprivation in the Birketvedt et al. (2002) study may have led to an increase in cortisol levels in the night eaters due to hunger-related stress, especially given the absence of food in the late evening and at night.

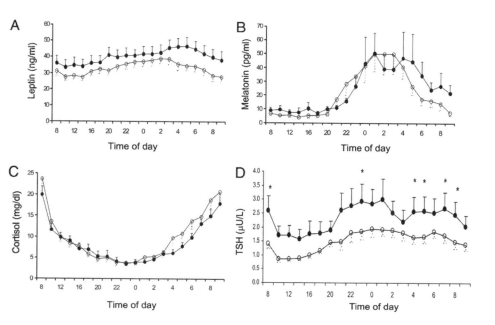

FIGURE 3.1. Twenty-four-hour profiles of (A) leptin, (B) melatonin, (C) cortisol, and (D) TSH in NES (•) and control subjects (○). Data are mean ± SE; $p < .05$, NES versus controls. From Allison et al. (2005). Copyright 2005 by the Endocrine Society. Reprinted by permission.

In a study of pre- and post-Roux-en-Y gastric bypass surgery in patients with NES (n = 4) and weight-matched controls (n = 4), Morrow, Gluck, Lorence, Flancbaum, and Geliebter (2008) found a relative elevation (p = .01) of afternoon (3:00 P.M.) fasting cortisol levels from 2 months to 5 months postsurgery in participants with NES, compared to a small decrease in controls despite similar weight loss. It was suggested that decreased food intake may have been a greater stressor for night eaters, possibly raising cortisol. The authors advised caution in interpreting the results due to the small sample size.

More recently, Geliebter, Carnell, and Gluck (2011) used a cold pressor test (CPT), a laboratory stressor, which entails submerging one hand for 2 minutes into a container with ice water to elevate cortisol. Twenty-eight overweight women (11 night eaters, 17 non-night eaters), were given a 1,254-kcal fixed breakfast meal and had a CPT stress test 2 hours later. Blood was drawn at −10 minutes (baseline), 0 minutes, and then at 2 minutes, immediately after hand withdrawal, and again at 5, 15, 30, 45, and 60 minutes afterward for cortisol. Baseline cortisol (p = .01) and cortisol area under the curve (AUC) were greater in night eaters compared to non-night eaters (p = .02), suggesting elevated levels of cortisol and higher cortisol levels following stress.

In a different study on the same sample (Carnell, Gluck, & Geliebter, 2011), the authors compared morning (fasting) cortisol as well as afternoon (nonfasting) cortisol levels between groups. Blood samples were taken at baseline (about 9:00 A.M. and again about 12:00 P.M., two hours after a fixed liquid meal). On another test day, participants arrived after a 1-mg dose of dexamethasone (DST) (which mimics cortisol) at 11:00 P.M. the night before, which normally should suppress morning cortisol. When it leads, however, to a cortisol level ≥ 5 µg/dl, this indicates decreased sensitivity to negative feedback, the likely result of an overactive HPA axis. There was a trend (p = .07) toward higher levels of cortisol after DST in the night eaters. Afternoon cortisol was significantly higher in night eaters than in non-night eaters (p = .01), but morning cortisol levels did not differ. The authors suggest that elevated cortisol levels in the afternoon may be a factor contributing to nighttime eating (Carnell et al., 2011).

Sleep Hormones

Although NES has been described as a condition of delayed circadian rhythms of food intake, the sleep–wake cycle is not altered (Goel, Stunkard, Rogers, Van Dongen, Allison, O'Reardon, et al., 2009).

Birketvedt et al. (1999) also measured plasma melatonin in their night and non-night eaters every 2 hours for 24 hours. Melatonin levels were lower for both overweight and normal-weight night eaters than for controls from 10:00 P.M. to 6:00 A.M. ($p < .001$). In the control groups, the obese participants had a higher melanocortin concentration than the nonobese participants between 2:00 A.M. to 4:00 A.M. ($p < .001$).

The results showed that night eaters had lower levels of melatonin during the sleeping phase of the circadian rhythm, which may help account in part for their sleep disturbance and night eating. It has been suggested that night eaters tend to eat foods high in carbohydrate content in order to increase their melanocortin levels. The rationale is that carbohydrate ingestion leads to higher plasma tryptophan, which is then converted to serotonin and melatonin (Birketvedt et al., 1999).

In contrast, a study by Allison et al. (2005) found no significant differences between groups in plasma melatonin (Figure 3.1, panel B). The differing results between Birketvedt et al. (1999) study and Allison et al. (2005) may also be a result of the latter study's inclusion of ad libitum snacks. Similarly, the circadian rhythms of melatonin did not differ in amplitude (Goel et al., 2009), although it was delayed by 1.1 hours in the group with NES, $t(25) = 2.17$, $p = .04$. The authors suggested that the delay was due to some light exposure when the night eaters arose to eat.

In randomized crossover of two conditions in seven healthy non-night eating volunteers, Qin et al. (2003) examined the effects of an imposed 3-week nocturnal lifestyle on plasma melatonin, leptin, glucose, and insulin. The control group consumed three fixed meals per day at 7:00 A.M., 1:00 P.M., and 7:00 P.M., and slept from 10:30 P.M. until 6:30 A.M. The experimental group slept in a shorter and delayed period from 1:30 A.M. to 8:30 A.M., ate no breakfast, but had the same fixed lunch and dinner, and could eat freely after dinner until bedtime. Blood was drawn on the twenty-second day from 9:00 A.M. to 6:00 A.M. every 3 hours. In the control diurnal group, melatonin increased 5.3 times to the usual peak (3:00 A.M.) from the nadir (3:00 P.M.) whereas in the experimental group melatonin increased only threefold. The smaller rise in plasma melatonin, resulting from decreased sleep and nighttime eating in the night eaters, suggested that abnormal sleep–eating patterns may contribute to the development or maintenance of night eating. Moreover, helping a person make changes in sleep and eating schedules may improve night eating behaviors.

Appetite-Related Hormones

Ghrelin

The hormone ghrelin is mainly secreted by the stomach and has been shown to increase hunger and food intake in animals and humans. Ghrelin increases before meals and decreases afterward. Somewhat surprisingly, concentration of ghrelin tends to be decreased in obese individuals (Geliebter, Gluck, & Hashim 2005). Relevance to obesity and eating disorders makes ghrelin a hormone of interest in the study of NES. Rosenhagen et al. (2005) examined mean ghrelin concentrations at three periods in a 27-year-old female night eater, which was 1,051 pg/ml at baseline, 977 pg/ml 8 weeks later when in remission during selective serotonin reuptake inhibitor (SSRI) treatment (citalopram, 100 mg/day for 16 weeks), and 1,013 pg/ml after relapse, without a change in BMI. Three healthy women served as controls, and their mean ghrelin concentrations were much lower: 372 pg/ml, 402 pg/ml, and 338 pg/ml. The authors also administered exogenous ghrelin to a healthy participant, which led to nocturnal eating, whereas a lower dose of ghrelin promoted sleep. The authors suggested that the high dose of ghrelin disrupted sleep due to increased hunger, despite ghrelin's soporific effects. A drawback of this study, however, is the very small sample.

Allison et al. (2005) also measured ghrelin levels, as well as cortisol and melatonin. Ghrelin did not differ between NES and non-NES, although in the same sample, Goel et al. (2009) observed a 5.2-hour delay, $t(26) = 4.15$, $p < .001$, and a 50% decrease in ghrelin amplitude, $t(26) = 2.45$, $p = .02$, in NES, which may be related to the delayed meal intake in night eaters. In the two other studies of ghrelin in night eaters, Geliebter et al. (2011) found that, following a CPT stress test, ghrelin was elevated among both people with NES and controls ($p = .04$). Ghrelin peaks, however, were higher in people with NES ($p = .03$), although the time of the peak did not differ, implying an intact ghrelin circadian rhythm. The elevated ghrelin peak in people with NES following stress may be a contributor to the increased nighttime eating. In the other study, Carnell et al. (2011) found that ghrelin levels during the morning and the evening did not differ between groups, possibly due to having only overweight participants, who tend to have lower ghrelin levels, or due to the absence of a stressor.

Leptin

Leptin is an anorexigenic hormone that is produced almost entirely by adipose tissue. It usually peaks during the night and has a morning nadir. The study by Birketvedt et al. (1999) showed that leptin was higher in the overweight than the normal-weight groups in both night eaters and non-night eaters. However, in a study of only lean participants (Qin et al., 2003), plasma leptin followed a similar pattern to that of melatonin, with a peak at 3:00 A.M. and a nadir at 9:00 A.M. In the diurnal lifestyle group, leptin increased 2.2-fold from nadir to peak, but increased only 1.4-fold in the nocturnal lifestyle group. Plasma leptin was significantly lower in the nocturnal lifestyle group between 9:00 P.M. and 6:00 A.M. In contrast, Allison et al. (2005) did not find significant differences between groups for leptin (Figure 3.1, panel A); however, there was a 1-hour phase delay in those with NES (Goel et al., 2009). This, coupled with the ghrelin 5-hour phase delay, makes for a combined 6-hour ghrelin–leptin phase delay in the NES circadian rhythm.

Insulin and Glucose

Insulin release varies according to the availability of glucose in order to ensure provision of energy as well as to prevent depleting energy storage. Insulin and glucose have a positive phase relationship, and both peak in the morning and fall during the night. In the Birketvedt et al. (1999) study, glucose and insulin did not differ between the night and non-night eaters among either the overweight or normal-weight groups. This may be because both groups consumed the fixed meals at the same times, and both insulin and glucose respond to food intake. In the Qin et al. (2003) study, the glucose concentration in the diurnal group showed three peaks consistent with mealtimes. In the nocturnal group, however, there were increases at 12:00 A.M., 3:00 A.M., and 6:00 A.M. ($p < .01$), compared to increases at 9:00 A.M. and noon ($p < .01$) in the diurnal group. Plasma insulin for the diurnal group peaked at the same times as glucose, but in the nocturnal group, it peaked at 9:00 P.M. and 12:00 A.M. The authors attributed this circadian difference to an irregular meal schedule of the nocturnal group. Similarly, in the Allison et al. (2005) study, night eaters had significantly higher levels of insulin at night, which coincided with eating times. These results differ from the Birketvedt et al. (1999) study, likely due to the night eaters' receiving ad libitum evening snacks. Goel et al. (2009) found that in the group with NES, glucose exhibited a phase delay of 12.4 hours, $t(28) = 2.04$, $p < .001$, and insulin had a phase delay of 2.8 hours, $t(28) = 3.2$, $p = .004$. The authors considered these results to be a consequence of the nighttime caloric intake.

Central Nervous System

Serotonin

The neurotransmitter serotonin has elicited much interest in research on NES due to its involvement in both sleep and appetite. Spaggiari et al. (1994) examined sleep in 10 night eaters and found no abnormalities in levels of glucose, insulin, cortisol, and growth hormone. Polysomnography revealed a total of 65 intrasleep awakenings, of which 55% led to food ingestion. Seven participants were treated with *d*-fenfluramine daily, with a range of 6 to 15 months, and of those, five exhibited a 50% reduction in nighttime eating episodes. Friedman et al. (2002) found improved NES symptoms with phototherapy (which indirectly also targets serotonin). O'Reardon, Stunkard, et al. (2003) conducted a trial in 17 night eaters (12 female; 18–65 years old; body mass index ≥ 27) given 50 mg of sertraline for the first 2 weeks, and then adjusted individually to a maximum of 200 mg for the remaining 10 weeks. Participants kept diaries that included detailed information about ingestions, getting out of bed at night, nighttime eating, as well as bedtime and waking times. The diaries were analyzed at the beginning, and at 6 and 12 weeks. Depression (Hamilton Depression Rating Scale [HDRS] and the Beck Depression Inventory [BDI]), and night eating (Night Eating Questionnaire [NEQ] and Night Eating Symptom Scale [NESS]), eating disorders (Eating Disorder Examination [EDE]), Clinical Global Impression Improvement (CGI-I), and weight loss were assessed. Participants reduced their number of awakenings from 2 to 0.8 per night ($p < .01$), and their nighttime ingestions from 1.5 per night to 0.5 per night ($p < .01$), with a reduction in intake after supper from 52% to 26% ($p < .01$). In addition, the CGI-I improved from 4 to 2.6 ($p < .01$). There were significant improvements in depression and night eating symptoms, but the improvements were not correlated. The authors concluded that SSRIs were effective in treating night eating but cautioned that the study was limited by its small sample size and unblinded nature.

O'Reardon et al. (2006) conducted a double-blind, randomized, placebo-controlled 8-week sertraline trial, which included 34 participants (14 overweight and three normal weight in each group). Night eaters qualified if they consumed 50% or more of their daily caloric intake after 8:00 P.M. The participants, who were seen every other week and weighed, kept food diaries. The sertraline dosage was adjusted according to effectiveness. At each meeting, participants completed the NESS, the BDI, and the Quality of Life Enjoyment and Satisfaction Questionnaire. The CGI-I and severity scales and the HDRS were completed by the study physician.

The sertraline group improved significantly more than the placebo group on most measures from baseline to week 8. At 8 weeks, 12 of the sertraline group had a score of ≤ 2 on the CGI, seven of whom were considered in remission, $F(4, 113) = 6.7$, $p < .001$. In the placebo group, only three responded to the treatment. The sertraline group's night eating symptoms score was reduced by 18 versus 5 points in the placebo group, $F(4, 112) = 8.0$, $p < .0001$. Nighttime ingestions in the sertraline group decreased by 81% as compared to only 14% in the placebo group, $F(4, 80) = 3.7$, $p = .01$. Nighttime awakenings also decreased more for the sertraline group than for the placebo group (74% vs. 14%), although the difference did not reach significance. The sertraline group reduced caloric intake after the evening meal by 68% versus 29% for the placebo group (week 8: $t(106) = 2.0$, $p = .047$).

Using single photon emission computed tomography (SPECT) to compare serotonin transporter (SERT) availability, Lundgren et al. (2008) studied six night eaters and six control subjects. They found that night eaters had significantly more serotonin reuptake in the raphe nucleus of the midbrain than did the controls, $F(1, 7) = 23.7$, $p < .01$, and this reuptake was associated with elevated SERT and thus reduced serotonin availability. Lundgren et al. (2009), using SPECT, also compared SERT in NES and major depressive disorder (MDD) and found significantly higher SERT binding in the midbrain and temporal lobes of patients with NES than in participants with MDD. The authors caution that these results do not indicate a new diagnostic marker for either disorder, but it demonstrates a distinction between the two disorders.

Finally Stunkard, Allison, Lundgren, and O'Reardon (2009) developed a biobehavioral model of NES (Figure 3.2), suggesting that a combination of stress and genetic susceptibility results in increased reuptake of serotonin, which leads to dysregulation of the eat–sleep cycle and reduced satiety at night. The model hypothesizes that interventions targeting the serotonin system restore homeostasis to satiety and circadian rhythm. More research is needed to verify and further develop this model.

Implications for Assessment and Treatment of NES

The limited research described above suggests that it may be premature to assess NES based solely on neuroendocrine levels. Several recommendations, however, can be made for the biological treatment of NES. Birketvedt et al. (1999) suggested administration of exogenous melatonin from

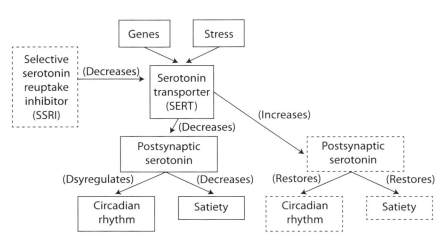

FIGURE 3.2. The putative interaction of stress and genetic vulnerability is depicted in the solid boxes at the top of the figure. The interaction gives rise to increased serotonin transporter (SERT) in the solid box, which decreases postsynaptic serotonin dysregulating circadian rhythm and decreasing satiety (solid boxes). Administration of selective serotonin reuptake inhibitors (SSRIs) (dotted box) decreases SERT, which increases postsynaptic serotonin, restoring circadian rhythm and satiety (dotted boxes). The solid boxes depict the interaction between genes and stress, resulting in elevated serum transporter. The result is decreased postsynaptic serotonin, leading to dysregulated circadian rhythm and decreased satiety. Dotted boxes show that the administration of SSRIs decreases serotonin transporters, leading to increased postsynaptic serotonin and restoration of circadian rhythm and satiety. From Stunkard, Allison, Lundgren, and O'Reardon (2009). Copyright 2009 by the International Association for the Study of Obesity. Reprinted by permission.

their findings of a blunted nighttime peak in melatonin in NES. However, there have been inconsistent responses to administration of nighttime melatonin in NES patients (Birketvedt & Florholmen, 2006). Similarly, they suggested further study of leptin as a treatment based on their findings of a blunted nighttime peak of leptin. Finally, they recommended consideration of treatment with CRH receptor antagonists, given the association of elevated CRH with diminished leptin and melatonin levels.

Qin et al. (2003) suggested that a nocturnal lifestyle may lead to some of the endocrine changes evident in NES, namely an attenuated peak in evening melatonin and leptin. Behavioral treatment, therefore, may help patients conform to a normal diurnal sleep–eating schedule. The improvement in night eating symptoms in the randomized placebo-controlled trial of sertraline (O'Reardon et al., 2006) suggests that this antidepressant is a promising treatment for NES. SSRIs may increase the availability of serotonin in the hypothalamus, responsible for the normal cycling of circadian rhythms. However, SSRIs may not be a viable treatment for some, as evidenced by the lack of response in almost half of the treatment group.

Areas for Future Research

NES remains an understudied condition, although it is attracting more interest. It remains unproven whether a blunted peak in melatonin contributes to nighttime awakenings, or if a blunted peak in leptin helps to prevent suppression of hunger during sleep. Although possible treatments for NES may include exogenous administration of melatonin, leptin, and/ or CRH receptor antagonists (Birketvedt et al., 1999), placebo-controlled trials need to be performed. To date, there are also no adequate studies on the long-term effects/benefits of SSRIs on NES. Further research is also needed on SERT availability in NES to provide convincing evidence that the serotonergic system is playing a major role in the maintenance of NES. One pilot study showed elevated SERT uptake in individuals with NES, and another study showed greater SERT binding in NES than MDD (Lundgren et al., 2009); however, these studies are the only ones of their kind, and are in need of replication and/or expansion.

Given the evidence involving melatonin and serotonin's effects on NES symptoms, another medication worthy of further study as a possible treatment for NES is agomelatine, an antidepressant, which acts as a melatonin receptor agonist as well as a serotonin receptor (5-HT_{2C}) antagonist (Millan et al., 2003; Yous et al., 1992). The burgeoning research on the biological aspects of NES shows promise of eventually leading to successful treatments.

References

Allison, K. C., Ahima, R. S., O'Reardon, J. P., Dinges, D. F., Sharma, V., Cummings, D. E., et al. (2005). Neuroendocrine profiles associated with energy intake, sleep, and stress in the night eating syndrome. *Journal of Clinical Endocrinology, 90,* 6214–6217.

Allison, K. C., Lundgren, J. D., O'Reardon, J. P., Geliebter, A., Gluck, M. E., Vinai, P., et al. (2010). Proposed diagnostic criteria for night eating syndrome. *International Journal of Eating Disorders, 43*(3), 241–247.

Birketvedt, G. S., & Florholmen, J. R. (2006). The night eating syndrome. In L. Malcom, D. P. Cardinali, & S. R. Pandi-Perumal (Eds.), *Sleep and sleep disorders: A neuropsychopharmachological approach* (1st ed., pp. 251–255) New York: Springer.

Birketvedt, G. S., Florholmen, J., Sundsfjord, J., Osterud, B., Dinges, D., Bilker, W., et al. (1999). Behavioral and neuroendocrine characteristics of the night-eating syndrome. *Journal of the American Medical Association, 282,* 657–663.

Birketvedt, G. S., Sundsfjord. J., & Florholmen, J. R. (2002). Hypothalamic–pituitary–adrenal axis in the night eating syndrome. *American Journal of Physiology–Endocrinology and Metabolism, 282,* E366–E369.

Bjorntorp, P., & Rosmond, R. (2000). Neuroendocrine abnormalities in visceral obesity. *International Journal of Obesity and Related Metabolic Disorders, 24*(Suppl. 2), S80–S85.

Carnell, S., Gluck, M. E., & Geliebter, A. (2011). *Cortisol and ghrelin in overweight women with and without night eating: Morning and afternoon levels.* Unpublished manuscript.

Epel, E., Lapidus, R., McEwen, B., & Brownell, K. (2001). Stress may add bite to appetite in women: A laboratory study of stress-induced cortisol and eating behavior. *Psychoneuroendocrinology, 26*(1), 37–49.

Friedman, S., Even, C., Dardennes, R., & Guelfi, J. D. (2002). Light therapy, obesity, and night-eating syndrome. *American Journal of Psychiatry, 159,* 875–876.

Geliebter, A., Carnell, S., & Gluck M. E. (2011). *Cortisol and ghrelin concentrations following a cold pressor stress test in overweight night eaters.* Unpublished manuscript.

Geliebter, A., Gluck, M. E., & Hashim, S. (2005). Plasma ghrelin concentrations are lower in binge-eating disorder. *Journal of Nutrition, 135*(5), 1326–1330.

Goel, N., Stunkard, A. J., Rogers, N. L., Van Dongen, H. P., Allison, K. C., O'Reardon, J. P., et al. (2009). Circadian rhythm profiles in women with night eating syndrome. *Journal of Biological Rhythms, 24,* 85–94.

Lundgren, J. D., Amsterdam, J., Newberg, A., Allison, K. C., Wintering, N., & Stunkard, A. J. (2009). Differences in serotonin transporter binding affinity in patients with major depressive disorder and night eating syndrome. *Eating and Weight Disorders, 14*(1), 45–50.

Lundgren, J. D., Newberg, A. B., Allison, K. C., Wintering, N. A., Ploessl, K., & Stunkard A. J. (2008). 123I-ADAM SPECT imaging of serotonin transporter binding in patients with night eating syndrome: A preliminary report. *Psychiatry Research, 162,* 214–220.

Millan, M. J., Gobert, A., Lejeune, F., Dekeyne, A., Newman-Tancredi, A., Pasteau, V., et al. (2003). The novel melatonin agonist agomelatine (S20098) is an antagonist at 5-hydroxytryptamine$_{2C}$ receptors, blockade of which enhances the activity of frontocortical dopaminergic and adrenergic pathways. *Journal of Pharmacology and Experimental Therapeutics, 306,* 954–964.

Morrow, J., Gluck, M., Lorence, M., Flacbaum, L., & Geliebter, A. (2008). Night eating status and influence on body weight, body image, hunger, and cortisol pre- and post-Roux-en-Y gastric bypass (RYGB) surgery. *Eating and Weight Disorders, 13*(4), e96–e99.

O'Reardon, J. P., Allison, K. C, Martino, N. S., Lundgren, J. D., Heo, M., & Stunkard, A. J. (2006). A randomized placebo-controlled trial of sertraline in the treatment of the night eating syndrome. *American Journal of Psychiatry, 164,* 893–898.

O'Reardon, J. P., Ringel, B. L., Dinges, D. F., Allison, K. C, Rogers, N. L., Martino, N. S., et al. (2004). Circadian eating and sleeping patterns in the night eating syndrome. *Obesity Research, 12*(11), 1789–1796.

O'Reardon, J. P., Stunkard, A. J., & Allison, K. C. (2004). A clinical trial of sertraline in the treatment of night eating syndrome. *International Journal of Eating Disorders, 35,* 16–26.

Qin, L. Q., Li, J., Wang, Y., Wang, J., Xu, J. Y., & Kaneko, T. (2003). The effects of nocturnal life on endocrine circadian patterns in healthy adults. *Life Science, 73,* 2467–2475.

Rosenhagen, C. M., Uhr, M., Schüssler, P., & Steiger, A. (2005) Elevated plasma ghrelin levels in night-eating syndrome. *American Journal of Psychiatry, 162,* 813.

Spaggiari, M. C., Granella, F., Parrino, L., Marchesi, C., Melli, I., & Terzano, M. G. (1994). Nocturnal eating syndrome in adults. *Sleep, 17,* 339–344.

Stunkard, A. J., Grace, W. J., & Wolff, H. G. (1955). The night-eating syndrome: A pattern of food intake among certain obese patients. *The American Journal of Medicine, 19,* 78–86.

Stunkard, A. J., Allison, K. C., Lundgren, J. D., & O'Reardon, J. P. (2009). A biobehavioral model of the night eating syndrome. *Obesity Reviews, 10*(Suppl. 2), 69–77.

Yous, S., Andrieux, J., Howell, H. E., Morgan, P. J., Renard, P., Pfeiffer, B., et al. (1992). Novel naphthalenic ligands with high affinity for the melatonin receptor. *Journal of Medical Chemistry, 35,* 1484–1486.

Chapter 4

Circadian Rhythms Associated with Night Eating Syndrome

Jennifer D. Lundgren
Raymond Boston
Glenys K. Noble

The most central feature of night eating syndrome (NES) is a circadian-delayed pattern of food intake that manifests behaviorally as evening hyperphagia, nocturnal awakening accompanied by ingestions of food, or both. Human and animal models of wake–feeding and sleep–fasting circadian patterns may be useful in understanding the etiology and maintenance of NES. This chapter reviews the relevant human and animal literatures on circadian rhythm, as well as the literature on circadian eating, sleeping, and neuroendocrine patterns in persons with NES. Suggestions for a new model of evaluating circadian rhythm in relation to eating behavior will be proposed, and the clinical implications of circadian rhythm in persons with NES will be discussed.

Circadian Rhythms: An Overview

Mammals and most other species exhibit regular, rhythmic variation in physiology and behavior, corresponding approximately to a 24-hour cycle (Vitaterna, Takahashi, & Turek, 2001). This regular variability, termed circadian rhythm, is set by both the light–dark cycle and the wake–feed and sleep–fast cycles (Silva, Sato, & Margolis, 2010). The biological clocks that regulate circadian rhythm in mammals are located both centrally, in the suprachiasmatic nuclei (SCN) of the anterior hypothalamus, and peripherally, in the organs such as the liver, gut, pancreas, fat, and muscle (Silva et al., 2010; see Figure 4.1).

Genes and the proteins they encode control the biological clock and, hence, circadian rhythm. The earliest research on genetic mutations affecting circadian rhythm in animals was conducted in the 1970s with fruit flies (*Dosophila melanogaster*) (Konopka & Benzer, 1971; Wager-Smith & Kay, 2000). The first mammalian circadian gene, *Clock*, was discovered in mice in the 1990s (Vitaterna et al., 1994). Since then, several additional mammalian (primarily rodent) circadian genes have

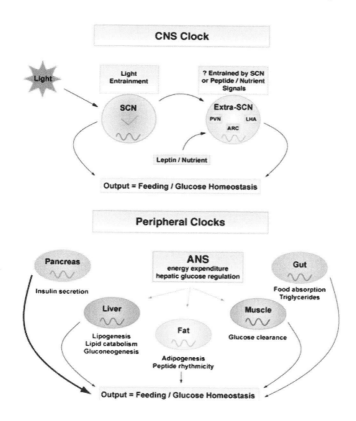

FIGURE 4.1. Central and peripheral circadian clocks. From Silva, Sato, and Margolis. (2010). Copyright 2010 by Cold Spring Harbor Laboratory Press. Reprinted by permission.

been discovered, including *mPer1, mPer2, mPer3, double-time, mCry1, mCry2,* and *BMAL1* (Vitaterna et al., 2001; Wager-Smith & Kay, 2000). Mutations in these genes result in a variety of circadian abnormalities such as lengthening or shortening of period, reduced amplitude, or loss in rhythm (Vitaterna et al., 2001). Less is known, however, about human circadian genes or genetic variation/modification (e.g., via epigenetic mechanisms) that can result in circadian disruption.

The central circadian clock, located in the SCN, is synchronized (entrained) by cues called zeitgebers. The primary zeitgebers for the SCN clock are light and food, but there is evidence that other stimuli, including temperature, exercise, and even social cues, can serve as synchronizing agents in the cellular circadian clocks throughout the body (Mistlberger & Skene, 2004; Vitaterna et al., 2001).

Light and food affect circadian rhythm through food-entrained oscillators (FEO) and light-entrained oscillators (LEO). Typically FEO and LEO cues are in synchrony, resulting in parallel behavioral and physiological processes. For example, most people fast while sleeping at night and consume food only while awake during the day. FEOs and LEOs can become desynchronized such that eating behavior does not occur during the normal light–dark and sleep–wake circadian cycles. When this happens, other cues entrain eating behavior, and the circadian rhythm at the cellular level can shift. For example, hormonal and neuroendocrine rhythms can be phase advanced or phase delayed. In the rodent literature, research has shown that food restriction to the daytime hours (when rodents are usually asleep and fasting) leads to anticipation of food and consequent food anticipatory activity (FAA) during this new feeding time (Mistlberger, 2009). Interestingly, the physiological rhythms become re-entrained as signals for feeding behavior at a new time, thereby reinforcing a phase-delayed or phase-advanced behavioral rhythm (Silver & Balsam, 2010). Examples include insulin, glucose, ghrelin, leptin, and thyroid-stimulating hormone (Silver & Balsam, 2010). It is quite possible, therefore, for feeding and sleeping cues to become desynchronized (through both endogenous and exogenous mechanisms), which could result in a dissociation of feeding and sleeping behavior, and consequent entrainment of new circadian rhythm at the cellular level.

Animal literature supports the importance of synchronization between light–dark, sleep–wake, and feeding cues and behavior, relative to species norms, on health (Arble, Ramsey, Bass, & Turek, 2010). One particular model of circadian dysregulation that could inform NES is the *Clock* mutant mouse (Turek et al., 2005). Turek and colleagues (2005) reported that *Clock* mutant mice had a clear diurnal activity pattern, such that they were more active during the dark phase, which is typical for mice. Compared to wild-type mice, however, they spent a higher percent of their total activity counts in the light phase. Their eating behavior was also quite different: only 53% of the 24-hour total food intake was consumed during the dark phase for the *Clock* mutant mice, compared to 75% of the total 24-hour food intake consumed during the dark phase for the wild-type mice. Energy intake and body weight increased significantly over a 10-week period for *Clock* mutant mice fed either a regular or a high-fat diet. *Clock* mutant, compared to wild-type mice (all fed a regular diet), had significantly higher levels of triglycerides, cholesterol, glucose, and leptin. This animal model has been quite influential in searching for circadian factors associated with obesity and metabolic syndrome, but importantly it also has the potential to inform NES research and treatment.

Preliminary evaluation of the *Clock* gene in persons with NES has not yielded potential mutations associated with the night eating behavioral phenotype (Stunkard, personal communication). This does not rule out the possibility, however, that circadian rhythm in persons with NES is dysregulated via other genetic mechanisms (e.g., additional genes or via epigenetic modulation). See Chapter 5 (Runfola, Root, & Bulik) of this book for a review of the genetics of NES.

Circadian Rhythm in NES

Although much of the general circadian rhythm research has been conducted with nonhuman mammals and invertebrates, the implications of these findings for NES suggest that it is quite possible for both endogenous (e.g., genetic mutation, epigenetic modulation) and exogenous (e.g., conditioned eating behavior) FEOs to re-entrain eating behavior during the nighttime hours, yet keep the sleep–wake circadian rhythm relatively stable. In addition, it would be expected that re-entrainment of eating behavior during the dark and sleep phases in humans could shift hormonal and neuroendocrine rhythm, which could physiologically reinforce the entrained eating behavior at an inappropriate time. It is important to note, however, that desynchrony of FEO and LEO is distinct from additional sleep homeostasis problems (e.g., insomnia, periodic limb movements), that may cause or maintain sleep difficulties in NES (Rosenwasser, 2010). See Chapter 9 (Howell & Crow) for a review of sleep and NES.

The literature on circadian abnormalities in persons with NES is small, but informative. Chapter 3 (Ungredda, Gluck, & Geliebter) reviews the neuroendocrine features of NES in detail, but the results vis-à-vis circadian rhythm are discussed below.

Behavioral Findings

Birketvedt and colleagues (1999) were the first to systematically study the circadian pattern of behavior, mood, and neuroendocrine features of NES. In their behavioral study, 10 overweight night eaters and 10 matched controls were assessed with 24-hour dietary records and actigraphy. Night eaters, compared to controls, consumed more calories (2,928 kcal vs. 2,332 kcal), reported more eating episodes (9.3 vs. 4.2), and exhibited a strikingly different pattern of cumulative caloric intake during a 24-hour period (6:00 A.M. to 5:59 A.M. the following morning). By 6:00 P.M., the group with NES had consumed only 37% of their total 24-hour caloric intake compared to 74% consumed by the control group. Although the controls completed much of their food intake by 8:00 P.M., the night eaters continued to eat until after midnight. Fifty-six percent of the night eaters' caloric intake was consumed between 8:00 P.M. and 5:59 A.M. the following morning, compared to only 15% for the control group. The group with NES reported more awakenings per night compared to the controls (3.6 vs. 0.3), and 52% of the awakenings were accompanied by food intake for the group with NES, whereas there were no nocturnal ingestions in the controls.

In parallel with the circadian-delayed food intake and sleep maintenance difficulty experienced by the group with NES, they also reported significant decreases in mood between 4:00 P.M. and 10:00 P.M. The control group's mood did not change during this time period. Although the controls did not continue to report mood data during the night (presumably because they were asleep), the group with NES continued to show decreases in mood until awakening the following morning. The mood ratings during awakenings in the middle of the night should be interpreted with caution, however, because it is unknown how the mood of controls would have changed had they reported their mood during their (less frequent) nighttime awakenings.

O'Reardon and colleagues (2004) replicated these behavioral findings in 46 overweight/obese night eaters and 43 matched controls, all of whom completed 24-hour food diaries and actigraphy. There was no significant difference in the total daily food intake of night eaters compared to controls (2,314 kcal vs. 2,420 kcal, respectively), but the pattern of food intake differed markedly. Similar to the Birketvedt and colleagues (1999) study, night eaters, compared to controls, consumed significantly less food during the first part of the day and significantly more food during the last part of the day. Despite the circadian delay in food intake, there was no corresponding delay in sleep. Sleep onset time and duration did not differ between groups, although night eaters reported non-significantly later sleep offset times of approximately 25 minutes. With regard to sleep homeostasis, night eaters reported more awakenings per night compared to controls (1.5 vs. 0.5, respectively), and only night eaters reported nocturnal ingestions of food (1.2/night vs. 0.0/night for the controls). Interestingly, nighttime arousals (during which the participant actually got out of bed) occurred earlier after quiescence for night eaters compared to controls (2 hours and 8 minutes vs. 3 hours and 13 minutes). These latter findings suggest that the circadian rhythm of sleep is intact, but that sleep homeostasis is disrupted in NES.

Lundgren and colleagues (Lundgren, Allison, O'Reardon, & Stunkard, 2008) found a circadian delay in eating behavior in a sample of 19 normal weight (body mass index < 25 kg/m²) persons with NES compared to 22 weight- and age-matched controls. Similar to the previous two studies, food intake was assessed with 24-hour dietary recalls, averaged over 1 week. The pattern of cumulative caloric intake beginning at 6:00 A.M. and ending at 5:59 A.M. the following morning differed such that the night eaters' early intake was less than that of controls and steadily increased throughout the day and into the night. At the end of the 24-hour period (5:59 A.M.), the night eaters had consumed significantly more calories than controls (2,284 kcal vs. 1,856 kcal). The time to 75% of caloric intake between groups differed as well, with the night eaters' median time to 75% intake at 11:00 P.M. and the controls' time to 75% intake at 7:00 P.M., yielding a 4-hour delay for the night eaters. In proportion to their total daily food intake, night eaters, compared to controls, reported significantly more evening food consumption, more nocturnal awakenings, more nocturnal ingestions of food, and less morning hunger.

Only one study has used polysomnography to assess sleep patterns of persons with NES compared to healthy controls (Rogers et al., 2006). In this report, Rogers and colleagues (2006) present findings on sleep architecture, rather than a circadian analysis of sleep per se. Their findings support O'Reardon and colleagues' (2004) study showing that there is not a circadian delay in sleep timing that corresponds to the delay in food intake. Specifically, there were no significant differences in sleep onset or sleep offset times. There were, however, several differences in sleep architecture such that night eaters showed less stage 2 sleep, a lower percent of stage 2 sleep in relation to total sleep time, reduced sleep efficiency, reduced total sleep time, and trends toward more awakenings and increased percent time in REM sleep. The authors did not report on circadian differences in the timing of sleep stages, so it is unclear whether the sleep architecture differences between groups represent circadian differences in sleep stage rhythm or whether these differences are due to problems with sleep homeostasis related to an underlying sleep disorder. See Chapter 9 (Howell & Crow) for a detailed overview of sleep in NES, with a particular emphasis on the relationship among NES, restless legs syndrome, and sleep-related eating disorder.

Neuroendocrine Findings

In addition to Birketvedt and colleagues' (1999) behavioral study, they also report on an inpatient study conducted in Norway. Twelve female night eaters (obese and non-obese) and 21 matched controls (obese and non-obese) were admitted to an inpatient clinical research center for 24 hours, after an 8-hour overnight fast (participants were admitted at 8:00 A.M.). Blood was drawn every 2 hours for the duration of their hospital stay. While in the inpatient setting, participants were provided four meals of 300 kcal each at 8:00 A.M., 12:00 P.M., 4:00 P.M., and 8:00 P.M. They were allowed to move freely until 11:00 P.M., at which time lights were turned off and they went to bed. No participants were allowed to eat after 8:00 P.M. Several neuroendocrine variables were assessed, including plasma melatonin, plasma leptin, plasma cortisol, blood glucose, and plasma insulin.

Glucose and insulin levels did not differ between NES and control groups before or after food intake. Plasma melatonin levels differed between NES and control groups, such that night eaters had an attenuated nocturnal rise in melatonin levels in comparison to controls. Plasma leptin levels also showed a lower nocturnal (midnight to 6:00 A.M.) rise in the NES groups (both obese and non-obese) compared to their weight-matched control groups. As expected, leptin levels were higher throughout the 24-hour period for obese participants, compared to non-obese participants, regardless of night eating status. Finally, cortisol levels were higher for night eaters compared to controls (independent of weight) from 8:00 A.M. until 2:00 A.M.

Using the same participants reported in the Rogers et al. (2006) study mentioned above, Allison and colleagues (2005) were unable to replicate the Birketvedt (1999) neuroendocrine findings. Specifically, levels of plasma melatonin, leptin, and cortisol did not differ across time between groups. There were group differences, however, for ghrelin and thyroid-stimulating hormone (TSH). Ghrelin levels were significantly lower between 1:00 A.M. and 9:00 A.M. for night eaters compared to controls, and TSH was higher in night eaters compared to controls throughout the day. Glucose and insulin levels were higher at night for night eaters compared to controls, and corresponded with night eating behavior for the NES group. Of note, participants in this study were allowed to consume food ad libitum, whereas the Birket-vedt (1999) participants were provided only with 1,200 kcal distributed evenly at four time periods during the waking hours (8:00 A.M. to 8:00 P.M.).

As a follow up to the Allison and colleagues (2005) report, Goel and colleagues (2009) re-analyzed the neuroendocrine data to compare the circadian rhythm, in particular the phase and amplitude, of these hormones in the NES and control groups. In comparison with matched controls, the group with NES showed a phase delay of 1.1 hours for melatonin and 1 hour for leptin. Glucose showed an inverted circadian rhythm of 12.4-hour delay/11.6-hour advance, and there was a 2.8-hour delay for insulin. Ghrelin showed a phase advance of 5.2 hours in night eaters compared to controls. Night eaters, compared to controls, had significantly lower amplitude for cortisol (25.7% lower), ghrelin (49.6% lower), and insulin (57.7% lower), and a higher amplitude for TSH (30.9% higher).

In summary, studies of persons with NES compared to matched controls show striking circadian differences in both food intake and neuroendocrine variables. It is unknown, however, whether there are primary endogenous factors that initially entrain the delayed food intake or if there are exogenous/behavioral conditioning factors that initially entrain the delay in food intake, or both. More research is also needed to understand whether and how the ghrelin phase advance and melatonin and leptin phase delays reinforce the delayed eating behavior once it is initially entrained. Of note, the circadian rhythm of sleep does not appear to be disrupted in NES. Sleep onset and duration are intact, but more studies are needed to examine potential circadian advances and delays in sleep architecture, given the differences in sleep architecture noted above (i.e., Rogers et al., 2006).

The circadian delay in eating behavior found in persons with NES is the most consistently noted, and in fact the defining feature, of the syndrome. There are several ways to study and classify normative and non-normative eating behavior. Often mathematical or statistical models (e.g., item response theory, latent class analysis) are used to quantify and compare behavior. Below, new models for studying and classifying circadian eating patterns are presented. Of note, these models were developed by Raymond Boston (University of Pennsylvania) and Glenys Noble (Charles Sturt University).

New Models for Evaluating
Circadian Eating Behavior in Humans

Models are the ideal tools for exploring and understanding departures from normality (Beersma, 2005) and, accordingly, they warrant serious consideration as devices to explore DSM candidacy for diseases and syndromes. Later we present models of circadian food intake in healthy controls and we show how aberrant states lead to changes in the model, hence providing areas of health-state discrimination.

One approach uses moderately sophisticated analytic intake models and one is entirely empirical and may well serve best as a guide to the structure of the analytic approaches. The data serving as the basis for model testing and refinement come from NES and non-NES samples including Striegel-Moore et al. (2006; Striegel-Moore, Franko, & Garcia, 2009) and data from Stunkard's laboratory. Specifically, 148 night eaters (100 female, and 129 overweight/obese) and 68 healthy controls (51 female, and 45 overweight/obese) who completed 24-hour food diaries for 7 consecutive days at the University of Pennsylvania. For analysis the food diary data were converted to hourly cumulative intake and based on the averages of the daily accumulations. Boston, Moate, Allison, Lundgren, and Stunkard (2008) have reported the use of these data for testing of the methods described in the deconvolution model below.

Deconvolution Model

An approach to modeling the hourly observations of daily accumulation of caloric intake that was initially explored assumed that each ingestion could be represented as a Gaussian pulse. This assumes that the meal intake is symmetrical and the data themselves define (1) when the peak intake rate is reached, (2) the magnitude of the peak intake rate, and (3) the duration of each intake pulse. We allowed three such intake pulses, one for each meal, and based on the work of Cutler (1978a, 1978b), we accepted that the shape and "boundedness" (Abramowitz & Stegun, 1964) of the Gaussian pulse will be molded to shapes and features best describing the observed accumulated intake. The equation for each meal, then, is

$$\mathrm{Meal}(t) = P1\exp[-P2(t - P3)^2] \tag{4.1}$$

where $P1$ is the maximum caloric intake rate (kcal/hour^{-1}), $P2$ is a spread factor defining the "meal duration" (hours^{-2}), and $P3$ is the time at which the peak intake is reached (hours, clock time). We see that the meal intake is symmetrical, since replacing $(t - P3)$ by $\pm d$ leads to the same function (Meal $\pm d$). In Figure 4.2 we present (1) the intake given by Equation 4.1 and (2) the model capturing the role of Equation 4.1 in describing our overall intake.

Allowing the intake to be given by Equation 4.1, the rate of accumulation of calories is then

$$\mathrm{UC\mathring{a}l}(t) = \mathrm{Meal}(t) \tag{4.2}$$

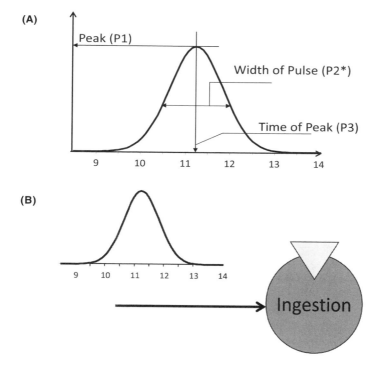

FIGURE 4.2. (A) Features of a Gaussian pulse; (B) Gaussian pulse being delivered into a system compartment. Triangle over the circle denotes a sampling site.

Questions remain; for example, how do we define the daily caloric intake, how do we determine the total intake of each meal, hence for each day, and where do values for *P1*, *P2*, and *P3* come from? As indicated, the intake model capturing the circadian intake comprises three functions of the form of Equation 4.1, and allowing *UB*, *UL*, and *UD* to describe each intake component (where *B*, *L*, and *D* denote breakfast, lunch, and dinner), we have

$$UB(t) = P1\exp[-P2(t - P3)^2]$$
$$UL(t) = P4\exp[-P5(t - P6)^2]$$
$$UD(t) = P7\exp[-P8(t - P9)^2]$$

(4.3)

We use the same intake definition convention to define intake patterns for each study group.

Figure 4.3 shows this model with night eater and control dietary recall data. As the figure illustrates, the peak amplitude and spread of eating episodes for breakfast, lunch, and dinner differ markedly between groups.

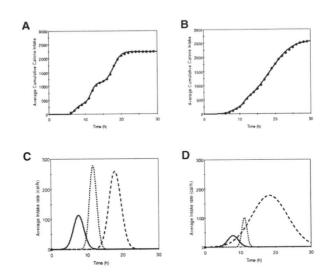

FIGURE 4.3. Use of the sum of three Gaussian curves to describe the average cumulative caloric intake of control subjects (panel A) and patients with NES (panel B). Panel C (control subjects) and panel D (night eaters) depict the individual Gaussian curves that describe the average rate of eating during each of three separate meals. From Boston, Moate, Allison, Lundgren, and Stunkard (2008). Copyright 2008 by the American Society for Nutrition. Reprinted by permission.

Empirical Characterization of Data

Differentiation of the data yielding new observations with units [calories/minute] will provide yet another perspective on the food intake data. Figure 4.4 shows a sample of trellis plots of intakes from four groups: normal-weight controls, overweight controls, normal-weight NES, and overweight NES. Of note are (1) the within-person variability of responses, (2) the between-group variability of responses, and (3) the variability in total intake within and between groups.

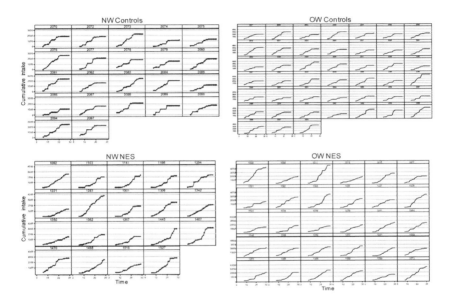

FIGURE 4.4. Trellis plots showing the diversity of responses from data for representative subjects from each of the four study groups. NW Controls, normal-weight controls; OW Controls, overweight controls; NW NES, normal-weight NES; OW NES, overweight NES.

Figure 4.5 shows the fit of Equation 4.3 to the intake data from our four groups (upper panels) and the predicted intake pattern at each intake for the four groups. Outstanding features here are the size and extent of the evening meal for the NES groups. Compare the morning and midday meals for the control groups with the same meals for the NES groups. It is interesting that although the eating patterns are quite different, the net accumulation of food for the day is not so different. This suggests that circadian energy control probably operates close to normally (by weight) with the NES subjects.

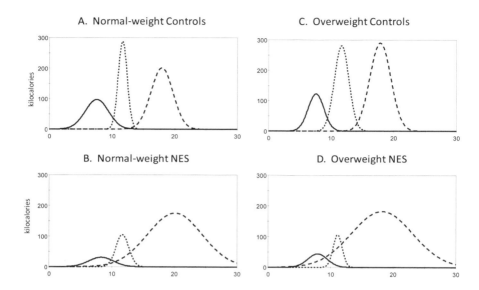

FIGURE 4.5. Plots of Equation 4.3 fitted to intake data for each of the four study groups (upper panels), and estimated intake pattern for each study group of the three intakes pulses (lower panels). Lines represent predicted values from model fits.

Another way to quantitatively capture differences in intake patterns between NES and control groups is to examine the fraction of calories remaining to be consumed as time during the day (eating period) advances. This is a function much like a Kaplan–Meier survival curve (Kaplan & Meier, 1958). It starts at one, at the beginning of the day, and falls monotonically to zero at the time when the entire intake has been consumed. The advantage of this function above simple cumulative intake plots is that it places all groups (in our case) on an identical scale. In Figure 4.6 we show plots of such a function for each of our study groups.

The lines on this plot help us observe the following: (1) at a time when both the control groups (normal weight and overweight) have consumed very close to half their total intake both NES groups have only consumed approximately one-quarter of their total intake (line *a*), and (2) at a time when the control groups have only 25% of their intake remaining to be consumed the NES groups have still to consume 50% of their intake.

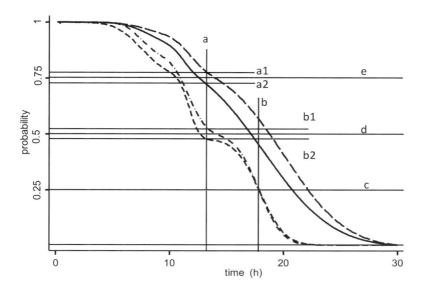

FIGURE 4.6. Plots of the probability that more calories remain to be consumed as a function of time into the eating period (day). – –, normal-weight controls; — —, normal-weight NES; –•–, overweight controls; — — — — — —, overweight NES. Line *a* coincides with (approximately) 50% of total consumption by the control groups; line *b* coincides with (approximately) 75% of total consumption by the control groups.

Model Summary

Two different quantitative models for the analysis of circadian intake, one based on dynamic considerations and the other based on statistical modeling, have been presented. Each is able to describe, and account for, intake differences in our four study populations quite precisely. We imagine that the deployment of these methods would be in instances where groups of patients, in different treatment, demographic, or health strata are studied in regard to their intake, and these methods of investigation would offer group discrimination (or study strata separation) based on investigation of mean group responses. The value of these mathematical models is that they quantify differences in the circadian pattern of food intake in persons with NES compared to healthy controls with more normative eating patterns and provide a novel analysis of eating behavior.

In this chapter, we have thus far provided a basic overview of circadian rhythms, a more detailed review of the circadian eating, sleep, and neuroendocrine studies conducted with persons with NES, and we presented two mathematical models for future research to better quantify and describe normative and non-normative circadian patterns of eating behavior. The clinical implications of circadian rhythm for the treatment of NES are significant, and are reviewed below.

Clinical Implications of Circadian Rhythm in Persons with NES

For decades, behavioral literature in both animals and humans has shown that eating behavior can be conditioned through both classical (Pavlovian) and operant (Skinnerian) mechanisms. For example, dogs in Pavlov's digestive physiology experiments became classically conditioned to salivate in the presence of many environmental stimuli that cued food. In addition, eating can become reinforced (via operant conditioning) if it is followed by a pleasant response–reward (e.g., reduction in negative affect). It is likely, therefore, that one of the mechanisms by which night eating (both evening hyperphagia and nocturnal ingestions of food) is developed and/or maintained is through conditioning. For example, a person who has difficulty staying asleep might initially eat to help herself fall back to sleep. If this coping strategy works, the night eating could become a regular sleep aid. Over time, as the night eating is paired with environmental cues such as watching television or reading, or even the sight of one's kitchen, these cues could stimulate eating at night.

Recently, the animal literature has shown that conditioned eating behavior can modify endogenous circadian rhythms (Mistlberger, 2009). It is likely in persons with NES that as eating behavior is delayed, neuroendocrine rhythm is re-entrained accordingly. In treatment, therefore, it is important to (1) explain that circadian rhythm both affects and is affected by behavior and (2) it is possible to restore circadian rhythm by re-establishing a normative eating and sleep schedule. As outlined in Allison's cognitive-behavioral therapy (CBT) treatment manual (Chapter 14), there are several strategies to help the patient with NES resume regular eating patterns. These include encouraging the consumption of breakfast, even if one is not hungry, and modifying environmental stimuli to reduce the likelihood of conditioned eating at night (e.g., posting a "kitchen is closed" sign or locking one's refrigerator).

There are also pharmacological interventions that target circadian hormones (e.g., melatonin), which may prove beneficial in the treatment of NES. Agomelatine, a novel melatonin agonist (MT_1 and MT_2 receptors) and serotonin antagonist ($5\text{-}HT_{2c}$ receptor) developed by Servier Laboratories is currently being tested in Europe for the treatment of depression (de Bodinat et al., 2010; Kasper et al., 2010). Kasper and colleagues (2010) found that agomelatine was more effective than sertraline in improving activity (measured by actigraphy), sleep, depression, and anxiety over 6 weeks. Agomelatine was better tolerated than sertraline, as evidenced by lower rates of withdrawal and adverse events. Given the circadian disruption, and evidence suggesting that the serotonin system is involved in NES (see Ungredda, Gluck, & Geliebter, Chapter 3, and Patel, O'Reardon, & Cristancho, Chapter 12), it is possible that this drug may prove beneficial in the treatment of NES.

Areas for Future Research

Circadian rhythm research for NES is in its infancy, and several areas need further exploration. First, studies are needed to determine whether the circadian rhythm disturbances noted in eating, sleep, and neuroendocrine factors originate in endogenous factors (e.g., genes), exogenous factors (e.g., learning and conditioning), or a combination of both. Second, more research in the area of sleep, both circadian sleep patterns and sleep homeostasis, is necessary to determine the role of sleep disruption in the etiology and maintenance of NES. Third, effective interventions, both behavioral and pharmacological, that target circadian rhythm should be developed and tested.

In conclusion, circadian rhythm is crucial to the survival of nearly all species. Although organisms are quick to adapt to changes in rhythm to ensure homeostasis, research suggests that desynchrony in rhythms can result in poor health outcomes. Persons with NES exhibit circadian-delayed food intake, intact circadian sleep patterns (but with some evidence of sleep homeostasis and sleep architecture problems), and associated circadian dysregulation of neuroendocrine factors. Interventions (e.g., CBT, sertraline) are available to restore normative eating and sleeping patterns and potentially resynchronize circadian rhythm. Future research is necessary to better understand the role of circadian rhythm in the etiology and maintenance of NES.

References

Abramowitz, M., & Stegun, I. A. (1964). *Handbook of mathematical functions with formulas, graphs and mathematical tables.* New York: Dover.

Allison K. C., Ahima, R. S., O'Reardon, J. P., Dinges, D. F., Sharma, V., Cummings, D. E., et al. (2005). Neuroendocrine profiles associated with energy intake, sleep and stress in the night eating syndrome. *Journal of Clinical Endocrinolology and Metabolism, 90*(11), 6214–6217.

Arble, D. M., Ramsey, K. M., Bass, J., & Turek, F. W. (2010). Circadian disruption and metabolic disease: Findings from animal models. *Best Practice and Research: Clinical Endocrinology and Metabolism, 24,* 785–800.

Beersma, D. G. M. (2005). Why and how do we model circadian rhythms? *Journal of Biological Rhythms, 20*(4), 304–313.

Birketvedt, G. S., Florholmen, J., Sundsfjord, J., Osterud, B., Dinges, D., Bilker, W., et al. (1999). Behavioral and neuroendocrine characteristics of the night-eating syndrome. *Journal of the American Medical Association, 282*(7), 657–663.

Boston, R. C., Moate, P. J., Allison, K. C., Lundgren, J. D., & Stunkard, A. J. (2008). Modeling circadian rhythms of food intake by means of parametric deconvolution: Results from studies of the night eating syndrome. *American Journal of Clinical Nutrition, 87*(6), 1672–1677.

Cutler, D. J. (1978a). Numerical deconvolution by least squares: Use of prescribed input functions. *Journal of Pharmacokinetic Biopharmacology, 6,* 227–241.

Cutler, D. J. (1978b). Numerical deconvolution by least squares: Use of polynomials to represent the input function. *Journal of Pharmacokinetic Biopharmacology, 6,* 227–241.

de Bodinat, C., Guardiola-Lemaitre, B., Mocaër, E., Renard, P., Munoz, C., & Millan, M. J. (2010). Agomelatine, the first melatonergic antidepressant: Discovery, characterization and development. *Nature Reviews Drug Discovery, 9*(8), 628–642.

Goel, N., Stunkard, A. J., Rogers, N. L.,Van Dongen, H. P. A., Allison, K. C., O'Reardon, J. P., et al. (2009). Circadian rhythm profiles in women with night eating syndrome. *Journal of Biological Rhythms, 24*(1), 85–94.

Kaplan, E. L., & Meier, P. (1958). Nonparametric estimations from incomplete observations. *Journal of American Statistical Association, 53,* 457–481.

Kasper, S., Hajak, G., Wulff, K., Hoogendijk, W. J. G., Monejo, A. L., Smeraldi, E., et al. (2010). Efficacy of the novel antidepressant agomelatine on the circadian rest–activity cycle and depressive and anxiety symptoms in patients with major depressive disorder: A randomized, double-blind comparison with sertraline. *Journal of Clinical Psychiatry, 71*(2), 109–120.

Konopka, R. J., & Benzer, S. (1971). Clock mutants of Drosophila melanogaster. *Proceedings of the National Academy of Sciences, 68,* 2112–2116.

Lundgren, J. D., Allison, K. C., O'Reardon, J. P., & Stunkard, A. J. (2008). A descriptive study of non-obese persons with night eating syndrome and a weight-matched comparison group. *Eating Behaviors, 9,* 343–351.

Mistlberger, R. E. (2009). Food-anticipatory circadian rhythms: Concepts and methods. *European Journal of Neuroscience, 30,* 1718–1729.

Mistlberger, R. E., & Skene, D. J. (2004). Social influences on mammalian circadian rhythms: Animal and human studies. *Biological Reviews, 79,* 533–556.

O'Reardon, J. P., Ringel, B. L., Dinges, D. F., Allison, K. C., Rogers, N. L., Martino, N. S., et al. (2004). Circadian eating and sleeping patterns in the night eating syndrome. *Obesity Research, 12*(11), 1789–1796.

Rogers, N. L., Dinges, D. F., Allison, K. C., Maislin, G., Martino, N., O'Reardon, J. P., et al. (2006). Assessment of sleep in women with night eating syndrome. *Sleep, 29*(6), 814–819.

Rosenwasser, A. M. (2010). Circadian clock genes: Non-circadian roles in sleep, addiction, and psychiatric disorders? *Neuroscience and Biobehavioral Reviews, 34,* 1249–1255.

Silva, C. M., Sato, S., & Margolis, R. N. (2010). No time to lose: Workshop on circadian rhythms and metabolic disease. *Genes and Development, 24,* 1456–1464.

Silver, R., & Balsam, P. (2010). Oscillators entrained by food and the emergence of anticipatory timing behaviors. *Sleep and Biological Rhythms, 8*(2), 120–136.

Striegel-Moore, R. H., Franko, D. L., & Garcia, J. (2009). The validity and clinical utility of night eating syndrome. *International Journal of Eating Disorders, 42*(8), 720–738.

Striegel-Moore, R. H., Franko, D. L., May, A., Ach, E., Thompson, D., & Hook, J. M. (2006). Should night eating syndrome be included in the DSM? *International Journal of Eating Disorders, 39*(7), 544–549.

Turek, F. W., Joshu, C., Kohsaka, A., Lin, E., Ivanova, G., McDearmon, E., et al. (2005). Obesity and metabolic syndrome in circadian *Clock* mutant mice. *Science, 308,* 1043–1045.

Vitaterna, M. H., King, D. P., Chang, A., Kornhauser, J. M., Lowrey, P. L., McDonald, J. D., et al. (1994). Mutagenesis and mapping of a mouse gene, Clock, essential for circadian behavior. *Science, 264,* 719–725.

Viaterna, M. H., Takahashi, J. S, & Turek, F. W. (2001). Overview of circadian rhythms. *Alcohol Research and Health, 25*(2), 85–93.

Wager-Smith, K., & Kay, S. A. (2000). Circadian rhythm genetics: From flies to mice to humans. *Nature Genetics, 26,* 23–27.

Chapter 5

Behavioral and Molecular Genetics of Night Eating Syndrome

Cristin D. Runfola
Tammy L. Root
Cynthia M. Bulik

Current thinking about eating disorders conceptualizes them as resulting from multiple genetic, epigenetic, and environmental interactions. As eating disorders are complex traits, it is not surprising that identification of genetic contributions is similarly complex. By definition, complex traits are not caused by one single gene, but rather a number of genes, each with a small to moderate effect in combination with environmental factors. Although a considerable body of research has focused on the genetics of eating disorders in general, the genetics of night eating syndrome (NES) has received less attention.

In this chapter, we review existing family, twin, and molecular genetic studies of night eating. Given that this area of research is relatively new, we also contextualize the findings with a brief discussion of genetic studies of associated clinical features, including binge eating, depression, and sleep disturbance. Second, we discuss the ways in which genetic epidemiological studies may inform classification, assessment, and treatment of NES. Finally, we present directions for future research to enhance the field.

Family Studies of Night Eating and NES

Assessing risk to offspring through family studies is typically the first step in determining genetic and environmental risk for disease. Family studies are able to address whether a particular disorder or trait runs in families; they are unable, however, to ascertain the mechanism behind the familial pattern and the extent to which any observed familial aggregation is due to genetic or environmental factors. To date, only two studies have examined familial risk for night eating behavior (Lamerz et al., 2005; Lundgren, Allison, & Stunkard, 2006). In the first German study, risk for night eating among 5- to 6-year-old children of mothers who endorsed night eating was nearly eight times greater than among children of mothers who did not endorse night eating. In this study, night eating in the children was based on parental report of the child getting up late in the evening or during the night to consume large amounts of high-calorie food more than once a week for at least 3 months (Lamerz et al., 2005). Similar estimates were obtained in an American study examining NES among first-degree adult relatives (Lundgren et al., 2006). In this study, when NES was defined as consuming at least 25% of daily caloric intake after dinner and/or nocturnal awakenings with food ingestion at least three times per week, risk was nearly five times greater in relatives of individuals with NES than in relatives of unaffected individuals (Lundgren et al., 2006). These findings are consistent with family studies of other eating disorders characterized by binge eating, which show a higher lifetime prevalence of eating disorders among relatives of bulimia nervosa (Hudson, Pope, Jonas, Yurgelun-Todd, & Frankenburg, 1987; Lilenfeld et al., 1998; Strober, Freeman, Lampert, Diamond, & Kaye, 2000) and binge-eating disorder probands compared to controls (Lilenfeld, Ringham, Kalarchian, & Marcus, 2008). The above two studies provide suggestive evidence that a familial vulnerability to night eating symptoms and syndromes may exist.

Twin Studies of Night Eating and NES

Twin Study Designs

In contrast to family studies, twin studies allow us to parse out the genetic (i.e., heritability) from environmental (i.e., shared and nonshared) liability to specific traits or phenotypes. Heritability refers to the proportion of phenotypic variation attributable to genetic factors. Common or shared environmental effects result from etiological influences to which both members of a twin pair are exposed regardless of zygosity (e.g., childhood socioeconomic status, [SES]) and serve to increase twin similarity. Unique or nonshared environmental effects are events occurring to one twin but not the other (e.g., one twin develops influenza and the other does not) and serve to decrease twin similarity. Monozygotic (MZ) twins share 100% of their genes and dizygotic (DZ) twins share on average 50%. When certain assumptions are met (Kendler, 1993), higher concordance among MZ than DZ twins suggests that genetic factors influence liability to expression of the phenotype. The greater the heritability estimate relative to the shared and nonshared environmental contributions, the more genetic factors are thought to contribute to phenotypic individual differences. Univariate twin modeling is used to estimate heritability of a single disorder, whereas more complex models can estimate heritability of more than one disorder simultaneously and/or assess group differences (see Kendler, 1993, for more specifics on twin modeling). For ease in interpretation, we present a graphical representation of a univariate twin model in Figure 5.1. Twin studies themselves are limited in that they are not able to determine which genes influence the phenotype under study. Molecular genetic methods are required to identify specific gene variants that actually influence specific traits or disorders.

Heritability of Night Eating and NES

Twin studies of night eating are in their infancy. The only study (Root et al., 2010) that examined the genetic and environmental influences of night eating reported moderate heritability for both males and females, suggesting familial aggregation of night eating is partly due to additive genetic factors. In this study of Swedish twins, night eating was defined as the presence of evening hyperphagia (consuming 25% or more of daily caloric intake after dinner) and/or nocturnal ingestions (waking up from sleep and eating) at least once per week, and was studied in the context of bivariate twin analysis with binge eating designed to determine the extent to which similar genetic and environmental etiological factors influence night eating and binge eating. The heritability of night eating was estimated to be .35 (95% confidence interval [CI]: .17, .52) in females and .44 (95% CI: .24, .61) in males. Heritability of binge eating was .70 (95% CI = .60, .77) in females and .74 (95% CI = .36, .93) in males. In the best-fitting models, the remaining variance for both night eating and binge eating was attributable to nonshared environmental influences.

A second question addressed by this investigation was the extent to which genetic and environmental factors that influence night eating and binge eating are shared. A moderate overlap in underlying genetic liabil-

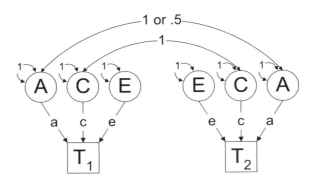

FIGURE 5.1. Graphical depiction of a univariate twin model (ACE model). The univariate ACE model parses the variance in liability to a trait (phenotype) due to additive genetic effects (A), family or common environment (C), and individual-specific or unique environment (E). T_1 represents twin 1 and T_2 represents twin 2. Because monozygotic (MZ) twins share all their genes and dizygotic (DZ) twins share about half their genes, the correction for additive genetic effects in MZ twins is 1 and in DZ twins is .5. Common environment (C) contributes equally to the correlation in MZ and DZ twins, as this includes environmental factors shared by both twin-pair members (e.g., social class during childhood). Individual-specific or unique environment (E) includes environmental factors to which only one member of a twin pair is exposed (e.g., traumatic life events) and serves to decrease similarity in twins. Lowercase letters represent path coefficients (a, c, or e). The square of the path coefficient (a^2, c^2, or e^2) determines the proportion of variance in liability to the studied disorder/trait accounted for by the latent variables. The heritability estimate is determined by multiplying the difference between MZ and DZ twin correlations by two, and is an indication of the extent to which genetic factors influence liability to a studied trait (phenotype).

ity was found (.66 genetic correlation [95% CI: .48, .96]), suggesting that although some genetic factors influence both night eating and binge eating, there also appear to be unique genetic factors that influence liability to each trait independently (Root et al., 2010).

No other twin studies of night eating are available with which to compare the findings of Root and colleagues (2010). Relative to binge eating, in which heritability estimates range from .43 to .82 (Bulik, Sullivan, & Kendler, 1998; Mitchell et al., 2010; Reichborn-Kjennerud et al., 2003; Root et al., 2010; Sullivan, Bulik, & Kendler, 1998b), heritability of night eating is lower. While this offers some form of comparison, we need to interpret these findings with caution, as the Root et al. (2010) study was a single assessment design and unable to examine the potential impact of measurement unreliability issues on the heritability estimate. Measurement reliability for binge eating assessed at 5-year intervals is at best moderate (k = 0.34) (Bulik et al., 1998), and heritability estimates for latent vulnerability to binge eating are substantially higher when measurement error is considered. Thus heritability estimates that rely on a single assessment may result in underestimations of the influence of genetic factors. Future studies should use multiple assessment periods in twin measurement models to estimate the variance due to measurement error, and to determine the resulting additive genetic and shared environmental influence on night eating after controlling for this error.

It is clear that additional targeted work is required before firm conclusions can be drawn. The aforementioned family studies offer preliminary support for familial aggregation of night eating phenotypes and the single twin study suggests genetic influences on night eating. Clear and consistent definitions of night eating and additional studies examining genetic and environmental factors, with both family and twin studies across males and females, are necessary. Twin studies have the potential to further refine diagnostic criteria for NES. For example, item–factor models can be used (1) to determine how strongly individual NES symptoms (observed variables or items) are related to the diagnosis of NES (latent trait) and (2) to identify specific symptoms (i.e., items) of NES that are most strongly influenced by genetic factors (Mazzeo et al., 2010; Neale, Lubke, Aggen, & Dolan, 2005). Such symptom-level approaches elucidate item-specific variance components that may differentially affect "sum score" heritability estimates (i.e., heritability estimates for the latent trait of NES derived from the summation of individual item scores that corresponded to individual NES symptoms); disregard for item-specific variance may result in over- or underestimation of the heritability estimate (Neale et al., 2005). Thus future twin studies using item–factor models may help refine the phenotype of NES by clarifying sources of variation for the individual components of NES and may inform refinements to the diagnostic criteria.

Molecular Genetic Studies of Dysregulated Eating Approaches

In order to identify actual genetic variants that influence NES and related phenotypes, molecular genetic approaches are required. To date, however, there have been no molecular genetic studies of night eating behavior in humans. In the absence of human data, we will review related bodies of literature to provide both context and direction. In this section, we present a basic primer on molecular genetic approaches. Second, we review molecular genetic studies of two syndromes that are commonly comorbid with NES and that are characterized by eating dysregulation, namely, bulimia nervosa (BN) and binge-eating disorder (BED). Night eating has been reported in about 9% of individuals with BN (Tzischinsky & Latzer, 2004) and in 15 to 20% of individuals with BED (Stunkard et al., 2009). We review both candidate gene studies focusing on pathways and mechanisms hypothesized to play a role in dysregulated eating as well as agnostic genome-wide approaches. Third, we review animal models that have explored the genetics of the relevant eating-related phenotype of hyperphagia, a core feature of NES.

Molecular Genetic Study Designs

Molecular genetic studies afford greater precision in identifying either chromosomal regions that may harbor risk loci for a trait or disorder or to identify genetic variants that may be associated with a specific trait. Both human and animal models can be applied to identify loci that influence syndromes or phenotypes related to the disorder. Linkage and association studies are the two most common molecular genetic study designs.

Linkage studies examine patterns of heredity in either large multiply affected families or large samples of affected sibling or relative pairs by genotyping genetic markers across the genome with the goal of identifying chromosomal regions with DNA segments that tend to be inherited together. These identified chromosomal regions narrow the search area of the genome that is more likely to contain disease-causing variants in a gene for a particular phenotype. This information can then be used to create a priori hypotheses needed to conduct association studies by identifying the candidate genes (located under the identified linkage peaks) potentially involved in risk. In contrast, association studies involve comparing a sample of affected individuals (e.g., individuals with NES) to a sample of unaffected individuals (e.g., individuals without NES) to determine the relevant genes influencing the phenotype.

Association studies involve genotyping single nucleotide polymorphism (SNP)—variations in the genome that are altered across individuals—in anywhere from one SNP in a prespecified candidate gene (i.e., candidate gene association study) to millions of SNPs (i.e., genome-wide association study [GWAS]). Whereas candidate-gene association studies require hypothesis-driven testing about the specific genes implicated in the phenotype under study, GWAS scan the entire genome to identify the common disease–common variant (CDCV) without an a priori hypothesis on disease etiology, rendering it an ideal technique for identifying genetic influences in psychiatric disorders. More advanced methodologies involving high-throughput sequencing (Lupski et al., 2010) and copy number variations are also gaining in popularity and feasibility (Carter, 2007; Medvedev, Stanciu, & Brudno, 2009). For interested readers, a more thorough description of GWAS methodology is described elsewhere (Psychiatric GWAS Consortium Steering Committee, 2009).

Molecular Genetic Studies of BN and BED

The genes studied thus far in BN and BED samples can be classified mostly into serotonergic (e.g., serotonin 2A receptor [5-HT2A]) and dopaminergic systems (e.g., dopamine D2 receptor [DRD2]) and systems involved in feeding and body weight regulation (e.g., brain-derived neurotrophic factor [BDNF]), melanocortin 4 receptor [MC4R]). As functional pathophysiology of serotonin, dopamine, and endocrine systems are found in individuals with night eating (Lundgren, Newberg et al., 2008; Stunkard & Lu, 2010), this review will focus on the candidate gene, linkage, and GWAS molecular studies of these systems in BN and BED (see Table 5.1).

Candidate Gene Studies of BN and BED

Serotonergic System. Serotonin (5-hydroxytryptamine [5-HT]) is a neurotransmitter involved in the regulation of body weight, appetite, mood, and sleep. Associations have been observed between the *5-HT2A* (Nishiguchi et al., 2001; Ricca et al., 2002) and *5-HTTLPR* genotypes and alleles (e.g., G, A, G/A) and BN (Di Bella, Catalano, Cavallini, Riboldi, & Bellodi, 2000). One study (Monteleone, Tortorella, Castaldo, & Maj, 2006) reported an association between *5-HTTLPR* alleles and BED. However, other individual studies (Enoch et al., 1998; Hammer et al., 2009; Lauzurica et al., 2003; Nacmias et al., 1999; Ricca et al., 2002; Ziegler et al., 1999), and more robust meta-analytic studies failed to replicate these findings (Calati, De Ronchi, Bellini, & Serretti, 2010; Lee & Lin, 2010), suggesting that concrete conclusions cannot yet be drawn about the role of serotonergic genes in BN or BED.

Dopaminergic System. Dopamine is a neurotransmitter involved in pleasure and reward, including food reward mechanisms. A higher frequency of the short allele for the dopamine transporter (*DAT1*) gene of the vari-

TABLE 5.1. Association Studies of BN and BED for Three Systems Involved in Night Eating: Serotonergic, Dopaminergic, and Endocrine

System / gene	BN[a]	BED[b]	References
Serotonergic system			
Serotonin 2A receptor (*5-HT2A*)	Yes	NE	Nishiguchi et al. (2001)
	Yes	No	Ricca et al. (2002)
	No	NE	Enoch et al. (1998); Lauzurica et al. (2003); Nacmias et al. (1999); Ziegler et al. (1999); Calati et al. (2010); Lee et al. (2010); Hammer et al. (2009)
Serotonin transporter (*5-HTTLPR*)	Yes	NE	Di Bella et al. (2000)
	NE	Yes	Monteleone et al. (2006)
Dopaminergic system			
Dopamine D2 receptor (*DRD2*)	NE	Yes	Davis et al. (2008)
Dopamine transporter (*DAT1*)	Yes	NE	Shinohara et al. (2004)
Endocrine system			
Ghrelin gene	Yes	NE	Ando et al. (2006)
	No	Yes	Monteleone et al. (2006, 2007)
	No	No	Ando et al. (2010); Kindler et al. (2011)
Leptin gene	No	NE	Hinney et al. (1998)
	NE	No	Potoczna et al. (2004)

Note. NE, not examined. This table represents only association studies of BN and BED that were conducted in systems previously found to be implicated in night eating (sertonergic, dopaminergic, and endocrine).
[a] Significantly associated with BN.
[b] Significantly associated with BED.

able number of tandem repeats (VNTR) polymorphism was found in individuals with BN compared with controls (Shinohara et al., 2004), and increased *DRD2* was found in BED versus non-BED controls (Davis et al., 2008). Examining the phenotype of BED, another study indicated that the presence of a seven-repeat allele of the *DRD4* contributes to binge-eating behavior (Levitan et al., 2004). No replication studies exist, and the above studies consisted of small sample sizes, interfering with our ability to interpret results.

Endocrine System. Ghrelin is a hormone produced in the stomach and pancreas that stimulates hunger. Two studies suggest that the *Leu72Met* ghrelin gene variant may play a role in genetic susceptibility to BN (Ando et al., 2006) and BED (Monteleone, Tortorella, Castaldo, Di Filippo, & Maj, 2007). However, contradictory results also exist in BN samples (Monteleone, Tortorella, Castaldo, Di Filippo, & Maj, 2006), and other studies failed to find an association between binge eating and ghrelin gene polymorphisms (Ando et al., 2010; Kindler et al., 2011). In contrast to ghrelin, leptin is a hormone derived from adipose tissue that *inhibits* appetite, playing a role in regulating energy intake and expenditure. Two studies have looked at the role of leptin genes in BN and BED, with both yielding negative results (Hinney et al., 1998; Potoczna et al., 2004).

Other Genes Involved in Feeding and Regulation. Other studies examined the role of BDNF, *MC4R*, catechol-O-methyltransferase (COMT), proopiomelanocortin (POMC), neuropeptide Y, and glucocorticoid receptor genes (Cellini et al., 2010; Kindler et al., 2011; Potoczna et al., 2004; Scherag, Hebebrand, & Hinney, 2010). Results are either contradictory, lacking in replication, or are difficult to interpret due to small sample sizes.

Linkage and GWAS of BN and BED

One genome-wide linkage analysis study in 308 multiplex families with eating disorders identified through BN probands found significant linkage on chromosome 10p and suggestive linkage on chromosome 14q (Bulik et al., 2003). The subphenotype of BN with self-induced vomiting was also examined separately, with results yielding a stronger linkage signal on chromosome 10p. No GWAS in BN or BED samples exist to date, but such studies are eagerly awaited with the hope that these genome-wide scans will illuminate other genes not yet identified and clarify the role of previously reviewed genes in BN and BED.

Animal Models of Hyperphagia

There are no genetic studies examining the phenotype of night eating in human samples, but animal models of behavior have explored the genetics underlying the phenotype of hyperphagia, a core feature of NES.

These studies suggest circadian, melanocortin, and BDNF genes may play a role in night eating behavior.

Circadian Genes. The period gene 2 (*mPer2*) and circadian locomotor output cycles kaput (*Clock*) genes are both located in the suprachiasmatic nucleus and are implicated in the regulation of diurnal rhythms of behavior driven by the light–dark cycle of the environment. Studies show *mPer2* deficit (Yang et al., 2009) and *Clock* mutant mice (Turek et al., 2005) consume more fat and overall calories during the inactive period (i.e., evening hyperphagia phenotype) and fewer calories during the active period (i.e., morning anorexia phenotype) compared with nonmutant mice. This delay in circadian intake of food is a core feature of NES (Goel et al., 2009; O'Reardon et al., 2004), and studies show that those who have night eating typically consume more calorically dense and high-fat foods (Birketvedt et al., 1999). These data suggest the circadian system, and, more specifically, *mPer2* and *Clock* genes may play a role in evening hyperphagia in humans. The association between NES and the circadian system is more thoroughly reviewed in Chapter 4 (Lundgren, Boston, & Noble).

Melanocortin Genes. α-Melanocyte-stimulating hormone (αMSH) is a neuroendocrine peptide that binds to and activates melanocortin 3 and 4 receptors (MC3R, MC4R), which have been linked to obesity and binge eating in humans (Lee, 2009). One study (Yang et al., 2009) showed αMSH injections reduced light-period feeding (i.e., evening hyperphagia), total high-fat diet (HFD; 60% calories from fat) intake, and subsequently resulted in weight loss in *mPer2* deficit mice, effects not found in their counterparts. The other study (Sutton, Babin, Gu, Hruby, & Butler, 2008) showed that, at initial onset of the light period (nighttime in humans), injection of SHU9119, an *MCR* antagonist, increased food intake during that light period. These results suggest the possible role of attenuated αMSH in evening hyperphagia in NES.

Brain-Derived Neurotrophic Factor. BDNF has effects on key neurotransmitter systems—namely, serotonin—shown to be involved in night eating and other eating disorders. In one study (Unger, Calderon, Bradley, Sena-Esteves, & Rios, 2007), BDNF mutations in the ventromedial and dorsomedial hypothalamus were reported to contribute to hyperphagic behavior in mice. Another study (Lyons et al., 1999) found that partial deletion of endogenous BDNF lead to 5-HT abnormalities and was associated with hyperphagia in mice. Thus animal models suggest an association between *BDNF* gene variants and hyperphagia (Lyons et al., 1999; Unger et al., 2007).

In summary, human and animal studies of dysregulated eating are fairly equivocal, and it is difficult to draw concrete conclusions from them, due to small sample sizes (see Bulik & Tozzi, 2004; Hinney, Friedel, Remschmidt, & Hebebrand, 2004; Mathes, Brownley, Mo, & Bulik, 2009; Scherag et al., 2010; Slof-Op't Landt et al., 2005; Striegel-Moore & Bulik, 2007, for reviews). Serotonergic, dopaminergic, and melanocortin systems have the most evidence for their role in feeding behavior and weight regulation. Association studies can clarify the role of the specific genes underlying these systems with NES, and GWAS approaches can potentially shed light on genes not identified previously, opening up new areas of inquiry and guiding future research. While exploratory approaches such as GWAS are optimal, due to the scarcity of individuals with night eating, it may be difficult to obtain adequate sample sizes to achieve enough power to show GWAS significance. Large collaborative investigations would be needed to successfully conduct GWAS of night eating.

Genetics of Depression and Sleep

Again, to provide context in the absence of direct human data on NES, we briefly review what is known about molecular genetic factors influencing two commonly co-occurring issues: depression and sleep.

Genetics of Depression

Between 53 and 56% of individuals with night eating report a lifetime history of depression (de Zwaan, Roerig, Crosby, Karaz, & Mitchell, 2006; Lundgren, Allison, O'Reardon, & Stunkard, 2008). Shared genetic vulnerability has been found between BN and depression (Kendler et al., 1995; Wade, Bulik, Prescott, & Kendler, 2004), but no studies have looked at shared genetic vulnerability between night eating and depression. A meta-analysis (Sullivan, Neale, & Kendler, 2000) of genetic epidemiological family and twin studies of major depression reported a summary odds ratio of 2.84 and heritability estimate of .37, suggesting that depression is familial. Genome-wide linkage studies are inconsistent, and GWAS (Lewis et al., 2010; Muglia et al., 2010; Shi et al., 2011; Shyn et al., 2011; Sullivan et al., 2009; Wray et al., 2012) have yet to find SNPs achieving genome-wide significance in depression samples. One GWAS (Bosker et al., 2011) found four genes—*C5orf20, NPY, TNF,* and *SLC6A2*—implicated in depression, which replicated findings of previous research; however, the authors cautioned that there was only modest support for these genes (significance levels between .0034 and .039), and that further replication is needed before any firm conclusions can be drawn.

Genetics of Sleep

Sleep regulation and function are compromised in individuals with NES. As other chapters in this book (Lundgren, Boston, & Noble, Chapter 4; Howell & Crow, Chapter 9) review the NES sleep literature in detail, below we briefly present the status of genetic research on sleep disturbance, and on sleep disorders that have some comorbidity with NES.

Sleep is strongly influenced by genetic factors. Twin studies demonstrate high heritability (up to .90) of sleep architecture (i.e., the structural components of sleep such as stage changes) and sleep regulation (i.e., sleep onset, latency, and efficiency) (Cirelli, 2009; Tafti, 2009). Sleep disturbances including increased nighttime awakenings (O'Reardon et al., 2004), reduced sleep efficiency (Tzischinsky & Latzer, 2004; Vetrugno et al., 2006), and reduced total sleep time (Rogers et al., 2006) are more likely to occur in those who endorse night eating behavior compared with those who do not. Regarding these specific phenotypes, twin studies in MZ and DZ adult twin pairs document a heritability of .44 for both sleep duration and sleep quality (Gedda & Brenci, 1983). Various genes are identified as contributors to sleep in humans (see Tafti, 2009, for review), including polymorphisms on the *Clock* gene. In rodents, *Clock* genes have been implicated in circadian feeding behavior strikingly similar to that observed in patients with NES (Turek et al., 2005).

Various sleep disorders are familial (Dauvilliers & Tafti, 2008; Tafti, 2009), including bruxism (Hublin, Kaprio, Partinen, & Koskenvuo, 1998), restless legs syndrome, and insomnia, which are also reported to occur in individuals with NES (Provini et al., 2009; Vetrugno et al., 2006). Molecular genetic studies have identified chromosomal regions and genes that may be implicated in restless legs syndrome and chronic primary insomnia (see Dauvilliers & Tafti, 2008; Tafti, 2009, for reviews). To our knowledge, there are no GWAS to date in the sleep literature.

In short, genetics play a role in both depression and sleep problems, which are frequent presenting complaints of individuals with NES. With rapid emergence of new technology, we will have unprecedented opportunities to explore the extent to which shared genetic and neurobiological mechanisms influence regulation of sleep, appetite, and mood—all of which are core components of NES.

Genetics of Night Eating: Informing Classification, Assessment, and Treatment

As genetic research in night eating is scant and eating disorder researchers are still learning about the numerous ways in which genes and environment interact to influence behavior, at present there are questions about how best to translate this knowledge into clinical practice. Below we discuss how current and future genetic research in night eating can inform and improve classification, assessment, and potential treatment.

Classification

Definitions of night eating have varied markedly in the literature, and debate still exists regarding how to best conceptualize the disorder in the *Diagnostic and Statistical Manual of Mental Disorders* (DSM; American Psychiatric Association, 2010). In future editions, NES is proposed to fall under the eating disorders umbrella in the eating disorder not otherwise specified (EDNOS) category. The DSM-5 Eating Disorder Work Group (American Psychiatric Association, 2010) describes NES as consisting of either evening hyperphagia (excessive food intake after the evening meal) or nocturnal ingestions (eating after awakening from sleep). Detailed criteria including frequency thresholds were not provided due to the limited research on the disorder. However, criteria proposed by Allison et al. (2010) include not only the obligatory criteria of evening hyperphagia and/or nocturnal ingestions, but three of five component features, including morning anorexia, sleep disturbance, depressed mood, a belief one needs to eat in order to sleep, and a strong desire to eat at night, while also offering threshold criteria for most component features. We propose that genetic research will aid in refining night eating definitions and clarify where and how to best capture this behavior in the DSM. Twin studies focusing on NES diagnostic categories are first needed, but may comprise heterogeneous samples, limiting our ability to accurately detect genetic influences in night eating. Multivariate twin modeling and item–factor models would allow for independent analyses of the component parts of NES to determine whether there is empirical support for their inclusion in the diagnostic criteria. Specifically, multivariate analysis would afford an exploration of shared genetic etiology between night eating and associated symptoms (e.g., depressed mood, sleep disturbance), and item–factor models (Neale, Aggen, Maes, Kubarych, & Schmitt, 2006) would allow for symptom-level examination of the differential contributions of these symptoms to a diagnosis. Therefore, item–factor models help parse out the individual heritability of specific symptoms of a disorder (e.g., nocturnal ingestions for NES), which may illuminate promising subphenotypes and endophenotypes that can help refine the NES phenotype (Bulik, Hebebrand, et al., 2007).

Twin research can also inform criterion threshold and frequency cutoffs for night eating (i.e., episodes of nocturnal eating per week required for a diagnosis). This approach can inform the optimal symptom thresholds for defining a clinical syndrome. Sullivan, Bulik, and Kendler (1998a) used this model to examine the optimal frequency criterion for binge eating in BN, and found empirical support for a threshold of once per week, as opposed to the arbitrary twice per week threshold currently required for a diagnosis of BN (American Psychiatric Association, 2000). This example illustrates how similar models can be applied to NES to refine and establish an empirically based set of criteria that will best capture the syndrome as it occurs in the population.

More granular studies of sub- and endophenotypes may also reduce heterogeneity of study samples. Putatively, there are more genes involved in a disorder than in a sub- or endophenotype, rendering it more difficult to detect contributing genetic loci with diagnostic syndromes such as NES. Subphenotypes are subgroups of a disorder that are more homogenous in their symptom presentation (e.g., BN with self-induced vomiting). Endophenotypes can be a specific trait (e.g., obsessionality), behavior, or biological marker associated with the disorder or latent phenotype (e.g., BN). Although proposed DSM-5 criteria for NES do not include subtypes (American Psychiatric Association, 2010), the two core features of NES—evening hyperphagia and nocturnal ingestions of food—may differ in their presentation and clinical profile, and could represent different subtypes of this syndrome. Sub- and endophenotypic research is an advantageous approach for clarifying diagnostic criteria (Bulik, Slof-Op't Landt, van Furth, & Sullivan, 2007).

Assessment

Refinement of the diagnostic system and definition for NES will improve our ability to screen and assess night eating and related behaviors. With the knowledge that night eating co-occurs with binge eating and has at least partial shared genetic etiology (Root et al., 2010), we know that the presence of one behavior (e.g., night eating) should signal the provider to consistently screen for the presence of the other (e.g., binge eating). Furthermore, this knowledge tells us that other relatives of the proband may be at risk for binge eating or night eating behavior, and relatives can be warned about this to provide ongoing screening for both behaviors in their offspring or other family members. Improved screening may identify symptoms of the disorder earlier, increasing chances for early intervention and treatment. We know that early intervention in other eating disorders is predictive of a less severe course and better treatment outcome (Herzog, Keller, & Lavori, 1988; van Son, van Hoeken, van Furth, Donker, & Hoek, 2010), and this may be true for night eating as well. Therefore, improved screening may improve efforts to prevent insidious, chronic cases of night eating.

Treatment and Prevention

Although this chapter focuses solely on the genetic epidemiology of night eating, we know that genes interact with the environment to influence behavior in other eating disorders. With a greater understanding of the genetic and environmental factors that contribute to night eating, we expect that, in the future, we will be able to draw from this research to improve treatment for night eating, specifically by enhancing psychoeducation, psychotherapy, prevention, and psychopharmacology.

An important component of the treatment of NES is psychoeducation for the patient and family. Often the patient and family members are curious about disease etiology and are concerned about their potential role in contributing to the disorder onset or course. Parents may erroneously believe that they are to blame for causing the illness in their offspring. Furthermore, other involved members, such as spouses, siblings, and friends, may become discouraged by the recovery process and the individual's inability simply to "snap out of it." Indeed, anecdotal evidence suggests individuals with night eating are often told to "just stop eating at night." Psychoeducation for family members and friends about the role of genetics and biology in the contribution and maintenance of night eating and associated clinical symptoms (depression, sleep disturbance), could improve understanding of the disorder, decrease blame, and increase compassion for the affected member. Specifically, involved loved ones may benefit from learning about how genetic factors may make one vulnerable to night eating, depression, and sleep issues, and how certain environmental factors can interact with genetics to elicit and maintain the behavior (e.g., poor sleep hygiene in insomnia). In turn, the patient might benefit from more supportive interactions from loved ones, as well as greater understanding of how s/he can arrange the environment to combat biology most effectively (Mazzeo & Bulik, 2009). This approach could empower the patient to address night eating and associated features (depression, sleep disturbance), resulting in greater motivation for treatment.

Ultimately, we expect that genetic research will lead to more targeted treatment approaches for all eating disorders. If we know that someone is at greater genetic risk for developing a behavior or disorder or for responding sensitively to a particular environment shown to put others with similar features at risk for a disorder, we can provide the patient with skills to arrange and cope with risky environmental conditions. An example of how biology can be used to inform treatment interventions is exemplified in guidelines for the treatment of sleep disorders. It has been recommended (Sin, Ho, & Chung, 2009) that providers treating patients with sleep disturbance educate their patients about the impact of environmental factors, such as sleep hygiene (e.g., going to bed at the same time every night) and diet manipulation (eliminating caffeine from your diet), on biology and sleep, and inform the patient of the role of genetics in differential responses to caffeine consumption in sleep (Yang et al., 2009). By providing scientific evidence for treatment recommendations, the patient receives a more thorough, sound rationale for treatment, which is not only in line with evidence-based practice, but may be important for increasing motivation for treatment (Pettersen, Rosenvinge, & Wynn, 2011). The identification of genetic mechanisms implicated in night eating may also shed light on new neurobiological areas to target through drug treatment.

Prevention

Future research examining the genetic and environmental interplay in night eating will clarify our understanding of *"which* risk factors are particularly potent for *which* individuals with *what* specific genetic vulnerability to eating disorders" (Mazzeo & Bulik, 2009, p. 11). This will improve our ability to establish personalized, targeted prevention and intervention treatment approaches for night eating, grounded in biologically based research (Bulik, Hebebrand, et al., 2007).

Areas for Future Research

Genetic research in night eating is scant. Our knowledge of the etiology of night eating can be greatly enriched though future family, twin, and molecular genetic studies in night eating. The importance of this research cannot be overemphasized, as it will unveil genetic and environmental etiological factors, providing needed guidance for efforts at improving the classification and treatment of NES.

References

Allison, K. C., Lundgren, J. D., O'Reardon, J. P., Geliebter, A., Gluck, M. E., Vinai, P., et al. (2010). Proposed diagnostic criteria for night eating syndrome. *International Journal of Eating Disorders, 43*(3), 241–247.

American Psychiatric Association. (2000). *Diagnostic and statistical manual of mental disorders* (4th ed., text rev.). Washington, DC: Author.

American Psychiatric Association. (2010). DSM-5 development. Retrieved January 2, 2011, from *www.dsm5.org/Pages/Default.aspx*.

Ando, T., Komaki, G., Naruo, T., Okabe, K., Takii, M., Kawai, K., et al. (2006). Possible role of preproghrelin gene polymorphisms in susceptibility to bulimia nervosa. *American Journal of Medical Genetics. Part B, Neuropsychiatric Genetics, 141B*(8), 929–934.

Ando, T., Komaki, G., Nishimura, H., Naruo, T., Okabe, K., Kawai, K., et al. (2010). A ghrelin gene variant may predict crossover rate from restricting-type anorexia nervosa to other phenotypes of eating disorders: A retrospective survival analysis. *Psychiatric Genetics, 20*(4), 153–159.

Birketvedt, G. S., Florholmen, J., Sundsfjord, J., Osterud, B., Dinges, D., Bilker, W., et al. (1999). Behavioral and neuroendocrine characteristics of the night-eating syndrome. *Journal of the American Medical Association, 282*(7), 657–663.

Bosker, F. J., Hartman, C. A., Nolte, I. M., Prins, B. P., Terpstra, P., Posthuma, D., et al. (2011). Poor replication of candidate genes for major depressive disorder using genome-wide association data. *Molecular Psychiatry, 16*(5), 516–532.

Bulik, C. M., Devlin, B., Bacanu, S. A., Thornton, L., Klump, K. L., Fichter, M. M., et al. (2003). Significant linkage on chromosome 10p in families with bulimia nervosa. *American Journal of Human Genetics, 72*(1), 200–207.

Bulik, C. M., Hebebrand, J., Keski-Rahkonen, A., Klump, K. L., Reichborn-Kjennerud, T., Mazzeo, S. E., et al. (2007). Genetic epidemiology, endophenotypes, and eating disorder classification. *International Journal of Eating Disorders, 40*(Suppl.), S52–S60.

Bulik, C. M., Slof-Op't Landt, M. C. T., van Furth, E. F., & Sullivan, P. F. (2007). The genetics of anorexia nervosa. *Annual Review of Nutrition, 27*(1), 263–275.

Bulik, C. M., Sullivan, P. F., & Kendler, K. S. (1998). Heritability of binge-eating and broadly defined bulimia nervosa. *Biological Psychiatry, 44*(12), 1210–1218.

Bulik, C. M., & Tozzi, F. (2004). Genetics in eating disorders: State of the science. *CNS Spectrums, 9*(7), 511–515.

Calati, R., De Ronchi, D., Bellini, M., & Serretti, A. (2010). The 5-HTTLPR polymorphism and eating disorders: A meta-analysis. *International Journal of Eating Disorders, 44*(3), 191–199.

Carter, N. P. (2007). Methods and strategies for analyzing copy number variation using DNA microarrays. *Nature Genetics, 39*(7), S16–S21.

Cellini, E., Castellini, G., Ricca, V., Bagnoli, S., Tedde, A., Rotella, C. M., et al. (2010). Glucocorticoid receptor gene polymorphisms in Italian patients with eating disorders and obesity. *Psychiatric Genetics, 20*(6), 282–288.

Cirelli, C. (2009). The genetic and molecular regulation of sleep: From fruit flies to humans. *Nature Reviews Neuroscience, 10*(8), 549–560.

Dauvilliers, Y., & Tafti, M. (2008). The genetic basis of sleep disorders. *Current Pharmaceutical Design, 14*(32), 3386–3395.

Davis, C., Levitan, R. D., Kaplan, A. S., Carter, J., Reid, C., Curtis, C., et al. (2008). Reward sensitivity and the D2 dopamine receptor gene: A case–control study of binge eating disorder. *Progress in Neuro-Psychopharmacology and Biological Psychiatry, 32*(3), 620–628.

de Zwaan, M., Roerig, D. B., Crosby, R. D., Karaz, S., & Mitchell, J. E. (2006). Nighttime eating: A descriptive study. *International Journal of Eating Disorders, 39*(3), 224–232.

Di Bella, D., Catalano, M., Cavallini, M. C., Riboldi, C., & Bellodi, L. (2000). Serotonin transporter linked polymorphic region in anorexia nervosa and bulimia nervosa. *Molecular Psychiatry, 5*(3), 233–234.

Enoch, M. A., Kaye, W. H., Rotondo, A., Greenberg, B. D., Murphy, D. L., & Goldman, D. (1998). 5-HT2A promoter polymorphism-1438G/A, anorexia nervosa, and obsessive–compulsive disorder. *The Lancet, 351*(9118), 1785–1786.

Gedda, L., & Brenci, G. (1983). Twins living apart test: Progress report. *Acta Geneticae Medicae Et Gemellologiae, 32*(1), 17–22.

Goel, N., Stunkard, A. J., Rogers, N. L., Van Dongen, H. P. A., Allison, K. C., O'Reardon, J. P., et al. (2009). Circadian rhythm profiles in women with night eating syndrome. *Journal of Biological Rhythms, 24*(1), 85–94.

Hammer, C., Kapeller, J., Endele, M., Fischer, C., Hebebrand, J., Hinney, A., et al. (2009). Functional variants of the serotonin receptor type 3A and B gene are associated with eating disorders. *Pharmacogenet Genomics 19*(10), 790–799.

Herzog, D. B., Keller, M. B., & Lavori, P. W. (1988). Outcome in anorexia nervosa and bulimia nervosa: A review of the literature. *Journal of Nervous and Mental Disease, 176*(3), 131–143.

Hinney, A., Bornscheuer, A., Depenbusch, M., Mierke, B., Tölle, A., Middeke, K., et al. (1998). No evidence for involvement of the leptin gene in anorexia nervosa, bulimia nervosa, underweight or early onset extreme obesity: Identification of two novel mutations in the coding sequence and a novel polymorphism in the leptin gene linked upstream. *Molecular Psychiatry, 3*(6), 539–543.

Hinney, A., Friedel, S., Remschmidt, H., & Hebebrand, J. (2004). Genetic risk factors in eating disorders. *American Journal of PharmacoGenomics, 4*(4), 209–223.

Hublin, C., Kaprio, J., Partinen, M., & Koskenvuo, M. (1998). Sleep bruxism based on self-report in a nationwide twin cohort. *Journal of Sleep Research, 7*(1), 61–67.

Hudson, J. I., Pope, H. G., Jonas, J. M., Yurgelun-Todd, D., & Frankenburg, F. R. (1987). A controlled family history study of bulimia. *Psychological Medicine: A Journal of Research in Psychiatry and the Allied Sciences, 17*(4), 883–890.

Kendler, K. S. (1993). Twin studies of psychiatric illness: Current status and future directions. *Archives of General Psychiatry, 50*(11), 905–915.

Kendler, K. S., Walters, E. E., Neale, M. C., Kessler, R. C., Heath, A. C., & Eaves, L. J. (1995). The structure of the genetic and environmental risk factors for six major psychiatric disorders in women: Phobia, generalized anxiety disorder, panic disorder, bulimia, major depression, and alcoholism. *Archives of General Psychiatry, 52*(5), 374–383.

Kindler, J., Baller, U., de Zwaan, M., Fuchs, K., Leisch, F., Grun, B., et al. (2011). No association of the neuropeptide Y (Leu7Pro) and ghrelin gene (Arg-51Gin, Leu72Met, Gin90Leu) single nucleotide polymorphisms with eating disorders. *Nordic Journal of Psychiatry, 65*(3), 203–207.

Lamerz, A., Kuepper-Nybelen, J., Bruning, N., Wehle, C., Trost-Brinkhues, G., Brenner, H., et al. (2005). Prevalence of obesity, binge eating, and night eating in a cross-sectional field survey of 6-year-old children and their parents in a German urban population. *Journal of Child Psychology and Psychiatry, 46*(4), 385–393.

Lauzurica, N., Hurtado, A., Escartí, A., Delgado, M., Barrios, V., Morandé, G., et al. (2003). Polymorphisms within the promoter and the intron 2 of the serotonin transporter gene in a population of bulimic patients. *Neuroscience Letters, 352*(3), 226–230.

Lee, Y., & Lin, P. (2010). Association between serotonin transporter gene polymorphism and eating disorders: A meta-analytic study. *International Journal of Eating Disorders, 43*(6), 498–504.

Lee, Y. S. (2009). The role of leptin-melanocortin system and human weight regulation: Lessons of experiments of nature. *ANNALS Academy of Medicine Singapore, 38*(1), 34–44.

Levitan, R. D., Masellis, M., Basile, V. S., Lam, R. W., Kaplan, A. S., Davis, C., et al. (2004). The dopamine-4 receptor gene associated with binge eating and weight gain in women with seasonal affective disorder: An evolutionary perspective. *Biological Psychiatry, 56*(9), 665–669.

Lewis, C. M., Ng, M. Y., Butler, A. W., Cohen-Woods, S., Uher, R., Pirlo, K., et al. (2010). Genome-wide association study of major recurrent depression in the U.K. population. *American Journal of Psychiatry, 167*(8), 949–957.

Lilenfeld, L. R., Kaye, W. H., Greeno, C. G., Merikangas, K. R., Plotnicov, K., Pollice, C., et al. (1998). A controlled family study of anorexia nervosa and bulimia nervosa: Psychiatric disorders in first-degree relatives and effects of proband comorbidity. *Archives of General Psychiatry, 55*(7), 603–610.

Lilenfeld, L. R., Ringham, R., Kalarchian, M. A., & Marcus, M. D. (2008). A family history study of binge-eating disorder. *Comprehensive Psychiatry, 49*(3), 247–254.

Lundgren, J. D., Allison, K. C., O'Reardon, J. P., & Stunkard, A. J. (2008). A descriptive study of non-obese persons with night eating syndrome and a weight-matched comparison group. *Eating Behaviors, 9*(3), 343–351.

Lundgren, J. D., Allison, K. C., & Stunkard, A. J. (2006). Familial aggregation in the night eating syndrome. *International Journal of Eating Disorders, 39*(6), 516–518.

Lundgren, J. D., Newberg, A. B., Allison, K. C., Wintering, N. A., Ploessl, K., & Stunkard, A. J. (2008). 123/-ADAM SPECT imaging of serotonin transporter binding in patients with night eating syndrome: A preliminary report. *Psychiatry Research: Neuroimaging, 162*(3), 214–220.

Lupski, J. R., Reid, J. G., Gonzaga-Jauregui, C., Rio Deiros, D., Chen, D. C., Nazareth, L., et al. (2010). Whole-genome sequencing in a patient with Charcot-Marie-Tooth neuropathy. *New England Journal of Medicine, 362*(13), 1181–1191.

Lyons, W. E., Mamounas, L. A., Ricaurte, G. A., Coppola, V., Reid, S. W., Bora, S. H., et al. (1999). Brain-derived neurotrophic factor-deficient mice develop aggressiveness and hyperphagia in conjunction with brain serotonergic abnormalities. *Proceedings of the National Academy of Sciences of the United States of America, 96*(26), 15239–15244.

Mathes, W. F., Brownley, K. A., Mo, X., & Bulik, C. M. (2009). The biology of binge eating. *Appetite, 52*(3), 545–553.

Mazzeo, S. E., & Bulik, C. M. (2009). Environmental and genetic risk factors for eating disorders: What the clinician needs to know. *Child and Adolescent Psychiatric Clinics of North America, 18*(1), 67–82.

Mazzeo, S. E., Mitchell, K. S., Bulik, C. M., Aggen, S. H., Kendler, K. S., & Neale, M. C. (2010). A twin study of specific bulimia nervosa symptoms. *Psychological Medicine, 40*(7), 1203–1213.

Medvedev, P., Stanciu, M., & Brudno, M. (2009). Computational methods for discovering structural variation with next-generation sequencing. *Nature Methods, 6*(11), S13–S20.

Mitchell, K. S., Neale, M. C., Bulik, C. M., Aggen, S. H., Kendler, K. S., & Mazzeo, S. E. (2010). Binge-eating disorder: A symptom-level investigation of genetic and environmental influences on liability. *Psychological Medicine, 40*(11), 1899–1906.

Monteleone, P., Tortorella, A., Castaldo, E., Di Filippo, C., & Maj, M. (2006). No association of the Arg51Gln and Leu72Met polymorphisms of the ghrelin gene with anorexia nervosa or bulimia nervosa. *Neuroscience Letters, 398*(3), 325–327.

Monteleone, P., Tortorella, A., Castaldo, E., Di Filippo, C., & Maj, M. (2007). The Leu72Met polymorphism of the ghrelin gene is significantly associated with binge eating disorder. *Psychiatric Genetics, 17*(1), 13–16.

Monteleone, P., Tortorella, A., Castaldo, E., & Maj, M. (2006). Association of a functional serotonin transporter gene polymorphism with binge eating disorder. *American Journal of Medical Geneics Part B: Neuropsychiatric Genetics, 141B*(1), 7–9.

Muglia, P., Tozzi, F., Galwey, N. W., Francks, C., Upmanyu, R., Kong, X. Q., et al. (2010). Genome-wide association study of recurrent major depressive disorder in two European case–control cohorts. *Molecular Psychiatry, 15*(6), 589–601.

Nacmias, B., Ricca, V., Tedde, A., Mezzani, B., Rotella, C. M., & Sorbi, S. (1999). 5-HT2A receptor gene polymorphisms in anorexia nervosa and bulimia nervosa. *Neuroscience Letters, 277*(2), 134–136.

Neale, M. C., Aggen, S. H., Maes, H. H., Kubarych, T. S., & Schmitt, J. E. (2006). Methodological issues in the assessment of substance use phenotypes. *Addictive Behaviors, 31*(6), 1010–1034.

Neale, M. C., Lubke, G., Aggen, S. H., & Dolan, C. V. (2005). Problems with using sum scores for estimating variance components: Contamination and measurement noninvariance. *Twin Research and Human Genetics, 8*(6), 553–568.

Nishiguchi, N., Matsushita, S., Suzuki, K., Murayama, M., Shirakawa, O., & Higuchi, S. (2001). Association between 5HT2A receptor gene promoter region polymorphism and eating disorders in Japanese patients. *Biological Psychiatry, 50*(2), 123–128.

O'Reardon, J. P., Ringel, B. L., Dinges, D. F., Allison, K. C., Rogers, N. L., Martino, N. S., et al. (2004). Circadian eating and sleeping patterns in the night eating syndrome. *Obesity, 12*(11), 1789–1796.

Pettersen, G., Rosenvinge, J. H., & Wynn, R. (2011). Eating disorders and psychoeducation: Patients' experiences of healing processes. *Scandinavian Journal of Caring Sciences, 25*(1), 12–18.

Potoczna, N., Branson, R., Kral, J. G., Piec, G., Steffen, R., Ricklin, T., et al. (2004). Gene variants and binge eating as predictors of comorbidity and outcome of treatment in severe obesity. *Journal of Gastrointestinal Surgery, 8*(8), 971–982.

Provini, F., Antelmi, E., Vignatelli, L., Zaniboni, A., Naldi, G., Calandra-Buonaura, G., et al. (2009). Association of restless legs syndrome with nocturnal eating: A case–control study. *Movement Disorders, 24*(6), 871–877.

Psychiatric GWAS Consortium Steering Committee. (2009). A framework for interpreting genome-wide association studies of psychiatric disorders. *Molecular Psychiatry, 14*(1), 10–17.

Reichborn-Kjennerud, T., Bulik, C. M., Kendler, K. S., Røysamb, E., Maes, H., Tambs, K., et al. (2003). Gender differences in binge-eating: A population-based twin study. *Acta Psychiatrica Scandinavica, 108*(3), 196–202.

Ricca, V., Nacmias, B., Cellini, E., Di Bernardo, M., Rotella, C. M., & Sorbi, S. (2002). 5-HT2A receptor gene polymorphism and eating disorders. *Neuroscience Letters, 323*(2), 105–108.

Rogers, N. L., Dinges, D. F., Allison, K. C., Maislin, N. M., O'Reardon, J. P., & Stunkard, A. J. (2006). Assessment of sleep in women with night eating syndrome. *Sleep, 29*(6), 747–748.

Root, T. L., Thornton, L. M., Lindroos, A. K., Stunkard, A. J., Lichtenstein, P.,

Pedersen, N. L., et al. (2010). Shared and unique genetic and environmental influences on binge eating and night eating: A Swedish twin study. *Eating Behaviors, 11*(2), 92–98.

Scherag, S., Hebebrand, J., & Hinney, A. (2010). Eating disorders: The current status of molecular genetic research. *European Child and Adolescent Psychiatry, 19*(3), 211–226.

Shi, J., Potash, J. B., Knowles, J. A., Weissman, M. M., Coryell, W., Scheftner, W. A., et al. (2011). Genome-wide association study of recurrent early-onset major depressive disorder. *Molecular Psychiatry, 16*(2), 193–201.

Shinohara, M., Mizushima, H., Hirano, M., Shioe, K., Nakazawa, M., Hiejima, Y., et al. (2004). Eating disorders with binge-eating behaviour are associated with the s allele of the 3'-UTR VNTR polymorphism of the dopamine transporter gene. *Journal of Psychiatry and Neuroscience, 29*(2), 134–137.

Shyn, S. I., Shi, J., Kraft, J. B., Potash, J. B., Knowles, J. A., Weissman, M. M., et al. (2011). Novel loci for major depression identified by genome-wide association study of sequenced treatment alternatives to relieve depression and meta-analysis of three studies. *Molecular Psychiatry, 16*(2), 202–215.

Sin, C. W. M., Ho, J. S. C., & Chung, J. W. Y. (2009). Systematic review on the effectiveness of caffeine abstinence on the quality of sleep. *Journal of Clinical Nursing, 18*(1), 13–21.

Slof-Op't Landt, M. C. T., van Furth, E. F., Meulenbelt, I., Slagboom, P. E., Bartels, M., Boomsma, D. I., et al. (2005). Eating disorders: From twin studies to candidate genes and beyond. *Twin Research and Human Genetics, 8*(5), 467–482.

Striegel-Moore, R. H., & Bulik, C. M. (2007). Risk factors for eating disorders. *American Psychologist, 62*(3), 181–198.

Strober, M., Freeman, R., Lampert, C., Diamond, J., & Kaye, W. (2000). Controlled family study of anorexia nervosa and bulimia nervosa: Evidence of shared liability and transmission of partial syndromes. *The American Journal of Psychiatry, 157*(3), 393–401.

Stunkard, A. J., Allison, K. C., Geliebter, A., Lundgren, J. D., Gluck, M. E., & O'Reardon, J. P. (2009). Development of criteria for a diagnosis: Lessons from the night eating syndrome. *Comprehensive Psychiatry, 50*(5), 391–399.

Stunkard, A. J., & Lu, X. Y. (2010). Rapid changes in night eating: Considering mechanisms. *Eating and Weight Disorders, 15*(1–2), e2–e8.

Sullivan, P. F., Bulik, C. M., & Kendler, K. S. (1998a). The epidemiology and classification of bulimia nervosa. *Psychological Medicine, 28*(3), 599–610.

Sullivan, P. F., Bulik, C. M., & Kendler, K. S. (1998b). The genetic epidemiology of binging and vomiting. *British Journal of Psychiatry, 173*, 75–79.

Sullivan, P. F., de Geus, E. J. C., Willemsen, G., James, M. R., Smit, J. H., Zandbelt, T., et al. (2009). Genome-wide association for major depressive disorder: A possible role for the presynaptic protein piccolo. *Molecular Psychiatry, 14*(4), 359–375.

Sullivan, P. F., Neale, M. C., & Kendler, K. S. (2000). Genetic epidemiology of major depression: Review and meta-analysis. *American Journal of Psychiatry, 157*(10), 1552–1562.

Sutton, G. M., Babin, M. J., Gu, X., Hruby, V. J., & Butler, A. A. (2008). A derivative of the melanocortin receptor antagonist SHU9119 (PG932) increases food intake when administered peripherally. *Peptides, 29*(1), 104–111.

Tafti, M. (2009). Genetic aspects of normal and disturbed sleep. *Sleep Medicine, 10*, S17–S21.

Turek, F. W., Joshu, C., Kohsaka, A., Lin, E., Ivanova, G., McDearmon, E., et al. (2005). Obesity and metabolic syndrome in circadian Clock mutant mice. *Science, 308*(5724), 1043–1045.

Tzischinsky, O., & Latzer, Y. (2004). Nocturnal eating: Prevalence, features and night sleep among binge eating disorder and bulimia nervosa patients in Israel. *European Eating Disorders Review, 12*(2), 101–109.

Unger, T. J., Calderon, G. A., Bradley, L. C., Sena-Esteves, M., & Rios, M. (2007). Selective deletion of BDNF in the ventromedial and dorsomedial hypothalamus of adult mice results in hyperphagic behavior and obesity. *The Journal of Neuroscience: The Official Journal of the Society for Neuroscience, 27*(52), 14265–14274.

van Son, G. E., van Hoeken, D., van Furth, E. F., Donker, G. A., & Hoek, H. W. (2010). Course and outcome of eating disorders in a primary care–based cohort. *International Journal of Eating Disorders, 43*(2), 130–138.

Vetrugno, R., Manconi, M., Ferini-Strambi, L., Provini, F., Plazzi, G., & Montagna, P. (2006). Nocturnal eating: Sleep-related eating disorder or night eating syndrome? A videopolysomnographic study. *Sleep, 29*(7), 949–954.

Wade, T. D., Bulik, C. M., Prescott, C. A., & Kendler, K. S. (2004). Sex influences on shared risk factors for bulimia nervosa and other psychiatric disorders. *Archives of General Psychiatry, 61*(3), 251–256.

Wray, N. R., Pergardia, M. L., Blackwood, D. H. R., Penninx, B. W. J. H., Gordon, S. D., Nyholt, D. R., et al. (2012). Genome-wide association study of major depressive disorder: New results, meta-analysis, and lessons learned. *Molecular Psychiatry, 17*(1), 36–48.

Yang, S., Liu, A., Weidenhammer, A., Cooksey, R. C., McClain, D., Kim, M. K., et al. (2009). The role of mPer2 Clock gene in glucocorticoid and feeding rhythms. *Endocrinology, 150*(5), 2153–2160.

Ziegler, A., Hebebrand, J., Görg, T., Rosenkranz, K., Fichter, M. M., Herpertz-Dahlmann, B., et al. (1999). Further lack of association between the 5-HT2A gene promoter polymorphism and susceptibility to eating disorders and a meta-analysis pertaining to anorexia nervosa. *Molecular Psychiatry, 4*(5), 410.

PART III

RELATION TO OTHER CLINICAL SYNDROMES

.

Chapter 6

The Relationship
of Night Eating Syndrome
with Obesity, Bariatric Surgery,
and Physical Health

Susan L. Colles
John B. Dixon

As additional research is undertaken and new data have come to light, night eating syndrome (NES) is emerging as a distinct pattern of non-normative eating behavior. To further determine its clinical significance, exploration of key associated factors is vital. This chapter reviews the literature underpinning three areas that have shown some, albeit inconsistent relationship to NES. First, the often contradictory literature on night eating and obesity is considered. Following, the potential effect of night eating among individuals who undergo bariatric surgery is discussed, along with suggestions for clinical practice. Finally, several studies have recently investigated the relationship between NES and aspects of physical health including diabetes, the metabolic syndrome, and oral health. These studies are reviewed, and suggestions for future research made.

The Association between NES and Obesity

To date, the evidence linking NES and obesity is largely based on research prevalence estimates showing consistently higher rates of night eating among overweight and obese treatment seekers, compared to samples from the general community. Prevalence estimates in community samples have generally been found in the vicinity of 1 to 2% (Rand & Kuldau, 1986; Rand, Macgregor, & Stunkard, 1997; Striegel-Moore et al., 2005; Striegel-Moore, Franko, Thompson, Affenito, & Kraemer, 2006). This contrasts to markedly higher figures collected from obese groups seeking medical or surgical weight loss. Table 6.1 lists studies that assessed NES rates among populations of weight loss candidates. Prevalence estimates vary greatly, reported in the range of 6 to 64% (median 14.5%). Table 6.2 lists studies that assessed characteristics of NES among various populations of bariatric surgery candidates. Within these reports, prevalence estimates also spanned from 1.9 to 55%.

This marked variability in the prevalence of NES among groups of obese treatment-seekers is most likely due to inconsistent research methods and varied diagnostic criteria; nevertheless, most studies assessed components of evening hyperphagia, trouble getting to sleep or staying asleep, and morning anorexia. Furthermore, although subjects were mainly selected cohorts of obese, middle-aged women, and these findings are not directly comparable and cannot be generalized to wider groups, they do provide evidence that, among obese treatment seekers, rates of NES are potentially high and certainly greater than in the general community.

Yet while these figures offer some support to the notion that NES is associated with obesity, the relationship, and the nature of the relationship, remains controversial. Epidemiological studies do not support that these conditions are associated (Rand et al., 1997; Striegel-Moore et al., 2006). Numerous cross-sectional studies also lack consistency. Some investigations among obese cohorts report no connection between NES and obesity (Adami, Campostano, Marinari, Ravera, & Scopinaro, 2002; Ceru-Bjork, Andersson, & Rossner, 2001; Gluck, Geliebter, & Satov, 2001; Napolitano, Head, Babyak, & Blumenthal, 2001; Rand, et al., 1997), while others report a positive relationship (Aronoff, Geliebter, & Zammit, 2001; Colles, Dixon, & O'Brien, 2007). No doubt this contradictory literature is in part due to differences in NES diagnostic criteria, small body mass index (BMI) ranges within homogenous populations, and inadequate power to detect group differences. One cross-sectional study to demonstrate a strong, independent association between NES

TABLE 6.1. Studies That Assessed the Prevalence of NES in Obese Subjects Seeking Nonsurgical Obesity Treatment

	Sample			NES assessment criteria						%NES
Study	Sample	n (%F)	Mean BMI	Mean age (years)	Morning anorexia	Evening hyperphagia	Poor sleep onset or maintenance	Mood disturbance	Wake to eat	Method	(n) (%F)
Ceru-Bjork et al. (2001)	Obesity clinic	194 (76)	40	44	No appetite in the morning	Largest food intake after 7:00 P.M.	Trouble getting to or staying asleep	No	No	Q	6% (11) (82%)
Stunkard et al. (1996)	Obesity clinic	79 (100)	35	39	No appetite for breakfast	≥ 50% food intake after 7:00 P.M.	Trouble getting to or staying asleep	No	No	CI	8.9% (7) (all F)
Calugi et al. (2009)	Obesity clinic	266	~43	~51	No	≥ 25% of total daily calories after dinner	No	No	*And/* or ≥ 3 times/ week in last 3 months	Q & CI	10.1% (27) (70%)
Stunkard (1959)	Obesity clinic	100	NR	NR	Morning anorexia with little food intake at breakfast	> 25% energy intake after evening meal	Sleeplessness > midnight at least half the time	No	No	Q	12% (12) (NR)

(continued)

TABLE 6.1. (continued)

		Sample		NES assessment criteria						
Study	Sample	n (%F)	Mean BMI	Mean age (years)	Morning anorexia	Evening hyperphagia	Poor sleep onset or maintenance	Mood disturbance	Wake to eat	Method	%NES (n) (%F)
Stunkard et al. (1996)	Obesity clinic	102 (100)	38	39	No appetite for breakfast	50% or more food intake after 7:00 P.M.	Trouble getting to or staying asleep	No	No	CI	13.7% (14) (all F)
Gluck et al. (2001)	Weight loss	76 (70)	37	44	Skipping breakfast > 4 days/ week	50% or more food intake after 7:00 P.M.	Difficulty falling or staying asleep > 4 days/week	No	No	Q	14% (11) (73%)
Stunkard et al. (1996)	Obese drug trial	40 (100)	36	40	No appetite for breakfast	50% or more food intake after 7:00 P.M.	Trouble getting to/ staying asleep	No	No	CI	15% (6) (all F)
Adami et al. (2002)	Cons/surg	166 (78)	44	NR	Morning anorexia	25% energy intake after the evening meal	Trouble falling or staying asleep most nights	No	No	CI	15.7% (26) (69%)

88

Napolitano et al. (2001)	Long-term obesity	83 (53)	41	48	No appetite in the morning	50% or more food intake after 7:00 P.M.	No	No	No	CI	43.4% (36) (50%)
Aronoff et al. (2001)	Metab clinic	110 (62)	55	48	No appetite for breakfast	50% or more food intake after 7:00 P.M.	Trouble getting to/ staying asleep	No	No	CI	51% (56) (41%)
Stunkard, Grace, & Wolff (1955)	Obesity clinic	25 (92)	NR	35	Morning anorexia with low food intake at breakfast	> 25% energy intake after evening meal	Sleeplessness > midnight at least half the time	No	No	CI	64% (16) (NR)

Note: Sample: (%F), percentage of the NES group who were female; NR, not reported; Cons/surg, mixed medical–surgical treatment group; Metab clinic, metabolic clinic. Method: Q, self-report questionnaire; CI, clinical interview.

TABLE 6.2. Studies That Assessed the Preoperative Prevalence of NES or Night Eating Behaviors among Bariatric Surgery Candidates

Study	Study type	Sample			NES assessment criteria					
		n (%F)	Mean BMI	Mean age (years)	Morning anorexia	Evening hyperphagia	Poor sleep onset or maintenance	Mood disturbance	Wake to eat	%NES (n) (%F)
Allison et al. (2006)	C/S; CI & Q	210 (82)	50	44	No	> 25% energy intake after the evening meal	No	No	Awakening after sleep onset and eating ≥ 3 nights/week	1.9% (4) (NR)
Adami et al. (1999)	P; CI	63 (76)	47	38	Morning anorexia	50% energy intake after 7:00 P.M.	Trouble getting to sleep or staying asleep	No	No	8% (5) (NR)
Powers et al. (1999)	P; CI	116 (83)	53	40	Morning anorexia	25% energy intake > evening meal	Trouble sleeping	No	No	10% (12) (91%)
Kuldau & Rand (1986)	C/S; CI & Q	174 (84)	NR	36	Poor appetite, not eating until later in day	Eating throughout evening without enjoyment	Having difficulty going to sleep	Feeling tense, upset, or anxious as bedtime neared	No	15% (26) (NR)
Adami et al. (2002)	C/S; CI	166 (78)	44	NR	Morning anorexia	25% energy intake after evening meal	Trouble sleeping	No	No	16% (26) (69%)

Study	Study type	Sample (%F)								
Colles et al. (2007)	C/S; CI & Q	180 (141)	45	45	No appetite for breakfast	Consume ≥ 50% of total energy intake after 7:00 P.M.	Trouble getting to sleep or staying asleep ≥ 3 nights/week	No	No	19.4% (35) (NR)
Rand & Kuldau (1993)	C/S; CI	253 (75)	≥ 40	~37	Morning anorexia, not eating until later in day	Eating later in day, with no enjoyment	Having difficulty sleeping	Feeling tense and/or upset	No	26% (65) (NR)
Rand et al. (1997)	R; CI	111 (93)	NR	~41	Morning anorexia or delay of eating	Excessive evening eating	Insomnia	Evening tension and/ or feeling upset	No	31% (34) (NR)
Hsu, Sullivan, & Benotti (1997)	R; CI	27 (100)	49	39	No	No	No	No	≥ 1/week for at least 3/12	33% (9) (all F)
Hsu et al. (1996)	R; CI	24 (100)	49	48	No	No	No	No	No set frequency or time frame	42% (10) (all F)
Latner et al. (2004)	R; phone interview	65 (100)	54	40	No	No	No	No	≥ 2/week for 3/12	55% (36) (all F)

Note. Study type: P, prospective; C/S, cross-sectional; R, retrospective; CI, clinical interview; Q, self-report questionnaire. Sample: (%F), percentage of the NES group who were female; NR, not reported.

and BMI countered some of these limitations by recruiting a comparatively large sample of 431 subjects, with BMI values ranging from 17.7 to
66.7 kg/m² (Colles et al., 2007). When assessed in a binary logistic regression model, data from this study showed a strong independent association between NES and BMI ($p < .001$). Figure 6.1 shows the prevalence
of NES across the study subjects, and the increase in NES presence with
increasing BMI. The rate of NES was significantly different between each
BMI group, χ^2 (4, $n = 48$) = 22.71, $p < .001$.

While the above study describes a probable association between NES
and obesity, especially among treatment seekers, the nature of the NES–
obesity relationship requires further exploration. A few studies within
the last decade have looked for possible causal associations. Marshall et
al. (Marshall, Allison, O'Reardon, Birketvedt, & Stunkard, 2004) compared 40 night eaters of BMI > 30 kg/m² and 40 night eaters of BMI < 25
kg/m². Of these two groups the obese individuals with NES were significantly older. While the authors suggested this as evidence to support that
NES contributes to weight gain over time, it should be borne in mind that,

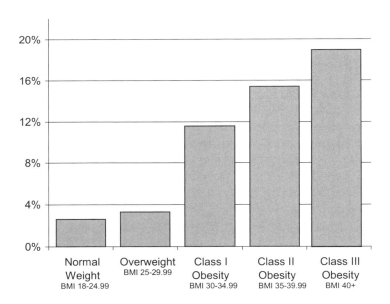

FIGURE 6.1. Distribution of 48 of 431 subjects with NES across all BMI categories. Across five BMI levels the prevalence of NES increased with increasing BMI. From Colles, Dixon, and O'Brien (2007). Reprinted by permission
of Nature Publishing Group.

among the general population, increasing weight is strongly associated with increasing age. Another prospective study involving 1,050 women from the Danish MONICA cohort found that obese women responding affirmatively to the question "Do you get up at night to eat?" gained significantly more weight over a 6-year period (mean 5.2 kg) compared to obese non-night eaters (mean weight gain 0.9 kg) (Andersen, Stunkard, Sorensen, Petersen, & Heitmann, 2004). No such association was found in men. The longitudinal design of this study provides a stronger argument that NES may be a risk factor for future obesity development.

Another longitudinal study that assessed change in body weight after an average of 3.4 years (in 59% of the original study group), found that nighttime eaters (those who ate between the hours of 11:00 P.M. and 5:00 A.M. from a computer-operated vending machine on any of three nights during an in-house clinical study) gained significantly more weight (mean 6.2 kg) compared to those who did not eat at night (mean 1.7 kg) (Gluck, Venti, Salbe, & Krakoff, 2008). Although these follow-up studies offer more support for a causal relationship between NES and obesity, as for most NES studies the use of variable research criteria and the inability to control for ongoing external variables and influences results in difficulty claiming causality.

Other studies to explore the association between obesity and NES have included a large psychiatric population, in which night eaters meeting a criterion of evening hyperphagia (more than one-third of calories after the evening meal) or nocturnal snacking (more than three times/week) were five times more likely to be obese than non-night eaters (Lundgren et al., 2006). More subjectively, patients attending sleep disorder clinics for problems that involve nocturnal eating often report weight gains directly linked to the onset of their sleep-related eating disorder (Schenck & Mahowald, 1994; Spaggiari et al., 1994).

It is certainly true that small, sustained increases in energy intake (that are not countered by similar increases in energy expenditure) lead to positive energy balance and, over time, weight gain. In this way, a consistent evening intake of high-carbohydrate snacks could drive weight gain. Another possibility is the suggestion that NES involves a general tendency to overeat. Controlled studies have recorded both increased (Birketvedt et al., 1999) and similar energy intakes among patients with NES (Allison et al., 2005; O'Reardon et al., 2004). In addition to the ongoing issue of variable NES diagnostic criteria, these inconsistent findings may be in part due to the inconsistent accuracy and sensitivity of most food intake quantitation methods, such that small differences in intake could easily be overlooked. To enhance food intake assessment (albeit in an unnatural eating environment), one recent study used a computer-operated vending machine to record food intake (Gluck et al., 2008). Of 160 healthy subjects living for 3 days in a clinical research unit, nighttime eaters (36% of the group) consumed significantly more calories over each day. In contrast, people with NES and non-NES subjects evaluated in a controlled laboratory setting consumed similar amounts of a daytime test meal despite those with NES reporting less hunger and greater preprandial feelings of fullness (Gluck et al., 2001). In addition to a time-delayed pattern of hunger and eating, NES has also been positively correlated with an irregular meal pattern and greater delays in eating when busy (Rand & Kuldau, 1986).

As a group, a number of the longitudinal and cross-sectional studies presented here offer some evidence to support the notion of a causal relationship between NES and obesity. Perhaps most compelling are the longitudinal studies that show significantly greater weight gain among night eaters compared to their non-NES counterparts; this greater tendency to gain weight results in the consistently higher proportion of night eaters found among obese persons seeking weight-loss treatment. These findings support the inclusion of assessment and, where necessary, management of NES among obese treatment seekers. Characteristics associated with NES can also be seen among normal-weight persons. Because of the seeming association between NES and obesity, identification and management of NES in persons of normal weight may deter future excessive weight gain.

Although a link between NES and obesity appears probable, the exact nature of this association is unclear. On examination, a range of potential variables may influence the relationship in a causal or counter-causal manner. Body weight through the course of one's life is influenced by a multitude of genetic, environmental, socioeconomic, and behavioral factors. In general, weight gain occurs when one or a range of these factors consistently promote an energy intake in excess of the body's requirement. With regard to NES, this excess intake could theoretically be driven via a number of pathways. Clearly, the intake of evening snacks is one probable means, as is the time-delayed pattern of night eating. Genetic or neuroendocrine factors may also play a role, and mood-related factors may also contribute. Figure 6.2 shows some of the possible mood and behavioral pathways through which NES may positively influence weight gain and obesity.

Other possibilities also lie in the reverse pathway, where weight gain and obesity tend to influence the presence of NES characteristics, for example, consideration that the lack of early food intake or restrained

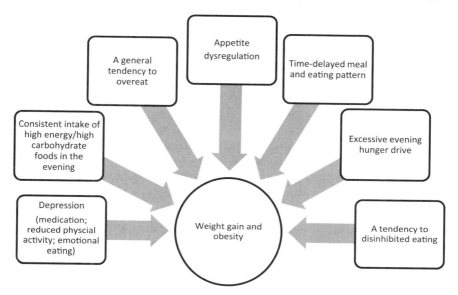

FIGURE 6.2. Possible pathways through which NES contributes to an increased risk of weight gain and obesity.

morning eating may lead to less regulated evening eating. Alternatively, the shame or guilt associated with weight gain may lead to a greater tendency to eat or overeat at night in the privacy of one's home. For these or any other causal pathways to be determined or better understood, a clearer comprehension of the etiology of NES is required.

NES in Bariatric Surgery Populations

Rising worldwide rates of obesity are leading increasing numbers of people to seek surgical weight loss therapies. With some of the highest NES prevalence estimates consistently recorded among obese persons seeking bariatric surgery, and more and more individuals opting for this intervention, it is important to consider the potential impact of NES on surgical outcomes.

Currently in the United States, the Roux-en-Y gastric bypass (RYGB) is the most common bariatric operation. Other surgical procedures in place include the adjustable gastric band (AGB) and sleeve gastrectomy. In brief, RYGB is an essentially irreversible operation that involves partial removal of the stomach (sleeve gastrectomy) and exclusion of the early part of the small intestine from the digestive process. Weight loss is predominantly achieved through a reduction in energy intake, decreased hunger, and enhanced feelings of satiety. Because a segment of small bowel is bypassed, a degree of nutrient and energy malabsorption can also occur. Adjustable gastric banding is a less invasive, reversible operation, involving placement of a flexible silicone band around the upper part of the stomach to produce a small pouch. The silicone band contains an inner inflatable balloon, connected by tubing to an access port, usually placed under the skin of the abdomen. Fluid can be injected into the port to inflate the balloon and squeeze the stomach to reduce to stomach's pouch size. Fluid can be injected into or removed from the balloon to increase or decrease the recipient's sense of the physical restriction. Gastric banding does not alter the digestion of nutrients, with weight loss occurring secondary to reduced intake. Sleeve gastrectomy involves partial removal of the stomach. Weight loss is induced via the physical restriction of energy intake consequent to the reduced stomach size. Figure 6.3 depicts the RYGB and AGB procedures.

Good evidence supports that RYGB and AGB facilitate excellent sustainable weight loss in the medium term (O'Brien, McPhail, Chaston, & Dixon, 2006), and successful surgical weight loss facilitates numerous concurrent improvements in physical health (Buchwald et al., 2004; Dixon & O'Brien, 2002) and well-being (Kolotkin, Meter, & Williams, 2001; van Gemert, Severeijns, Greve, Groenman, & Soeters, 1998). Sleeve gastrectomy has only been performed as a stand-alone operation for a short time, and while early evidence suggest that it can facilitate good weight loss, more detailed, longer-term data are required (Daskalakis & Weiner, 2009).

Association of NES with Surgical Outcomes

With the potentially high occurrence of night eating characteristics among bariatric candidates, it is important to consider possible impacts of this syndrome on surgical and lifestyle outcomes. It is certainly conceivable that the postoperative continuation of nighttime eating could confound weight loss success or maintenance. Other possible associates to NES, such as the propensity to background overeating, an inability to adhere to a structured meal pattern, plus a range of related behavioral, psychological, or biological traits may affect weight-loss success or other relevant measures such as feelings of well-being and quality of life.

A survey of the clinical practice of disordered eating among U.S. bar-

a) Roux-en-Y gastric bypass

b) Adjustable gastric banding

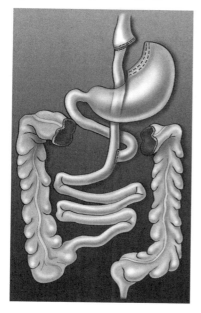 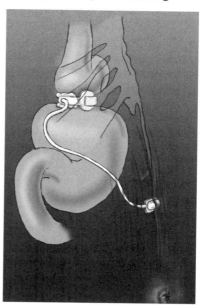

FIGURE 6.3. Visual representations of (a) Roux-en-Y gastric bypass and (b) adjustable gastric banding. Images reprinted with permission of the American Society for Metabolic and Bariatric Surgery. Copyright 2011. All rights reserved.

iatric clinics suggests that symptoms of night eating are assessed preoperatively in some settings, and that management of those identified with NES varies widely (Devlin, Goldfein, Flancbaum, Bessler, & Eisenstadt, 2004). Observing the limitation of a very small response rate (of 1,356 sent surveys, 150 responses were received; response rate 11.1%), the survey data indicated that around half of the clinics (52.7%) routinely assessed for preoperative NES. When a positive diagnosis was made, 28.7% of the clinic surgeons proceeded with surgery; 18.7% postponed surgery; 3.3% recommended against surgery. The remaining half of the clinics to assess for NES indicated that presurgical management of those identified with the syndrome was variable or unclearly defined. Based on the poor response rate to this survey it seems reasonable to assume that more than half of the currently operating bariatric clinics do not assess for preoperative symptoms of NES.

Despite the consistently high numbers of NES among studied surgical candidates, to date no research has assessed the efficacy of particular presurgical NES treatments, or the benefit to surgical outcomes. Furthermore, while characteristics of NES may or may not be assessed prior to surgery, the postoperative continuation or change in NES-related behaviors has barely been measured and described, and, of the few studies to do this, most have compared postsurgical changes to retrospective reports of presurgical behavior. In this vein, three small retrospective studies have described sizable reductions in "waking to eat" ranging from 67 to 83% around two postsurgical years (Hsu, Betancourt, & Sullivan, 1996; Latner, Wetzler, Goodman, & Glinski, 2004). Yet, in addition to their small sample size and the measurement limitation of retrospective baseline night snacks, these substantial reductions are based on very broad "night eating" criteria. In contradiction to these large declines, another retrospective study reported little change in NES prevalence from a preoperative 31% to 27% at 32 ± 30 months after gastric restrictive surgery (Rand et al., 1997).

Two prospective studies that offer more valid measurements of preoperative behaviors also show somewhat conflicting results (Adami, Meneghelli, & Scopinaro, 1999; Colles, Dixon, & O'Brien, 2008a). One study recorded four subjects who displayed a pattern of night eating (4/63, 6%) at 3 years following biliopancreatic diversion, which was similar to baseline (5/63, 8%) (Adami et al., 1999). At 12 months after AGB, the other investigation diagnosed NES in 10 of 129 subjects (7.8%), a significant reduction from 17.1% (20 subjects) at baseline (Colles et al., 2008a). The incidence and change in nocturnal snacking was also measured, commencing at 10 subjects (7.8%) at baseline, and reducing to four subjects (3.1%) by 12 postsurgical months. Of note in this study, only four of those diagnosed with postoperative NES were considered night eaters at baseline. An additional six subjects began experiencing this cluster of behaviors after surgery.

While it is important to clarify the possible implications that a presurgical diagnosis of NES (and other behavioral and psychological conditions) may have on postsurgical outcomes, the value of this has been brought into question (Colles et al., 2008a). Although more research is required, it seems possible that a patient's postsurgical behavior better predicts surgical outcomes, in particular weight loss, than behaviors measured preoperatively. At present however, attempts to measure postsurgical NES (and other eating-related behaviors) tend to be thwarted from many angles. Some of the issues are specific to the operation type, such as the fact the AGB has a tendency to produce morning anorexia where recipients don't feel able or driven to eat immediately after rising. Other issues are more general and include the lack of agreed-upon NES definition; how to reliably measure postoperative eating behavior given that different surgeries enforce various changes in eating habits, mood, and often also sleeping patterns; the generally poor follow-up of surgical recipients precipitated by lack of clinic staff, lack of follow-up emphasis, and by choice of the patients themselves. It is far easier and more convenient to assess presurgical behavior, and thus most and sometimes all behavioral and psychological assessment of bariatric candidates is only carried out before surgery.

Despite this, some studies have assessed aspects of postsurgical eating behavior and highlight some of the ways in which surgical intervention may alter characteristics of NES. Both gastric restrictive and reductive surgeries have been shown to reduce general measures of hunger and uncontrolled or disinhibited eating, while indicators of cognitive restraint and greater eating control are increased (Colles, Dixon, & O'Brien, 2008b; Karlsson, Sjostrom, & Sullivan, 1998). Theoretically, these postoperative changes may help to reduce evening eating and nighttime snacks and deter a general tendency to overeat. Although presently available research suggests no direct association between NES and obstructive sleep apnea (OSA) (Olbrich et al., 2009), sleep quality and the occurrence and severity of OSA also improve with weight loss (Dixon, Schachter, & O'Brien, 2001). Obtaining better postsurgical sleep may help to reduce nighttime awakenings and the ensuing tendency to snack. Weight loss following successful bariatric surgery also routinely shows marked improvements in quality of life, mood, and symptoms of depression (Dixon, Dixon, & O'Brien, 2003; Kolotkin et al., 2001). Although the nature of association between NES and low mood is uncertain, an overall improved disposition may counter the cycle of NES. Enhancements in mood (and concurrent weight loss and improvements in quality of life) may also reduce life stress, which has the potential to positively affect sleep quality and be a further positive reinforcement for healthy eating behavior.

The most frequently used outcome measure of "surgical success" is weight loss. Thus far, attempts to measure differences in postsurgical weight loss among patients with NES and non-NES patients are limited by heterogeneity in study design and methods. Of those to consider this outcome, one prospective study at an average of 5.5 years following gastric restrictive surgery found no weight difference between presurgical patients with NES and non-NES patients (Powers, Perez, Boyd, & Rosemurgy, 1999). Another prospective study that assessed NES at baseline and 12 months post-banding also found no differences in weight loss between preoperative patients with NES and non-NES patients (Colles et al., 2008a). Importantly, however, this study also assessed NES characteristics and weight loss following surgery. Although not significantly different to non-NES patients, at 12 months post-AGB the mean percentage of weight loss in night eaters was 16.9% compared to 21.1% in non-NES patients. The NES groups also showed a statistical trend toward fewer band adjustments ($p = .069$). One small retrospective study also found that more frequent postsurgical nocturnal eating in six of 65 subjects (11%) was associated with greater postsurgical BMI and less treatment satisfaction than in non-NES patients at an average of 16.4 months following RYGB (Latner et al., 2004). This group also observed no correlation between presurgical nocturnal eating and poorer postsurgical weight loss.

In short, the effect of presurgical NES, if any, on short-, medium-, and long-term surgical outcome remains to be determined, and the course of NES following obesity surgery is essentially unknown (Colles & Dixon, 2006). Yet for obese, depressed night eaters, no evidence supports that preoperative NES be a contraindication for surgery. In the case of intractable obesity, surgical intervention may be the last option to attain significant weight reduction and improvements in comorbid disease and quality of life. Furthermore, although scant, some evidence does suggest the limited utility of defining patients by their presurgical behavioral characteristics. Any of the common characteristics of NES—extensive evening snacking, sleep onset or sleep maintenance insomnia, and low mood—may alter after surgery, either as a direct effect of the intervention or indirectly with weight loss. To identify and assess for positive or negative change, ongoing postoperative review and clinical management are essential. Only in this way can outcomes including weight loss, physical and mental health and well-being, eating and lifestyle behaviors, and general adherence to treatment recommendations be optimized.

Suggestions for Management of the Bariatric Surgery Patient with NES

In the presurgical stage:

- Due to the potential for high levels of NES among bariatric surgery candidates, assessment of this cluster of behaviors should be part of routine preoperative psychological and behavioral assessment. Initial assessment may be carried out by self-report survey, but a definitive diagnosis should be confirmed during clinical interview.
- No currently available evidence supports the exclusion of those identified with NES from surgical intervention.

- The decision whether to commence treatment for NES prior to surgery should be undertaken on a case-by-case basis. Whenever preoperative NES treatment is indicated, the most appropriate treatment option should be decided according to available research, expert opinion, and patient preference.
- Identification of preoperative NES can also be useful to highlight those who are accustomed to the NES cluster of behaviors, and following surgery may be more prone to a time-delayed pattern of eating, low mood, or waking to eat. These individuals can be earmarked for additional postsurgical monitoring.

In the postsurgical stage:

- As it should be in the preoperative phase, following surgery the focus of the surgeon and related team of health care professionals should continue to be on patient care.
- While there are definite reasons to assess NES prior to surgery, it is important to note that, following surgery, either as a direct or indirect consequence, any of the behavioral or mood-related aspects of NES may spontaneously resolve.
- There is increasing evidence that postsurgical eating behaviors are more closely correlated with surgical outcomes than those measured prior to surgery.
- Rather than placing all emphasis on the presurgical period, continued assessment of postsurgical eating behavior (and other aspects of health, nutritional status, and well-being), followed by appropriate and timely intervention as required, is a surer way to help patients achieve and maintain good weight-loss outcomes and optimal physical and mental health.
- It is important for both the health practitioner and patient to realize that postsurgical follow-up and management should be a lifelong commitment.

NES and Impact on Physical Health

Over the last decade, as awareness of NES has grown, a small amount of research has focused on the effect of NES on aspects of physical and medical health. A few studies have considered the impact of NES on diabetic control and features of the metabolic syndrome. On the association between NES and the metabolic syndrome, one recent cross-sectional study of 266 obese treatment seekers observed no differences in weight and no correlation between those with NES (10.1%) and the presence of the metabolic syndrome assessed according to the modified Adult Panel Treatment-III proposal or any of its individual metabolic parameters (Calugi, Dalle Grave, & Marchesini, 2009). The authors suggested that elevated body weight, not NES, drives the observed metabolic abnormalities. In contrast however, are the findings of a study that involved survey assessment of 714 type I and type II diabetics, 9.7% of whom were identified as night eaters (Morse, Ciechanowski, Katon, & Hirsch, 2006). Most notably, the night eating group was less adherent to lifestyle advice and glucose monitoring, significantly more likely to be obese, to eat in response to negative emotions, have an $HbA_{1C} > 7\%$, and to suffer a higher rate of diabetic complications. One other study to assess NES across several large diabetic populations by clinical interview derived comparatively lower NES estimates at 3.8% (32/845), but offered no grouped evaluation of clinical or metabolic variables (Allison et al., 2007).

Two recent studies have considered the impact of night eating on oral health. Looking specifically at tooth loss, Lundgren, Williams, and Heitmann (2010) assessed data on 2,217 Danish subjects enrolled in the MONICA study. The group consisted of males and females ranging in age from 30 to 60 years, with an average BMI of 25.9 kg/m². After controlling for variables including age, education level, smoking status, carbohydrate intake, and diabetes diagnosis, those classified as night eaters on initial investigation were found to have lost significantly more teeth at follow-up 5 to 6 years later. In a community sample of 174 individuals attending an academic dental faculty practice, Lundgren et al. assessed the influence of evening hyperphagia (7.1% of study sample) and frequent nocturnal eating upon wakening (2.2% of study sample) on markers of oral health (Lundgren, Smith, et al., 2010). Using stepwise regression, nocturnal eating upon wakening significantly predicted missing teeth, periodontal pockets, and active carious lesions. Regression analysis also deemed the 2.2% who frequently ate upon wakening 4.4 times more likely (95% confidence interval [CI] = 1.2–15.4) to have a BMI ≥ 25.9 kg/m², compared to the remainder of the cohort. Evening hyperphagia (without nocturnal eating) was not significantly associated with poorer dental health or BMI.

While this small number of disparate studies does not allow conclusions, they do draw attention to the fact that NES and diabetes do co-occur, and that ongoing symptoms of NES may confound diabetes management, an issue with serious long-term side effects. The findings on dental health also underscore the possible increased risk of accelerated tooth loss and dental caries among those with NES, specifically those who frequently eat upon wakening, and highlight the need to encourage good oral hygiene in night eaters.

Areas for Future Research

While presently available data do indicate the potential for NES to negatively affect several physical health-related areas, clearly more study is required. Greater insights into issues surrounding causality and countercausality, and the exact nature of the NES–obesity relation need to be uncovered by prospective, longitudinal research. Investigation of the course and health implications of NES needs to be carried out within sizable cohorts that allow valid statistical comparisons of selected traits while controlling for differences in BMI and other potential confounders. Outcome variables of particular interest would include differences in weight and weight change over time (including during weight-loss therapy), and the prevalence and course of conditions such as diabetes and heart disease. Future research to address the nature of the NES–obesity relationship could include investigation into how factors such as the delayed sense of appetite and evening eating pattern affect a tendency to gain weight, how morning anorexia affects eating patterns for the remainder of the day, and the clearer characterization of nighttime snacks and general eating (and overeating) tendencies. Intervention studies that manipulate 24-hour eating patterns and assess concomitant changes in circulating hormones would also shed light on associations between the patterning of diurnal hormones and eating.

Much like the research surrounding NES and obesity, there are few currently available studies that explore the impact of NES on outcomes of obesity surgery, and they provide largely fragmented and inconclusive results. Future work needs to better define the relevance of preoperative NES and investigate the potential benefits of particular presurgical NES treatments on surgical outcome. Just as important is the need to more clearly characterize both favorable and unfavorable postsurgical eating behaviors and develop reliable methods to assess high-risk persons. In this way, both the behavioral and psychological aspects of NES can be tracked more effectively, and the course of postsurgical NES be accurately determined and described. Furthermore, because NES prevalence is consistently higher among obese treatment seekers, future research could also consider whether it is the presence of night eating or its associated features such as low mood and depression that produce a particular drive for treatment over and above the need to lose weight. Certainly among those with binge-eating disorder, related feelings of loss of control over eating are the most psychologically disturbing factor and may be one of the most significant driving forces to compel the individual to seek treatment (Colles, Dixon, & O'Brien, 2008c).

In order to validate and facilitate future investigation of the relationship between NES and obesity and its implications for bariatric surgical outcomes and health, it is of prime importance to focus efforts on better understanding the etiology of NES and to reach agreement on the most clinically significant features of NES and its resultant diagnostic criteria.

References

Adami, G. F., Campostano, A., Marinari, G. M., Ravera, G., & Scopinaro, N. (2002). Night eating in obesity: A descriptive study. *Nutrition, 18*(7–8), 587–589.

Adami, G. F., Meneghelli, A., & Scopinaro, N. (1999). Night eating and binge eating disorder in obese patients. *International Journal of Eating Disorders, 25*(3), 335–338.

Allison, K. C., Ahima, R. S., O'Reardon, J. P., Dinges, D. F., Sharma, V., Cummings, D. E., et al. (2005). Neuroendocrine profiles associated with energy intake, sleep, and stress in the night eating syndrome. *Journal of Clinical Endocrinolgy and Metabolism, 90*(11), 6214–6217.

Allison, K. C., Crow, S. J., Reeves, R. R., West, D. S., Foreyt, J. P., Dilillo, V. G., et al. (2007). Binge-eating disorder and night eating syndrome in adults with type 2 diabetes. *Obesity, 15*(5), 1287–1293.

Allison, K. C., Wadden, T. A., Sarwer, D. B., Fabricatore, A. N., Crerand, C. E., Gibbons, L. M., et al. (2006). Night eating syndrome and binge-eating disorder among persons seeking bariatric surgery: Prevalence and related features. *Surgery for Obesity and Related Diseases, 2*(2), 153–158.

Andersen, G. S., Stunkard, A. J., Sorensen, T. I., Petersen, L., & Heitmann, B. L. (2004). Night eating and weight change in middle-aged men and women. *International Journal of Obesity and Related Metabolic Disorders, 28*(10), 1338–1343.

Aronoff, N. J., Geliebter, A., & Zammit, G. (2001). Gender and body mass index as related to the night-eating syndrome in obese outpatients. *Journal of the American Dietic Association, 101*(1), 102–104.

Birketvedt, G. S., Florholmen, J., Sundsfjord, J., Osterud, B., Dinges, D., Bilker, W., et al. (1999). Behavioral and neuroendocrine characteristics of the night-eating syndrome. *Journal of the American Medical Association, 282*(7), 657–663.

Buchwald, H., Avidor, Y., Braunwald, E., Jensen, M. D., Pories, W., Fahrbach, K., et al. (2004). Bariatric surgery: A systematic review and meta-analysis. *Journal of the American Medical Association, 292*(14), 1724–1737.

Calugi, S., Dalle Grave, R., & Marchesini, G. (2009). Night eating syndrome in class II-III obesity: Metabolic and psychopathological features. *International Journal of Obesity, 33*(8), 899–904.

Ceru-Bjork, C., Andersson, I., & Rossner, S. (2001). Night eating and nocturnal eating: Two different or similar syndromes among obese patients? *International Journal of Obesity and Related Metabolic Disorders, 25*(3), 365–372.

Colles, S. L., & Dixon, J. B. (2006). Night eating syndrome: Impact on bariatric surgery. *Obesity Surgery, 16*(7), 811–820.

Colles, S. L., Dixon, J. B., & O'Brien, P. E. (2007). Night eating syndrome and nocturnal snacking: Association with obesity, binge eating, and psychological distress. *International Journal of Obesity, 31*(11), 1722–1730.

Colles, S. L., Dixon, J. B., & O'Brien, P. E. (2008a). Grazing and loss of control related to eating: Two high-risk factors following bariatric surgery. *Obesity, 16*(3), 615–622.

Colles, S. L., Dixon, J. B., & O'Brien, P. E. (2008b). Hunger control and regular physical activity facilitate weight loss after laparoscopic adjustable gastric banding. *Obesity Surgery, 18*(7), 833–840.

Colles, S. L., Dixon, J. B., & O'Brien, P. E. (2008c). Loss of control is central to psychological disturbance associated with binge-eating disorder. *Obesity, 16*(3), 608–614.

Daskalakis, M., & Weiner, R. A. (2009). Sleeve gastrectomy as a single-stage bariatric operation: Indications and limitations. *Obesity Facts, 2*(Suppl. 1), 8–10.

Devlin, M. J., Goldfein, J. A., Flancbaum, L., Bessler, M., & Eisenstadt, R. (2004). Surgical management of obese patients with eating disorders: A survey of current practice. *Obesity Surgery, 14*(9), 1252–1257.

Dixon, J. B., Dixon, M. E., & O'Brien, P. E. (2003). Depression in association with severe obesity: Changes with weight loss. *Archives of Internal Medicine, 163*(17), 2058–2065.

Dixon, J. B., & O'Brien, P. E. (2002). Health outcomes of severely obese type 2 diabetic subjects 1 year after laparoscopic adjustable gastric banding. *Diabetes Care, 25*(2), 358–363.

Dixon, J. B., Schachter, L. M., & O'Brien, P. E. (2001). Sleep disturbance and obesity: Changes following surgically induced weight loss. *Archives of Internal Medicine, 161*(1), 102–106.

Gluck, M. E., Geliebter, A., & Satov, T. (2001). Night eating syndrome is associated with depression, low self-esteem, reduced daytime hunger, and less weight loss in obese outpatients. *Obesity Research, 9*(4), 264–267.

Gluck, M. E., Venti, C. A., Salbe, A. D., & Krakoff, J. (2008). Nighttime eating: Commonly observed and related to weight gain in an inpatient food intake study. *American Journal of Clinical Nutrition, 88*(4), 900–905.

Hsu, L. K., Betancourt, S., & Sullivan, S. P. (1996). Eating disturbances before and after vertical banded gastroplasty: A pilot study. *International Journal of Eating Disorders, 19*(1), 23–34.

Hsu, L. K., Sullivan, S. P., & Benotti, P. N. (1997). Eating disturbances and outcome of gastric bypass surgery: A pilot study. *International Journal of Eating Disorders, 21*(4), 385–390.

Karlsson, J., Sjostrom, L., & Sullivan, M. (1998). Swedish obese subjects (SOS)—an intervention study of obesity. Two-year follow-up of health related quality of life (HRQL) and eating behavior after gastric surgery for severe obesity. *International Journal of Obesity, 22*, 113–126.

Kolotkin, R. L., Meter, K., & Williams, G. R. (2001). Quality of life and obesity. *Obesity Reviews, 2*(4), 219–229.

Kuldau, J. M., & Rand, C. S. W. (1986). The night eating syndrome and bulimia in the morbidly obese. *International Journal of Eating Disorders, 5*(1), 143–148.

Latner, J. D., Wetzler, S., Goodman, E. R., & Glinski, J. (2004). Gastric bypass in a low-income, inner-city population: Eating disturbances and weight loss. *Obesity Research, 12*(6), 956–961.

Lundgren, J. D., Allison, K. C., Crow, S., O'Reardon, J. P., Berg, K. C., Galbraith, J., et al. (2006). Prevalence of the night eating syndrome in a psychiatric population. *American Journal of Psychiatry, 163*(1), 156–158.

Lundgren, J. D., Smith, B. M., Spresser, C., Harkins, P., Zolton, L., & Williams, K. (2010). The relationship of night eating to oral health and obesity in community dental clinic patients. *General Dentistry, 58*(3), 134–139.

Lundgren, J. D., Williams, K. B., & Heitmann, B. L. (2010). Nocturnal eating predicts tooth loss among adults: Results from the Danish MONICA study. *Eating Behaviors, 11*(3), 170–174.

Marshall, H. M., Allison, K. C., O'Reardon, J. P., Birketvedt, G., & Stunkard, A. J. (2004). Night eating syndrome among nonobese persons. *International Journal of Eating Disorders, 35*(2), 217–222.

Morse, S. A., Ciechanowski, P. S., Katon, W. J., & Hirsch, I. B. (2006). Isn't this just bedtime snacking? The potential adverse effects of night-eating symptoms on treatment adherence and outcomes in patients with diabetes. *Diabetes Care, 29*(8), 1800–1804.

Napolitano, M. A., Head, S., Babyak, M. A., & Blumenthal, J. A. (2001). Binge-eating disorder and night eating syndrome: Psychological and behavioral characteristics. *International Journal of Eating Disorders, 30*(2), 193–203.

O'Brien, P., E., McPhail, T., Chaston, T. B., & Dixon, J. B. (2006). Systematic review of medium-term weight loss after bariatric operations. *Obesity Surgery, 16*(8), 1032–1040.

O'Reardon, J. P., Ringel, B. L., Dinges, D. F., Allison, K. C., Rogers, N. L., Martino, N. S., et al. (2004). Circadian eating and sleeping patterns in the night eating syndrome. *Obesity Research, 12*(11), 1789–1796.

Olbrich, K., Muhlhans, B., Allison, K. C., Hahn, E. G., Schahin, S. P., & de Zwaan, M. (2009). Night eating, binge eating, and related features in patients with obstructive sleep apnea syndrome. *European Eating Disorders Review, 17*(2), 120–127.

Powers, P. S., Perez, A., Boyd, F., & Rosemurgy, A. (1999). Eating pathology before and after bariatric surgery: A prospective study. *International Journal of Eating Disorders, 25*(3), 293–300.

Rand, C. S. W., & Kuldau, J. M. (1986). Eating patterns in normal weight individuals: Bulimia, restrained eating, and the night eating syndrome. *International Journal of Eating Disorders, 5*(1), 75–84.

Rand, C. S., & Kuldau, J. M. (1993). Morbid obesity: A comparison between a general population and obesity surgery patients. *International Journal of Obesity and Related Metabolic Disorders, 17*(11), 657–661.

Rand, C. S., Macgregor, A. M., & Stunkard, A. J. (1997). The night eating syndrome in the general population and among postoperative obesity surgery patients. *International Journal of Eating Disorders, 22*(1), 65–69.

Schenck, C. H., & Mahowald, M. W. (1994). Review of nocturnal sleep-related eating disorders. *International Journal of Eating Disorders, 15*(4), 343–356.

Spaggiari, M. C., Granella, F., Parrino, L., Marchesi, C., Melli, I., & Terzano, M. G. (1994). Nocturnal eating syndrome in adults. *Sleep, 17*(4), 339–344.

Striegel-Moore, R. H., Dohm, F. A., Hook, J. M., Schreiber, G. B., Crawford, P. B., & Daniels, S. R. (2005). Night eating syndrome in young adult women: Prevalence and correlates. *International Journal of Eating Disorders, 37*(3), 200–206.

Striegel-Moore, R. H., Franko, D. L., Thompson, D., Affenito, S., & Kraemer, H. C. (2006). Night eating: Prevalence and demographic correlates. *Obesity, 14*(1), 139–147.

Stunkard, A., Berkowitz, R., Wadden, T., Tanrikut, C., Reiss, E., & Young, L. (1996). Binge-eating disorder and the night-eating syndrome. *International Journal of Obesity and Related Metabolic Disorders, 20*(1), 1–6.

Stunkard, A. J. (1959). Eating patterns and obesity. *Psychiatric Quarterly, 33,* 284–295.

Stunkard, A. J., Grace, W. J., & Wolff, H. G. (1955). The night-eating syndrome: A pattern of food intake among certain obese patients. *American Journal of Medicine, 19*(1), 78–86.

van Gemert, W. G., Severeijns, R. M., Greve, J. W., Groenman, N., & Soeters, P. B. (1998). Psychological functioning of morbidly obese patients after surgical treatment. *International Journal of Obesity and Related Metabolic Disorders, 22*(5), 393–398.

Chapter 7

Night Eating Syndrome and Other Eating Disorders

Yael Latzer
Orna Tzischinsky

There is a continuous debate in the literature regarding the relationship between night eating syndrome (NES) and eating disorders (EDs). Some conceptualize NES as a subtype of obesity, while others treat this syndrome as a variant of other EDs, in particular bulimia nervosa (BN) and binge-eating disorder (BED). Still others see it as a separate syndrome among EDs. Finally, NES has been viewed as a variant of a sleep disorder, termed sleep-related eating disorder (SRED). SRED is reviewed in detail in Chapter 9 (Howell & Crow). Readers are encouraged to review Chapter 9, as a portion the literature on night eating behavior in patients with AN and BN has conceptualized the night eating behavior as SRED.

Little is known about the relationship between NES and EDs. Most of the research on NES has focused on overweight and obese patients, whereas only a few studies have examined NES among patients diagnosed with EDs, specifically those with BN or BED. To the best of our knowledge, only two case studies and few studies have been published on NES among patients with anorexia nervosa (AN). Likewise, few studies have been based on patients seeking treatment for EDs.

Thus the aim of this chapter is to describe the relationship of NES with other EDs. We review the existing literature regarding NES among patients with BED, BN, and AN, and discuss the research findings in light of the discrepancies and similarities. We also evaluate the research diagnostic criteria for NES proposed for the DSM-5 in light of the current review.

Eating Disorders

EDs are among the most prevailing public health problems, reaching epidemic proportions in many Western countries (Fairburn & Harrison, 2003). EDs include AN, BN, BED, and eating disorder not otherwise specified (EDNOS), also termed partial ED syndromes.

EDs likely reflect complex, interdependent, multidimensional causalities (Keel, Mitchell, Miller, Davis, & Crow, 1999) . Dieting behaviors may be propelled into a full-blown disorder by an interaction of antecedent genetic, biological, psychological, familial, and social conditions, accompanied by various environmental influences. EDs have been traditionally conceptualized as sociocultural-dependent syndromes, related primarily to the thin body ideal and of relevance predominantly in wealthier Western countries (American Psychological Association, 2001; Halmi, 2002; Hoek, 2006)

AN appears primarily during adolescence, whereas BN and BED appear primarily in young adults; all EDs occur mainly in females, with 5–10% of the patients being male (Hoek, 2006). The lifetime prevalence of AN, BN, and BED among females in Western countries is estimated to be between 0.3 and 1.20%, 1 and 1.5%, and 3 and 3.5%, respectively, and among males 0.3%, 0.7%, and 2%, respectively (Latzer, Merrick, & Stein, 2010). The prevalence of partial ED (EDNOS) syndromes is in the range of 3 to 22% (Shisslak, Crago, & Estes, 1995), depending on whether the disorders are diagnosed according to standardized clinical interviews (lower prevalence) or standardized questionnaires (higher prevalence). Although the prevalence rate for both AN and BN is lower in non-Western than in Western countries (there are yet no sufficient data for BED or EDNOS), it is gradually increasing in non-Western countries in recent years (Makino, Tsuboi, & Dennerstein, 2004). Both AN and BN have shown an increase in their incidence in the second half of the 20th century, particularly among young women (Hoek, 2006), although at least some studies argue that what is raised is actually the frequency of treatment use.

The standardized mortality ratios in AN are between 5 and 10 times greater than in normal controls, and considerably higher than those reported for most other psychiatric disturbances, being the highest in bingeing–purging type AN. By contrast, relatively low mortality rates (0.3–3 times greater than controls) have been reported in BN (Keel & Klump, 2003; Shisslak et al., 1995).

AN and BN are associated with a high rate of DSM-IV Axis I comorbidities. Between 40 and 70% of these patients have lifetime affective (mainly depressive) and anxiety (mainly obsessive–compulsive and social phobia) disorders, and similar rates of patients with bingeing–purging AN and BN have lifetime substance use disorders (SUDs) (Williamson, Gleaves, & Stewart, 2005; Wonderlich, Crosby, Mitchell, & Engel, 2007). AN and BN represent chronic disorders, with recovery occurring mostly after 4 to 10 years from the start of the illness (Fichter & Quadflieg, 2007; Keel & Klump, 2003).

Anorexia Nervosa

Diagnostic criteria of AN include a refusal to maintain weight at age and height recommendations, fear of gaining weight, body image disturbance, undue influence of weight and shape on self-evaluation, and amenorrhea in postmenarcheal females (in 33% of cases, AN appears prior to onset of menarche) (American Psychiatric Association, 2000; American Psychological Association, 2001). AN appears primarily during adolescence, although in recent years there has been increasing evidence of first appearance of AN both in younger children and at an older age. AN usually starts as a restricting subtype, with 30 to 60% of restricting patients progressing to bingeing–purging AN or BN (Fairburn & Harrison, 2003; Latzer, Witztum, & Stein, 2008).

Bulimia Nervosa

Diagnostic criteria for BN (American Psychiatric Association, 2000) include recurrent episodes of uncontrolled binge eating and compensatory behaviors to prevent weight gain. Compensatory behaviors often involve purging behaviors, such as self-induced vomiting (which represents around 85% of purging behaviors) and misuse of medications, particularly laxatives, but also nonpurging behaviors, such as fasting and excessive exercise. In addition to these symptoms, BN is also associated with body image disturbance, which manifests as undue influence of weight and shape on self-evaluation. The bingeing and purging behaviors in BN are not associated with low weight; that is, they do not occur exclusively during AN episode (Fairburn & Harrison, 2003; Latzer et al., 2008).

Binge-Eating Disorder

BED, a provisional diagnosis in the DSM-IV-TR (American Psychiatric Association, 2000), is defined by bingeing behaviors similar to those occurring in BN, but with no compensatory behaviors to prevent weight gain. Approximately 30% of overweight individuals are diagnosed with BED (Fairburn & Harrison, 2003; Latzer et al., 2008). Few studies relate to BN and BED as a similar phenomenon, and the etiology of binge eating in both diagnostic groups has been the subject of abundant speculation. Various etiological mechanisms have been proposed for the behavior of binge eating, as well as for the various eating disorder syndromes of which binge eating forms a part. For example, the restraint theory relates to the alternation of food intake restriction and subsequent binge eating (Herman & Polivy, 2005). Psychological factors play a prominent role in many of these theories. Indeed, the standard definition of binge eating includes psychological and psychiatric features, including lack of control over one's eating and psychiatric comorbidity.

Both BN and BED include the binge-eating episode, which is characterized by consumption of large quantities of food quickly and uncontrollably. Binge-eating behavior in both BN and BED often occurs during the evening hours, with the peak time between 7:00 P.M. and 9:00 P.M. (Smyth et al., 2009). In both diagnostic groups, the binge episode generally occurs in solitude due to embarrassment about the amount of food consumed at a more rapid pace than normal until there is a feeling of being uncomfortably replete (Fairburn & Harrison, 2003; Tzischinsky & Latzer, 2004). The question remains as to whether the subgroup of individuals who tend to have binge episodes during the evening and/or at nighttime require a separate diagnosis, presenting as NES or a variant of BN, BED, or AN binge–purge type (Latzer & Stein, 2010).

NES among Patients with EDs

Most of the studies conducted on the relationship between NES and EDs have been based on an overweight and obese female population with and without BED (Stunkard et al., 1996). The estimated prevalence of NES among patients with EDs ranges from 5 to 43.4%, depending on the sample population, the diagnostic categories, and the setting of recruitment (eating disorder, sleep disorder, or weight loss centers). Some studies have been conducted on NES in patients with AN (Lundgren et al., 2011; Schenck, Hurwitz, Bundlie, & Mahowald, 1991; Schenck, Hurwitz, O'Connor, & Mahowald, 1993; Tzischinsky & Latzer, 2004; Winkelman, 1998). Others have been conducted on NES in patients with BED (Adami, Campostano, Marinari, Ravera, & Scopinaro, 2002; Allison, Grilo, Masheb, & Stunkard, 2005; Berkowitz, Stunkard, & Stallings, 1993; Greeno, Wing, & Marcus, 1995; Grilo & Masheb, 2004; Lundgren et al., 2006; Mancini & Aloe, 1994; Napolitano, Head, Babyak, & Blumenthal, 2001; O'Reardon, Stunkard, & Allison, 2004; Stunkard et al., 2009; Tzischinsky & Latzer, 2004; Winkelman, 1998). Very little research has been conducted on NES among patients with BN (Birketvedt et al., 1999; Gupta, 1991; Lundgren et al., 2011; Lundgren, Shapiro, & Bulik, 2008; Tzischinsky & Latzer, 2004; Williamson, Lawson, Bennett, & Hinz, 1989; Winkelman, Herzog, & Fava, 1999; Winkelman, 1998). In addition, two case reports have described NES in this patient population (Guirguis, 1986; Roper, 1989).

NES among Patients with AN

To the best of our knowledge, only a few reports have presented NES among patients with AN. Three studies examined night eating behavior among patients seeking treatment for sleep disorders, but the night eating was conceptualized as SRED (Schenck et al., 1991; Schenck et al., 1993; Winkelman, 1998), and three examined patients seeking treatment for EDs (Lundgren et al., 2011; Tzischinsky & Latzer, 2004; Winkelman et al., 1999). In two separate reports, Schenck et al. (1991; Schenck et al., 1993) reviewed patients seeking treatment in a sleep disorder clinic over a 7-year period and found 38 patients with SRED. About 70% of the patients were diagnosed with sleepwalking, 13% with restless leg syndrome, and 10% with obstructive sleep apnea, all based on polysomnographic data. Only 5% had a diagnosis of current or past AN (not mentioned whether it was restricting or binge–purge type).

Winkelman (1998) conducted a sleeping and eating assessment of 23 patients who were seeking treatment for SRED at a sleep disorders center. The majority (83%) were female, with most of them suffering from the disorder chronically since adolescence for a mean duration of 15.8 years. Nearly all of the patients reported nocturnal ingestion (NI) (1 to 6 episodes per night) after sleep onset, and 66% reported bingeing during the night. Nearly 50% were diagnosed as having somnambulism, and more than 90% reported that they were half awake and unaware during the NI. Thirteen percent of the patients were diagnosed as having AN.

Using a larger sample, Winkelman et al. (1999) conducted another study on 700 patients who were seeking treatment for EDs, including 126 outpatients and 24 inpatients with EDs, 126 obese subjects, 207 individuals with depression, and 217 college students. They were assessed both for SRED, defined as waking to eat after sleep onset with altered awareness, and for simple NI, defined as waking to eat after sleep onset with full awareness. Results indicated that the prevalence of SRED was 16.7% in the inpatient group and 8.7% in the outpatient group. Of the patients with EDs with SRED, 33% were diagnosed as having AN.

Tzischinsky and Latzer (2004) assessed the prevalence of NES-NI among individuals seeking outpatient treatment for EDs. Their results showed that no patients with AN reported on NI episodes. The most recent research on NES among patients with EDs was conducted by Lundgren and colleagues (2011), who examined the prevalence and characteristics of NES in a sample of 68 inpatients being treated for EDs, including 32 with AN, 32 with BN, and 4 with EDNOS. NES was diagnosed in 25% of the total sample, and in 9.4% of patients with AN. Patients with AN reported only 1.1 NI per week as compared to patients with BN who reported 3.5 NI per week.

According to the literature, we may conclude that the percentage of AN patients with NES is very small. Most of them have additional sleep disorders and can be part of the SRED diagnostic subgroup or those without reported sleeping problems, but generally do not exhibit night eating behavior after sleep onset. It is not yet clear whether the patients with AN are the binge–purge type or the restricting type. In general, patients with AN were significantly less likely to report night eating behavior than patients with BN, and in particular were less likely to report evening hyperphagia (EH) (Lundgren et al., 2011; Winkelman et al., 1999).

NES among Patients with BN

The prevalence rate of NES among patients with BN who seek treatment for ED ranges from 9 to 47.1% (Lundgren et al., 2011; Tzischinsky & Latzer 2004; Winkelman, 1998). Only a few studies have been conducted on NES among patients with BN, mostly with patients seeking treatment for sleep disorders at a sleep center. Two case studies from the late 1980s provided initial reports on the clinical and psychological characteristics of patients with BN who also suffer from NES.

The first documented report was described by Guirguis (1986) in the case of a 32-year-old woman who described waking up three to four times every night, walking to the kitchen, and eating in an uncontrolled way. Most of the time she was not aware of her behavior until the following morning, when she discovered the evidence of empty food containers. She was then preoccupied with food and body shape the next day, starving herself and spending hours exercising in order to control her weight gain. According to the current diagnostic criteria, her problem would be described as SRED and BN nonpurging subtype.

Roper (1989) described a similar case of a 36-year-old woman who would wake up during the night, sleepwalk to the refrigerator, and eat anything in it, including raw meat, butter, and uncooked vegetables. Usually she was unaware of her night ingestion until the morning, when she found the discarded wrappers or food remains. The author described her binge-eating episodes as somnabulistic bulimia. It is hard to know from this report whether she had compensatory behavior after the binge episodes. However, it seems that, according to the current diagnostic criteria, her behavior would be considered characteristic of SRED among patients with BN. Gupta (1991) also reported on the phenomenon of SRED among patients with BN, with 31% describing their eating during the night with little or no awareness at least two to three times in the previous month.

In Winkelman et al.'s (1999) study, 13% of the patients were diagnosed with BN. The author suggested that SRED is a relatively homogeneous syndrome that combines somnambulistic and daytime eating disorders and thus deserves separate diagnostic criteria. This approach is supported by previous polysomnographic data showing that SRED is composed of patients with a number of underlying sleep disorders (Schenck et al., 1993; Spaggiari et al., 1994). In Winkelman et al.'s (1999) study, results showed that of the patients with SRED, 67% were diagnosed as having BN. There was variability reported in the degree of awareness of NES-NI episodes, and it is important to note that the question of awareness of SRED among patients with EDs is still unclear.

Tzischinsky and Latzer (2004) were the first to describe prevalence features and NES-NI among patients with BN. They recruited 10 patients with BN from an outpatient ED clinic who complained about having binge-eating episodes, both during the day and after sleep onset. The patients were monitored by an actigraph for 1 week and completed a subjective sleep report questionnaire. They reported high sleep disorders, including a low level of alertness, midsleep awakenings, and excessive daytime sleepiness. All of them were aware of the NI binge episodes. The number of binge episodes during the night ranged from two to four (see Figure 7.1), and the mean age of onset of NES-NI was 18.4 years.

The results showed that the prevalence of NES-NI among patients with BN was 9% of all patients with BN referred to the EDs clinic during a 3-year period. In addition, the results indicated that traumatic life

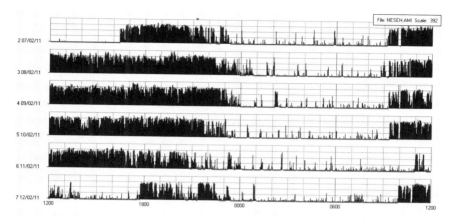

FIGURE 7.1. Nocturnal awakenings during 1 week of actigraphy monitoring of a patient diagnosed with BN.

events, in particular sexual and physical abuse (50% of the cases), coincided closely with the onset of NES-NI binge-eating episodes, as well as a high level of psychiatric comorbidity (82%), anxiety, or depression. EH was not assessed; however, about 50% of the patients with BN reported having binge–purge episodes during the evening before sleep onset.

In a small study of NES among individuals with BN enrolled in an outpatient cognitive-behavioral therapy intervention, 35.8% of patients reported EH and 38.7% reported NI during the previous month (Lundgren, Shapiro, et al., 2008). In this study, all participants reported awareness of their nocturnal eating episodes. In the most recent research related to NES among patients with EDs, Lundgren et al. (2011) found that patients with BN were more likely to be diagnosed with NES than were patients with AN (40.6% vs. 9.4%, respectively). Moreover, patients with BN were significantly more likely than patients with AN to report EH. Patients with BN reported 3.5 NI per week, as compared to those with AN, who reported only 1.1 NI per week.

In conclusion, patients with BN (binge–purge type) engage in compensatory behavior (e.g., self-induced vomiting, excessive exercise, dietary restriction) following binges. It may be possible that the delayed eating (i.e., breakfast skipping) found in NES patients is a kind of compensatory mechanism following the night eating episodes and not just a circadian delay in eating. It may also be possible that overeating during the evening hours represents a variant of BN and not a distinct entity of NES-EH (Lundgren et al., 2011). What is clear is that there is a subtype of patients with BN who also have NES-NI. The differences between BN with or without NES-NI need further exploration.

NES among Patients with BED

Extensive research has been conducted during the last 20 years trying to understand the relationship between NES and BED. Mancini and Aloe's (1994) case report, which was the first to describe the combination of obesity, BED, NI, and SRED, described a 41-year-old woman with BED whose NES and history of obesity and nightly sleepwalking was accompanied by compulsive eating behavior for nearly 22 years. Her eating consisted of NI of high-calorie food, often with sloppy meal consumption or preparation, and she was totally unaware of the night eating episodes.

Greeno et al. (1995) examined the prevalence of NES in 40 overweight women with BED and 39 overweight controls. They were monitored for negative mood or anxiety and NES-NI for an average of eight nights. Six women (15%) with BED reported NES-NI, while none of the control group had NES-NI. The amount of calories consumed during the NES-NI episodes varied widely, ranging from 141 kcal to more than 1,000 kcal. Two of the six participants reported that they were in control during their NES-NI episodes and that the episodes were not binges. Patients reported tiredness, but not poor mood or anxiety, during the NES-NI episodes. In this study, NES-NI was associated more with EDs than with being overweight. On the basis of these results, the authors suggested that NES should be evaluated and treated as part of the BED diagnosis among ED patients, differently from overweight and obese patients. Yet the question of whether NES-NI is a subtype of BED or a separate ED syndrome remains unclear.

Grilo and Masheb (2004) examined the frequency of NES-NI (based on waking up at night and eating) and its correlates in 207 adults (45 men and 162 women) with BED, using semistructured interviews and a battery of behavioral and psychological measures. Overall, 28% ($N = 58$) of the participants reported NES during the previous 28 days. Participants who reported NES had a significantly higher BMI, but otherwise differed little from those who did not report NES-NI. There were no significant differences in the number of days or number of episodes of binge eating between NES-NI and non–NES-NI, BED groups. Thus it is suggested that the ambiguity and overlap around the differences between BED and NES-NI need further exploration.

Other studies of patients with obesity who have additionally been assessed for BED have found that NES (defined as both NI and/or EH) and binge-eating behavior commonly co-occur. Although these behaviors may well overlap, it is suggested that NES and BED have different underlying behavioral constructs. Moreover, some researchers propose the concept that BED only, BED with NES, and NES only constitute a psychopathology continuum, with BED accompanied by NES having higher psychopathology and NES only having lower psychopathology (Napolitano et al., 2001; Stunkard et al., 1996).

Stunkard et al. (1996) assessed the prevalence of BED and NES in 231 women with obesity from three different groups (television sample, weight reduction sample, and medication trial sample). They used DSM-IV criteria for the diagnosis of BED and morning anorexia, evening hyperphagia, and insomnia for the diagnosis of NES. Results indicated that there was little overlap between the two disorders. The authors suggested that BED was far less frequent when using in-depth interview methods as compared to self-administered questionnaires, and they concluded that the frequency of NES is comparable to that of BED when using such methods.

With regard to psychological and behavioral characteristics associated with both NES (defined both as EH and/or NI) and BED, Napolitano et al. (2001) examined 42 males and 41 females who were seeking weight loss treatment. Individuals were classified into one of four groups: NES only (N = 23), BED only (N = 13), both NES and BED (N = 13), or healthy control group (N = 34). Results indicated that the prevalence of NES was 43.4%. Patients with NES scored significantly lower on disinhibition than patients with BED. In addition, individuals who met the criteria for both NES and BED scored significantly higher than NES-only patients on state and trait anxiety and disinhibition. Moreover, patients with BED presented significantly higher scores on disinhibition and hunger and anxiety, as compared to patients without BED and to patients with NES. Thus the authors suggested that NES may represent a subcategory among obese individuals, which also overlaps with BED. As such, individuals with NES may have less psychopathology than patients with BED and may indeed represent a separate subgroup.

Similar to Napolitano et al. (2001), Allison et al. (2005) also observed that individuals with BED have higher psychopathology, both in terms of eating patterns and emotional level, than individuals with NES. They compared eating patterns, disordered eating, and depressive symptoms in 177 individuals with BED, 69 individuals with NES, and 45 overweight individuals versus a comparison group without BED or NES. Participants with BED reported more binge-eating episodes, shape/weight concerns, disinhibition, and hunger than the NES and comparison groups. However, the NES group reported more eating pathology than the comparison participants. Therefore the researchers suggested that NES should be considered as a separate diagnostic subcategory from BED.

Colles, Dixon, and O'Brien (2007) investigated the clinical significance of NES and nocturnal snacking by exploring the relationship between NES and (1) obesity, (2) BED, and (3) psychological distress. They compared 180 bariatric surgery candidates, 93 members of a nonsurgical weight-loss support group, and 158 general community respondents (81 males, 350 females; mean age: 45.8 ± 13.3 years; mean body mass index [BMI, kg/m²]: 34.8 ± 10.8; and BMI range: 17.7–66.7). Nocturnal snacking (awakening to eat) was recorded. Validated questionnaires assessed BED, symptoms of depression, appearance dissatisfaction, and mental health-related quality of life. Results indicated that NES criteria were met by 11.1% of the total cohort. Individuals with comorbid NES and BED reported elevated psychological distress similar to other groups. NES alone was not associated with psychological distress. Those with NES-NI who consumed nocturnal snacks reported poorer mental health-related quality of life and greater depressive symptoms and hunger than others with NES.

In Tzischinsky and Latzer's (2004) study on the prevalence of NES-NI among outpatients from an ED clinic, 12 BED patients who complained about having binge-eating episodes after sleep onset were monitored by an actigraph for 1 week and completed a subjective sleep report questionnaire. They reported high sleep disorders, including a low level of alertness, midsleep awakenings, and excessive daytime sleepiness. Ten of the 12 patients were aware of the NI binge episodes. The number of binges during the night ranged from three to five (see Figure 7.2), and the mean age of onset of binges during the night was 28.7 years.

The results showed that the prevalence of NES-NI among patients with BED was 16% of all patients with BED referred to the ED clinic during a 3-year period. In addition, the results indicated that traumatic life events, in particular sexual and physical abuse (60% of the cases), coincided closely with the onset of NES-NI, as well as a high level of psychiatric comorbidity (64%), anxiety, or depression.

Similarly, Allison, Grilo, Masheb, and Stunkard (2007) found a higher prevalence of emotional and sexual abuse, emotional and physical neglect, and depression in BED and NES groups than in overweight individuals. These results emphasize that patients with BED and NES, in particular NES-NI, who are seeking treatment for EDs may have high

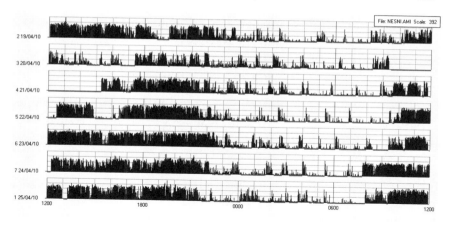

FIGURE 7.2. Nocturnal awakenings during 1 week of actigraphy monitoring for a patient diagnosed with BED.

rates of traumatic life events, as well as high levels of loneliness, psychological distress, and psychiatric comorbidity, thereby highlighting the need for further research on general psychopathology and the relationship with BED.

Several authors suggest that, although the behaviors of NES and BED may well overlap, the two diagnoses most likely have different underlying behavioral constructs. Adami et al. (2002) investigated the frequency of NES diagnosed among 166 patients with obesity and its relationship with BED. Results indicated that NES was more frequent among patients with BED than among patients without BED; however, disinhibition and hunger scores were higher among the patients with BED than among the patients without BED and individuals with NES. A similar conclusion was reached by de Zwaan, Burgard, Schenck, and Mitchell (2003), who suggested that subjects with NES do not show the same level of ED-related psychopathology that is typical for subjects with BED. Thus NES might represent a distinct entity, in which nighttime eating is not just a symptom of BED.

Furthermore, Sassaroli et al. (2009) showed that night eating behavior in patients with NES is associated with nocturnal mental anxiety, whereas as night eating behavior in patients with BED is associated with diurnal anxiety. No relationship was found between nocturnal mental anxiety and nighttime binges in patients with BED, suggesting that there are differences in the etiology of night eating behavior in both populations. Stunkard, Allison, Geliebter, Lundgren, Gluck, et al. (2009) also noted that BED is not associated with a circadian delay of food intake, which is characteristic of individuals with NES.

Even after 55 years from the initial research on NES, there is still considerable debate about whether NES represents a distinct entity or whether it is a variant of BED in which the binges occur in the evening after dinner or at night after sleep onset. According to the literature reviewed we may suggest carefully that NES-EH may be related to a variant of BED. However, patients with NES-NI with BED represent a distinct entity.

Discussion

In the 55 years since NES was first described, many studies have been conducted on this syndrome with a number of different populations. However, little is known about the relationship between NES and other EDs, including AN, BN, BED, and EDNOS. There is ongoing debate as to whether NES is a separate diagnostic syndrome or a subgroup of eating, sleeping, or overweight disorders. Different definitions for NES have been used and proposed. Initially, NES definition and diagnosis were viewed mainly in the context of the overweight and obese population seeking weight loss treatment, while patients with an ED diagnosis were excluded from the research. Thus the need for studying NES within the context of patients with ED has taken on increasing importance.

When NES has been documented in individuals diagnosed with ED, it has been mainly among patients with BED and BN. Only recently a few studies have related to patients with AN as well. Studies of patients with obesity who have additionally been assessed for BED have found that NES and binge-eating behavior commonly co-occur. However, some researchers suggest that although these behaviors may well overlap, NES and BED have different underlying behavioral constructs. Moreover, they suggest that BED only, BED with NES, and NES only constitute a psychopathology continuum, with BED accompanied by NES having higher psychopathology and NES only having lower psychopathology (Napolitano et al., 2001; Stunkard et al., 1996).

Although there appears to be a relationship between SRED, NES, and daytime ED, in particular patients with BN, the question of whether a new subgroup should be called SRED or NES is still unclear. Further research is needed to clarify this question, while emphasizing the differences between NES-NI and NES-EH among patients with BN. NES among patients with BN without SRED has been described only in the last decade by groups of researchers in Israel and Missouri who are experts in eating and sleep disorders.

The studies conducted on patients with BED with NES seeking treatment for ED raises the question of whether binge-eating behavior during evening hours relates to an EH diagnosis of NES or is a part of BED diagnosis (Lundgren, Allison, O'Reardon, & Stunkard, 2008; Tzischinsky & Latzer, 2004; Winkelman, 1998). It is important to note that binge-eating behavior frequently occurs during the evening hours (EH) among patients with BED. The behavioral and functional overlap between evening binge eating and EH continues to be problematic for the diagnosis of NES. We may suggest that BED with NES-NI should be viewed separately as a subtype of NES, while NES-EH should be considered as a variant of BED. In addition, as Stunkard et al. (Stunkard, Allison, Geliebter, Lundgren, Gluck, et al., 2009) noted, BED is not associated with a circadian delay of food intake, which is characteristic of NES-NI.

The findings show that there is not a clear answer as to whether the morning anorexia that exists among NES patients with EDs relates to the binge episodes during the evening or the night ingestions, rather than being necessarily related to the phase delay of the hunger–satiety cycle, as previously hypothesized. Furthermore, it remains unclear whether binge episodes, the amount of calories consumed, and the food types consumed are similar between BED alone, NES alone, and BED combined with NES. The same questions need to be answered with regard to BN and NES. In addition, the differences between the groups in terms of psychiatric comorbidity and psychological distress must also be determined.

As described in the review, various researchers support different perspectives on the relationships between NES and EDs. These differences may be explained by the varying methodologies and diagnostic definitions of NES used in the different studies. Moreover, there is a significant difference in the psychopathology and other clinical and personal characteristics between the NES-EH subtype and the NES-NI subtype.

An additional observation is that the level of awareness in the diagnostic criteria should be reconsidered, since most of the ED patients with night binge episodes report full awareness of the episodes as compared to those with SRED. The dichotomous classification of awareness/no awareness in the new proposed diagnostic criteria reflects the complexity of ED patients' actual experiences. Patients who seek treatment for sleep disorders are often found to complain about NES-NI and are partially or even fully aware of the NES-NI episodes. They are also usually diagnosed as suffering from sleep disorders, mainly somnambulism.

Areas for Future Research

The review of the literature of this chapter raised a number of questions that require further research:

1. Are the newly proposed NES criteria (Allison, Lundgren, O'Reardon, et al., 2010) clinically useful or valid in ED populations when many patients with BED, BN, and perhaps AN binge–purge type also meet the criteria for NES?
2. Are the nocturnal ingestions that occur among patients with ED a variant of BN or BED or a variant of SRED?
3. Is the evening hyperphagia that occurs among patients with ED a variant of BN or BED?
4. In what ways are the characteristics and behaviors (calorie consumption, type of food) of night eating among patients with ED similar or different from the night eating in overweight and obese populations, normal-weight populations, and SRED populations?
5. In what ways do the history of traumatic life events and the level of psychiatric and psychological comorbidity differ between the NES among patients with EDs, overweight and obese populations, normal-weight populations, and SRED populations?

The questions raised in this chapter and the prevalence of NES found among EDs suggest that even before answering these questions, it is important to routinely assess NES behavior in individuals seeking treatment for EDs. It is suggested that the NEQ be used for the basic evaluation of all patients with EDs.

In addition, it is suggested that cognitive-behavioral therapy (CBT) be employed in combination with SSRI medication (e.g., sertraline), which was found to be effective in a randomized placebo-controlled trial among individuals diagnosed with NES (O'Reardon et al., 2006). To date, the treatment studies for patients with NES have focused on weight-loss reduction (Ceru-Bjork, Andersson, & Rossner, 2001); SSRI medication (O'Reardon et al., 2006); light therapy (Friedman, Even, Dardennes, & Guelfi, 2002); psychotherapy (Oswald & Adam, 1986); controlled behavioral treatment (Pawlow, O'Neil, & Malcolm, 2003); and CBT (Allison, Lundgren, Moore, O'Reardon, & Stunkard, 2010). Most of those studies were conducted among individuals with obesity, SRED, post–bariatric surgery, and BED in a communal sample.

An initial clinical trial of CBT among patients with NES was recently conducted by Allison, Lundgren, Moore, et al. (2010). Significant improvements in the core aspects of NES and weight reduction suggested the need for a control treatment trial. It is important to note that this treatment trial was not focused mainly on ED patients with NES. A recent CBT preliminary trial was conducted in the ED clinic in Israel among patients who suffer from BED with NES. Three out of the five patients finished the CBT trial. They were female, ranging in age from 55 to 62, with a BMI range from 30.6 to 40.5. The treatment was based on a CBT protocol reported by Allison, Stunkard, and Thier (2004). Two sessions related to sleep hygiene were added to the basic protocol, and measurements of satiety and hunger were added to the diary provided to the patients during treatment. Preliminary results indicated improvements in three different dimensions: sleep habits, level of psychopathology, and weight. These preliminary results call for further research of this protocol in larger controlled samples with follow-up (Edelstein et al., 2010).

References

Adami, G. F., Campostano, A., Marinari, G. M., Ravera, G., & Scopinaro, N. (2002). Night eating in obesity: A descriptive study. *Nutrition, 18*(7–8), 587–589.

Allison, K. C., Stunkard, A. J., & Thier, S. L. (2004). *Overcoming the night eating syndrome: A step-by-step guide to breaking the cycle.* Oakland, CA: New Harbinger.

Allison, K. C., Grilo, C. M., Masheb, R. M., & Stunkard, A. J. (2005). Binge-eating disorder and night eating syndrome: A comparative study of disordered eating. *Journal of Consulting and Clinical Psychology, 73*(6), 1107–1115.

Allison, K. C., Grilo, C. M., Masheb, R. M., & Stunkard, A. J. (2007). High self-reported rates of neglect and emotional abuse, by persons with binge-eating disorder and night eating syndrome. *Behaviour Research and Therapy, 45*(12), 2874–2883.

Allison, K. C., Lundgren, J. D., Moore, R. H., O'Reardon, J. P., & Stunkard, A. J. (2010). Cognitive behavior therapy for night eating syndrome: A pilot study. *American Journal of Psychotherapy, 64*(1), 91–106.

Allison, K. C., Lundgren, J. D., O'Reardon, J. P., Geliebter, A., Gluck, M. E., Vinai, P., et al. (2010). Proposed diagnostic criteria for night eating syndrome. *International Journal of Eating Disorders, 43*(3), 241–247.

American Psychiatric Association. (2000). *Diagnostic and statistical manual of mental disorders* (4th ed. text rev.). Washington, DC: Author.

American Psychological Association. (2001). *Publication manual of the American Psychological Association.* Washington, DC: Author.

Berkowitz, R., Stunkard, A. J., & Stallings, V. A. (1993). Binge-eating disorder in obese adolescent girls. *Annals of the New York Academy of Sciences, 699,* 200–206.

Birketvedt, G. S., Florholmen, J., Sundsfjord, J., Osterud, B., Dinges, D., Bilker, W., et al. (1999). Behavioral and neuroendocrine characteristics of the night-eating syndrome. *Journal of the American Medical Association, 282*(7), 657–663.

Ceru-Bjork, C., Andersson, I., & Rossner, S. (2001). Night eating and nocturnal eating: Two different or similar syndromes among obese patients? *International Journal of Obesity and Related Metabolic Disorders, 25*(3), 365–372.

Colles, S. L., Dixon, J. B., & O'Brien, P. E. (2007). Night eating syndrome and nocturnal snacking: Association with obesity, binge eating, and psychological distress. *International Journal of Obesity, 31*(11), 1722–1730.

de Zwaan, M., Burgard, M. A., Schenck, C. H., & Mitchell, J. E. (2003). Night-time eating: A review of the literature. *European Eating Disorders Review, 11*(1), 7–24.

Edelstein, R., Rabin, O., Hason, M., Givon, M., Alon, S., Kabakov, O., et al. (2010). *CBT for patients with BED and NES*. Israeli Annual Conference of ATID Nutrition Association, Bar Ilan University.

Fairburn, C. G., & Harrison, P. J. (2003). Eating disorders. *Lancet, 361*(9355), 407–416.

Fichter, M. M., & Quadflieg, N. (2007). Long?term stability of eating disorder diagnoses. *International Journal of Eating Disorders, 40*(S3), S61–S66.

Friedman, S., Even, C., Dardennes, R., & Guelfi, J. D. (2002). Light therapy, obesity, and night-eating syndrome. *American Journal of Psychiatry, 159*(5), 875–876.

Greeno, C. G., Wing, R. R., & Marcus, M. D. (1995). Nocturnal eating in binge-eating disorder and matched-weight controls. *International Journal of Eating Disorders, 18*(4), 343–349.

Grilo, C. M., & Masheb, R. M. (2004). Nighttime eating in men and women with binge-eating disorder. *Behaviour Research and Therapy, 42*(4), 397–407.

Guirguis, W. R. (1986). Sleepwalking as a symptom of bulimia. *British Medical Journal (Clinical Research Ed.), 293*(6547), 587–588.

Gupta, M. A. (1991). Sleep related eating in bulimia nervosa: An underreported parasomnia disorder. *Sleep Research, 20,* 182.

Halmi, K. A. (2002). Eating disorders in females: Genetics, pathophysiology, and treatment. *Journal of Pediatric Endocrinology and Metabolism, 15*(Suppl. 5), 1379–1386.

Herman, C. P., & Polivy, J. (2005). Normative influences on food intake. *Physiology and Behavior, 86*(5), 762–772.

Hoek, H. W. (2006). Incidence, prevalence, and mortality of anorexia nervosa and other eating disorders. *Current Opinion in Psychiatry, 19*(4), 389.

Keel, P. K., Mitchell, J. E., Miller, K. B., Davis, T. L., & Crow, S. J. (1999). Long-term outcome of bulimia nervosa. *Archives of General Psychiatry, 56*(1), 63.

Keel, P. K., & Klump, K. L. (2003). Are eating disorders culture-bound syndromes? implications for conceptualizing their etiology. *Psychological Bulletin, 129*(5), 747–769.

Latzer, Y., Merrick, J., & Stein, D. (2010). Eating disorders: Diagnosis, epidemiology, etiology, and prevention. In Y. Latzer, J. Merrick, & D. Stein (Eds.),

Understanding eating disorders: Integrating culture, psychology and biology (pp. 1–11). Hauppauge, NY: Nova Science Publishers.

Latzer, Y., Witztum, E., & Stein, D. (2008). Eating disorders and disordered eating in Israel: An updated review. *European Eating Disorders Review, 16*(5), 361–374.

Lundgren, J. D., Allison, K. C., Crow, S., O'Reardon, J. P., Berg, K. C., Galbraith, J., et al. (2006). Prevalence of the night eating syndrome in a psychiatric population. *American Journal of Psychiatry, 163*(1), 156–158.

Lundgren, J. D., Allison, K. C., O'Reardon, J. P., & Stunkard, A. J. (2008). A descriptive study of non-obese persons with night eating syndrome and a weight-matched comparison group. *Eating Behaviors, 9*(3), 343–351.

Lundgren, J. D., McCune, A., Spresser, C., Harkins, P., Zolton, L., & Mandal, K. (2011). Night eating patterns of individuals with eating disorders: Implications for conceptualizing the night eating syndrome. *Psychiatry Research, 186*(1), 103–108.

Lundgren, J. D., Shapiro, J. R., & Bulik, C. M. (2008). Night eating patterns of patients with bulimia nervosa: A preliminary report. *Eating and Weight Disorders, 13*(4), 171–175.

Makino, M., Tsuboi, K., & Dennerstein, L. (2004). Prevalence of eating disorders: A comparison of Western and non-Western countries. *Medscape General Medicine, 6*(3), 49.

Mancini, M. C., & Aloe, F. (1994). Nocturnal eating syndrome: A case report with therapeutic response to dexfenfluramine. *Revista Paulista De Medicina, 112*(2), 569–571.

Napolitano, M. A., Head, S., Babyak, M. A., & Blumenthal, J. A. (2001). Binge-eating disorder and night eating syndrome: Psychological and behavioral characteristics. *International Journal of Eating Disorders, 30*(2), 193–203.

O'Reardon, J. P., Allison, K. C., Martino, N. S., Lundgren, J. D., Heo, M., & Stunkard, A. J. (2006). A randomized, placebo-controlled trial of sertraline in the treatment of night eating syndrome. *American Journal of Psychiatry, 163*(5), 893–898.

O'Reardon, J. P., Stunkard, A. J., & Allison, K. C. (2004). Clinical trial of sertraline in the treatment of night eating syndrome. *International Journal of Eating Disorders, 35*(1), 16–26.

Oswald, I., & Adam, K. (1986). Rhythmic raiding of refrigerator related to rapid eye movement sleep. *British Medical Journal, 292*(6520), 589.

Pawlow, L. A., O'Neil, P. M., & Malcolm, R. J. (2003). Night eating syndrome: Effects of brief relaxation training on stress, mood, hunger, and eating patterns. *International Journal of Obesity and Related Metabolic Disorders, 27*(8), 970–978.

Roper, P. (1989). Bulimia while sleepwalking, a rebuttal for sane automatism? *Lancet, 2*(8666), 796.

Sassaroli, S., Ruggiero, G. M., Vinai, P., Cardetti, S., Carpegna, G., Ferrato, N., et al. (2009). Daily and nightly anxiety among patients affected by night eating syndrome and binge-eating disorder. *Eating Disorders, 17*(2), 140–145.

Schenck, C. H., Hurwitz, T. D., Bundlie, S. R., & Mahowald, M. W. (1991). Sleep-related eating disorders: Polysomnographic correlates of a heterogeneous syndrome distinct from daytime eating disorders. *Sleep, 14*(5), 419–431.

Schenck, C. H., Hurwitz, T. D., O'Connor, K. A., & Mahowald, M. W. (1993). Additional categories of sleep-related eating disorders and the current status of treatment. *Sleep, 16*(5), 457–466.

Shisslak, C. M., Crago, M., & Estes, L. S. (1995). The spectrum of eating disturbances. *International Journal of Eating Disorders, 18*(3), 209–219.

Smyth, J. M., Wonderlich, S. A., Sliwinski, M. J., Crosby, R. D., Engel, S. G., Mitchell, J. E., et al. (2009). Ecological momentary assessment of affect, stress, and binge–purge behaviors: Day of week and time of day effects in the natural environment. *International Journal of Eating Disorders, 42*(5), 429–436.

Spaggiari, M. C., Granella, F., Parrino, L., Marchesi, C., Melli, I., & Terzano, M. G. (1994). Nocturnal eating syndrome in adults. *Sleep, 17*(4), 339–344.

Stunkard, A., Berkowitz, R., Wadden, T., Tanrikut, C., Reiss, E., & Young, L. (1996). Binge-eating disorder and the night-eating syndrome. *International Journal of Obesity and Related Metabolic Disorders, 20*(1), 1–6.

Stunkard, A. J., Allison, K. C., Geliebter, A., Lundgren, J. D., Gluck, M. E., & O'Reardon, J. P. (2009). Development of criteria for a diagnosis: Lessons from the night eating syndrome. *Comprehensive Psychiatry, 50*(5), 391–399.

Stunkard, A. J., Allison, K. C., Lundgren, J. D., & O'Reardon, J. P. (2009). A biobehavioural model of the night eating syndrome. *Obesity Reviews, 10*(Suppl. 2), 69–77.

Tzischinsky, O., & Latzer, Y. (2004). Nocturnal eating prevalence, features, and night sleep among binge-eating disorders and bulimia nervosa patients in Israel. *European Eating Disorders Review, 12*, 101–109.

Williamson, D. A., Gleaves, D. H., & Stewart, T. M. (2005). Categorical versus dimensional models of eating disorders: An examination of the evidence. *International Journal of Eating Disorders, 37*(1), 1–10.

Williamson, D. A., Lawson, O. D., Bennett, S. M., & Hinz, L. (1989). Behavioral treatment of night bingeing and rumination in an adult case of bulimia nervosa. *Journal of Behavior Therapy and Experimental Psychiatry, 20*(1), 73–77.

Winkelman, J., Herzog, D., & Fava, M. (1999). The prevalence of sleep-related eating disorder in psychiatric and non-psychiatric populations. *Psychological Medicine, 29*(06), 1461–1466.

Winkelman, J. W. (1998). Clinical and polysomnographic features of sleep-related eating disorder. *Journal of Clinical Psychiatry, 59*(1), 14–19.

Wonderlich, S. A., Crosby, R. D., Mitchell, J. E., & Engel, S. G. (2007). Testing the validity of eating disorder diagnoses. *International Journal of Eating Disorders, 40*(Suppl.), S40–S45.

Chapter 8

Night Eating Syndrome and Other Psychiatric Disorders

Melisa V. Rempfer
Meghan E. Murphy

Even in the earliest published description of night eating syndrome (NES), Stunkard, Grace, and Wolff (1955) highlighted its relationship with emotional functioning. In their observation of 20 obese individuals with night eating behaviors, Stunkard et al. (1955) noted that the eating pattern was particularly prominent during periods of life stress and served as a sensitive indicator of emotional distress among their sample. The psychological characteristics of persons with NES, however, as with other aspects of the syndrome, remained understudied for many decades (Vinai et al., 2008). In recent years, as research and clinical interest in NES have increased, additional studies have supported the link between nighttime eating patterns and various dimensions of psychopathology.

Interestingly, although there has been much debate throughout the years regarding the diagnostic criteria for NES, few criteria sets have included emotional or psychological features as part of the formal diagnostic picture. Although specific NES criteria have varied considerably, in recent years the diagnosis has typically focused on three symptoms: evening hyperphagia, nocturnal awakenings to eat, and morning anorexia (Allison et al., 2010). While some have proposed that anxiety and/or evening tension should be included as core diagnostic characteristics (e.g., Kuldau & Rand, 1986; Rand, Macgregor, & Stunkard, 1997), this practice has not been used widely. As such, diagnostic inconsistencies have contributed to the relatively underdeveloped literature on the psychiatric and emotional comorbidities of NES.

This chapter reviews the existing literature on NES and key dimensions of psychopathology. Most prominently, NES has been studied with regard to depression and anxiety (e.g., Boseck et al., 2007; de Zwaan, Roerig, Crosby, Karaz, & Mitchell, 2006; Sassaroli et al., 2009; Striegel-Moore et al., 2008). Indeed, there is noteworthy overlap among the diagnostic criteria for various mood and anxiety disorders and NES, namely with regard to appetite and sleep symptoms. Therefore, it may not be surprising that a substantial literature documents the association among these conditions. Although less is known regarding NES and substance abuse or serious mental illness (SMI), emerging research in these areas suggests their relevance (e.g., Lundgren et al., 2006; Lundgren, Allison, O'Reardon, & Stunkard, 2008). In addition, outside of these specific psychiatric conditions, there also has been limited NES research on various aspects of emotional functioning and other psychological traits. Each of these dimensions of psychopathology is reviewed below.

NES and Depression

Night eating has long been linked with emotional distress. The first published research on NES (Stunkard et al., 1955) noted a trend of depression in their participants when weight loss attempts were unsuccessful. More recently, Stunkard and other researchers have suggested depressed mood as one of the associated features of NES (Allison et al., 2010; Vinai et al., 2008). Due to this link, many researchers have investigated the relationship between depression and NES, and the majority has found the two to be correlated. Some researchers, however, have not found this relationship or have found that, after controlling for confounding variables such as comorbid binge eating or obesity, depression is no longer associated with NES. The following sections review the literature investigating the relationship between NES and depression. For an overview of research findings, see Table 8.1.

Much of the early NES research began in weight loss clinics. As a result, these studies included persons who were overweight or obese and who often had other patterns of disordered eating. These variables present confounds for investigating the role of depression in NES, as it is difficult to parse out whether the depression is related to obesity, NES, or some other eating disorder. Among these studies, Gluck, Geliebter, and Satoy

TABLE 8.1. Studies of NES Comorbidity

Study	Sample	Relevant findings
		Depression
Gluck et al. (2001)	76 overweight outpatients participating in a weight loss program	• Those with NES ($n = 11$) had higher rates of depressive symptoms than those without NES. • None reported severe or extreme levels of depression.
Calugi et al. (2009)	266 participants with obesity from an inpatient weight loss program	• Those with NES ($n = 27$) had higher depression scores than those without. • A majority of those with NES had levels of depression considered moderate (18.5%) or severe (44.4%).
Boseck et al. (2007)	14 self-defined night eaters	• More than half the sample met criteria for either lifetime (57.1%) or current (14.3%) mood disorder.
Birketvedt et al. (1999)	10 obese participants with NES; 10 matched controls	• During a 1-week behavioral study, self-reported mood was lower in those with NES compared to controls.
Allison et al. (2005)	15 females with NES; 14 female controls without NES	• Persons with NES reported more depressive symptoms than those without NES.
Striegel-Moore et al. (2008)	8,786 participants from the National Health and Nutrition Examination Survey–III (NHANES–III)	• Among participants who ate after 11:00 P.M., $n = 864$ were without depressive features and $n = 330$ exhibited depressive features.
de Zwaan et al. (2006)	106 community participants recruited via newspaper advertising identified as having nighttime eating problems	• Elevated rates of MDD, including 19% with current MDD and 56% with a lifetime history. • Twenty-eight percent of the sample were taking antidepressant medications. • Those with a history of MDD were more likely to be distressed by night eating than those without psychiatric history.
Lundgren et al. (2008)	19 nonobese participants with night eating; 22 non-obese controls	• Participants with night eating reported significantly higher levels of depressed mood than controls. • Those with NES were more likely to have a history of psychiatric disorders.
Thompson & DeBate (2010)	270 college students	• Significant correlation between depressive symptomatology and night eating behavior.

(continued)

TABLE 8.1. (continued)

Study	Sample	Relevant findings
Napolitano et al. (2001)	83 participants in a university-based weight loss program	• No significant differences in depressive symptoms among four groups: those with NES only (n = 23), those with BED only (n = 13), those with BED and NES (n = 13), and those without an eating disorder diagnosis (n = 34).
Powers et al. (1999)	116 preoperative patients undergoing bariatric surgery	• No statistically significant difference on depression symptoms between those with BED and those with NES. • Persons with BED demonstrated a trend toward more depressive symptoms than those with NES.
Colles et al. (2007)	431 total participants, including 180 bariatric surgery candidates, 93 members of a nonsurgical weight loss group, and 158 general community respondents	• NES alone was not associated with psychological distress. • However, those with NES who consumed nocturnal snacks had higher reported depressive symptoms than those in the NES without nocturnal snacking group.
Striegel-Moore et al. (2005)	Community cohort of black women with NES (n = 20) and without NES (n = 662)	• No significant differences between those with or without NES on measures of depression or general psychological distress. • No group differences in psychiatric comorbidity.
		Anxiety
de Zwaan et al. (2006)	106 community participants recruited via newspaper advertising identified as having nighttime eating problems (also reported above)	• Elevated rates of anxiety disorders in self-diagnosed participants with night eating, including generalized anxiety disorder (17%) and post traumatic stress disorder (18%).
Napolitano et al. (2001)	83 participants in a university-based weight loss program	• Individuals with comorbid BED and NES (n = 13) had significantly higher levels of state anxiety those with NES only (n = 23), those with BED only (n = 13), and those without an eating disorder diagnosis (n = 34).
Sassaroli et al. (2009)	202 obese participants from eating disorder treatment units	• Elevated anxiety levels among persons with BED and NES (n = 16), but only mild anxiety in those with NES alone (n = 13).

Lundgren et al. (2008)	19 non-obese participants with night eating; 22 non-obese matched controls (also reported above)	• 47.4% of the participants with NES met lifetime anxiety criteria while only 9.1% of the controls met the same criteria. • Participants with NES had more perceived stress than controls.
Rand & Kuldau (1986)	232 normal-weight volunteers from the general population	• General distress (psychoneuroticism) correlated to NES symptoms.

Substance abuse

Lundgren et al., 2006	399 psychiatric outpatients	• Higher rates of substance use disorder in those diagnosed with NES than those without NES.
Lundgren et al. (2008)	19 non-obese participants with night eating; 22 non-obese matched controls (also reported above)	• Higher rate of lifetime substance abuse/ dependence in participants with NES than controls.
Rand et al. (1997)	2,097 randomly selected adults from general population	• No significant differences in reports of alcohol abuse or dependence between those with NES and those without.
Striegel-Moore et al. (2008)	8,786 participants from the NHANES III (also reported above)	• Participants reporting night eating symptoms ($n = 2,068$) were more likely to have a lifetime history of marijuana or crack/cocaine use, but less likely than non-night eaters to engage in binge drinking in the last year (five or more drinks in a day).

Studies within psychiatric populations

Kruger et al. (1996)	61 participants with BPD I or II	• Elevated rate of night eating; 10 participants (16%) reported nighttime eating episodes 2 to 6 nights per week.
Lundgren et al. (2006)	399 psychiatric outpatients (also reported above)	• Elevated rates of NES in this psychiatric sample (12.3–15.6%). • Higher rates of atypical antipsychotics in those with NES compared to those without NES.
Lundgren et al. (2010)	68 overweight and obese individuals with serious mental illness enrolled in weight loss program	• Elevated rate of NES in this sample (25%).

(2001) investigated depression in a group of overweight persons participating in a weight loss program. Within this sample of 76 outpatients, 14% ($n = 11$) met diagnostic criteria for NES as defined by Stunkard and colleagues (1996). The participants endorsing NES reported significantly higher rates of depressive symptoms than those not endorsing NES on the Zung Depression Inventory; however, none of the participants with NES reported severe or extreme depression.

In an inpatient weight loss sample, Calugi, Grave, and Marchesini (2009) found that 27 of the 266 patients with obesity qualified for NES according to the Night Eating Syndrome History and Inventory (NESHI). As compared to the non-NES participants, patients with NES had significantly greater depressive symptoms on the Beck Depression Inventory (BDI). In addition, the majority of their BDI scores fell within the moderate to severely depressed range (18.5% and 44.4%, respectively). The depressive symptoms were the only factor that remained significantly related to NES when other factors were controlled for through logistic regression. Thus Calugi et al. suggest NES may be more important as an indicator of psychological distress as opposed to disordered eating.

Boseck et al. (2007) conducted ecological momentary assessments of 14 night eaters over a 2- to 3-day period and found affect to be the lowest when the individuals were waking in the night. In another continuous assessment study, Birketvedt et al. (1999) found mood to be significantly lower in the obese participants with NES as compared to their matched controls. In addition, Birketvedt et al. noted the same trend as Boseck et al., in that the mood of the participants with NES fell as the day progressed. Specifically, after 4:00 P.M. the mood of NES participants fell at a rate of 0.25 units (on a 10-unit scale) per hour, but the control participants exhibited no significant mood changes. Allison et al. (2005) found a significant difference in BDI scores between 15 females with NES and 14 female controls, such that the persons with NES reported more depressive symptoms. However, the researchers found no significant differences between the two groups in levels of stress hormones (cortisol and prolactin). In contrast, Birketvedt et al. (1999) found significant differences in cortisol levels between persons with NES and controls during the hours of 8:00 A.M. to 2:00 A.M.

One of the limitations of much of the NES research is that it has been conducted in obese populations, and obesity alone may be associated with certain psychological profiles or distress. In response to this critique, NES researchers have begun to investigate the syndrome in the general population. Striegel-Moore et al. (2008) utilized the National

Health and Nutrition Examination Survey–III (NHANES–III) to investigate night eating behaviors in persons ages 15 to 39 years. Of the 8,786 participants within this age category, 2,068 (25.1%) reported night eating on a *single* 24-hour dietary recall. In this study, night eating was defined rather generally as consuming 50% or more of your daily calories after 7:00 P.M. or consuming anything after 11:00 P.M. Within those endorsing night eating, latent class analysis identified four subtypes of night eating. Two subtypes were characterized by those who ate after 11:00 P.M. or consumed 50% or more of their calories after 7:00 P.M. This group represented the bulk of the sample. The remaining two subtypes were characterized by similar characteristics, but they also reported higher rates of depressive symptoms and the majority reported problems with sleep. Next, the authors investigated how the discriminating factors between the groups were related and found that individuals' nutrition profiles were more related to late night eating (consuming food after 11:00 P.M.), while lifetime history of marijuana use and overall health were more related to depressive symptomology.

A noteworthy strength of this research by Striegel-Moore and colleagues (2008) was that it included a large, national sample of the general population, but the authors used very lenient criteria for night eating classification, which may have accounted for a higher rate of false positives. In addition, the NES diagnosis was made based on a single 24-hour dietary recall, which more than a quarter of their sample completed for a Saturday. This may have influenced the findings because weekends may be associated with different eating patterns than typical weekdays. Once the researchers limited their night eating criteria to include only persons who ate after 11:00 P.M., their prevalence rates dropped to 14.5%, with 864 participants being night eaters without depressive features and 330 being night eaters with depression.

De Zwaan et al. (2006) also investigated NES within the general population by recruiting through newspaper advertisements. Like Striegel-Moore et al. (2008), de Zwaan and colleagues used broad criteria to identify people with NES, resulting in 106 of their 286 respondents qualifying as night eaters. Although the study results included all 106 participants, only 31 participants met the Stunkard et al. (1955) criteria for NES, while just 14 met the criteria proposed by Birketvedt et al. (1999). Within this sample, lifetime prevalence of major depressive disorder (MDD) as assessed by the Structured Clinical Interview for the DSM-IV (SCID) was quite high, with 56% of the participants meeting diagnostic criteria. Within this group, nearly 19% of these individuals met criteria for current MDD. In addition, 28% of the participants were currently taking antidepressant medications. Like de Zwaan et al. (2006), Boseck and colleagues (2007) also found elevated rates of lifetime mood disorders in their sample, with 57.1% meeting criteria for a past mood disorder, and 14.3% meeting current criteria for a mood disorder.

Upon further investigation, de Zwaan et al. (2006) found an interesting relationship among night eating, depression, and distress. First, a quarter of the participants did not report their night eating as troublesome. Surprisingly, this was not related to the frequency of the night eating but to a lifetime history of a psychological disorder, such that those with a history of MDD were more likely to be distressed by their night eating than those without a history of a psychiatric disorder.

As previously mentioned, one criticism of the NES literature is that many of the samples include people who are obese, which may confound the results when investigating psychiatric comorbidities of NES. In this study, de Zwaan and colleagues (2006) found no diagnostic differences between the participants who were obese (body mass index [BMI] > 30 kg/m²) and those who were not obese (BMI < 25 kg/m²). This suggests that the psychiatric comorbidities may be associated with night eating as opposed to obesity. However, more than a quarter of their sample reported nighttime awakenings due to insomnia, which suggests that, at least for a subgroup of persons, night eating behavior may be associated with primary sleep difficulties.

Lundgren et al. (2008) also conducted a descriptive study on NES in non-obese persons. In this study, the authors compared 19 non-obese night eaters and 22 non-obese controls on several measures, including the Night Eating Questionnaire (NEQ), the NESHI, a 10-day food and sleep recall, the SCID, and the BDI. Although exclusion criteria included several psychiatric disorders, including a lifetime history of bipolar disorder, psychotic disorder, current substance abuse or dependence, and current MDD of moderate or higher severity, there were still significant differences between groups on depressive symptoms, such that night eaters reported significantly higher levels of depressed mood. On lifetime psychiatric history, people with NES were significantly more likely than controls to meet diagnostic criteria for Axis I disorders. Specifically, 73.7% of the participants with NES met lifetime criteria for an Axis I disorder, while only 18.2% of the controls met diagnostic criteria. The majority of the NES participants had a lifetime prevalence of unipolar mood and anxiety disorders; these rates were significantly greater than the rates of unipolar mood and anxiety disorders in the control group. These findings replicate those of de Zwaan et al. (2006), in which people with NES had higher rates of unipolar mood disorders and anxiety disorders.

Thompson and DeBate (2010) investigated night eating and depression within a general college student population. Specifically, 270 college students completed a paper-and-pencil questionnaire including the BDI, the NEQ, and self-reported weight and height. The majority of their participants reported an average weight, while nearly 32% reported weights in the overweight or obese range. There were significant correlations between the BDI and six NEQ items and the total NEQ score, such that as depression symptoms increased so did night eating behaviors. Of the five NEQ items correlated with the BDI, half of the items represent associated features of depression, including insomnia and depressed mood; therefore, these items may represent some redundancy in the findings. In addition, late hours, high evening calorie consumption, and skipping breakfast are all characteristics of college students that may confound the findings. Another limitation is that, although there was a relationship among depression and the NEQ, less than 1% of the sample reported always eating when they woke in the night.

In contrast to these findings, there are several studies in which depression does not appear to be associated with NES (see Table 8.1). Napolitano, Head, Babyak, and Blumenthal (2001) investigated NES and binge-eating disorder (BED) in persons engaged in a university-based weight loss program. Within their sample of 83 participants, 23 were diagnosed with NES only, 13 with BED only, 13 with both BED and NES, and 34 had no eating disorder diagnosis. Participants completed a battery of assessments, including a depression questionnaire, but the researchers found no significant differences in depressive symptoms among the four groups. In another study, Powers, Perez, Boyd, and Rosemurgy (1999) investigated depression and other psychopathology in preoperative bariatric surgery candidates with either BED or NES and found no statistically significant differences between the two groups. However, the persons with BED demonstrated a trend toward higher depressive symptoms than the participants with NES.

Colles, Dixon, and O'Brien (2007) investigated psychological distress in persons with NES from three different recruitment sites: bariatric surgery candidates ($n = 180$), weight loss support group members ($n = 93$), and general community members ($n = 158$). Of these 431 respondents, 11% met criteria for NES according to the criteria proposed by Stunkard et al. (1996), 12% were identified as binge eaters (BE), and 4% met criteria for both NES and BE. Participants' current depressive symptoms were assessed using the BDI and their health-related quality of life was assessed via the Medical Outcomes Trust Short Form–36 (SF-36). NES-only and BE-only participants were matched with controls on age, gender, BMI, and recruitment origin. When comparing the NES-only group with their matched controls, there were no significant differences between groups on the psychological variables (BDI and SF-36), while the BE-only group reported significantly greater depressive symptoms, poorer psychological health, and greater social difficulties as compared to their matched controls.

Of the participants reporting NES, 40% also reported binge eating. This sample group was compared to the NES-only and BE-only groups. These comparisons revealed that the BE-only and BE and NES groups were similar in psychological distress, with both groups reporting moderate depressive symptoms, while the NES-only group was significantly lower in depressive symptoms. Within the NES samples, Colles et al. (2007) compared those with nocturnal snacking versus those without. The nocturnal snackers, regardless of comorbid BE, reported statistically higher levels of depression, poorer psychological health, and greater social difficulties than did the participants with NES without nocturnal snacking. In addition, an investigation of nocturnal snacking in the entire sample revealed it was significantly correlated with the BDI, such that participants with nocturnal snacking reported greater depressive symptoms. In addition, nocturnal snacking was positively correlated with psychological distress and social difficulties. This represents one of the few studies that investigated psychological distress in NES while controlling for binge eating; similar to other studies (Napolitano et al., 2001; Striegel-Moore et al., 2005), the psychological distress levels have been low when BED is controlled.

One of the major critiques of the NES research is that all of the samples have consisted of predominantly female, Caucasian participants. In the only study on NES in African American females, Striegel-Moore et al. (2005) found no significant differences in either psychiatric disorders or current mood and psychological distress between African American women with or without NES. In summary, although there are some conflicting reports (Napolitano et al., 2001; Colles et al., 2007), most studies on NES and depression suggest at least some degree of comorbidity. Furthermore, some research indicates that NES eating patterns may reflect mood fluctuations (Birketvedt et al., 1999; Boseck et al., 2007), and those persons with a history of depression may be more distressed by their night eating than those without comorbid depression. Nonetheless, research suggests that even in studies documenting a link between NES and depressed mood, a substantial proportion of persons with NES may have only mild (or no) depressive symptomatology (e.g., Allison et al., 2005; Striegel-Moore et al., 2008). More refined research methods are needed in order to parse out the specific pattern of relationships between NES and depression. For instance, NES diagnostic conceptualizations may differentiate those with more depressive profiles, namely, follow-up research examining the specific behavior of nocturnal eating (vs. evening hyperphagia) is needed.

NES and Anxiety

When compared to depression, the relationship between NES and anxiety has been relatively understudied. This is surprising, as psychological distress was more prominently highlighted than depression as an associated feature of NES when it was first introduced by Stunkard et al. (1955). The research in anxiety and NES has been inconsistent and mirrors the depression–NES literature, in that persons with comorbid NES and BED appear to have the most pronounced psychological distress.

Two studies have reported on anxiety disorder rates within NES samples drawn from the general population (de Zwaan et al., 2006; Lundgren et al., 2008). Both researchers used the SCID to assess lifetime history of psychiatric disorders. De Zwaan et al. (2006) found elevated rates of anxiety disorders in self-diagnosed participants with night eating, with generalized anxiety disorder (17%) and posttraumatic stress disorder (18%) being the most common diagnoses. These findings were replicated by Lundgren et al. (2008), who found people with NES were significantly more likely than controls to meet diagnostic criteria for a lifetime history of an anxiety disorder; specifically, 47.4% of the participants with NES met lifetime anxiety criteria while only 9.1% of the controls met the same criteria.

Napolitano et al. (2001) also investigated anxiety in persons enrolled in weight loss programs who met criteria for NES and BED. Within their sample of 83 participants, 23 were diagnosed with NES only, 13 with BED only, 13 with both BED and NES, and 34 had no eating disorder diagnosis. When comparing diagnostic groups, persons with comorbid BED and NES had significantly higher levels of state anxiety. This group (BED + NES) was also elevated on behavioral disinhibition and trait anxiety, but these differences were not statistically significant ($p = .08$). It is worth noting, however, this study was significantly underpowered, and larger sample sizes may have affected these trend-level findings.

In contrast to the early conceptualization of NES by Stunkard et al. (1955), Napolitano et al. (2001) found that the participants with only NES had significantly lower anxiety symptoms than those with dual diagnoses or with a diagnosis of BED alone. Thus the authors concluded it may be the combination of NES and BED that leads to an increase in anxiety symptoms; this is corroborated by their findings that the NES and BED group reported the highest levels of state and trait anxiety. Like several of the other studies, this study was limited in that the sample was self-selected. In addition, the majority of the participants were Caucasian, female, and were already seeking weight loss treatment.

In another study, Sassaroli and colleagues (2009) briefly assessed anxiety in persons with BED, NES, and comorbid BED and NES. Of the 202 obese patients recruited from eating disorder units in northern Italy, 54 met criteria for BED, 13 met criteria for NES, and 16 met criteria for both BED and NES. Within this eating disorders inpatient population, the participants with comorbid BED and NES were the only group who reported significantly elevated anxiety. The participants with NES reported mild anxiety, which was within the normal range.

In contrast to the research of Sassoroli et al. (2009) and Napolitano et al. (2001), Lundgren et al. (2008) found that within a non-obese sample, participants with NES reported significantly higher perceived stress than their matched controls. Another study (Rand & Kuldau, 1986) investigated disordered eating within a general population, non-obese sample and found psychoneuroticism, or general distress, to be most strongly correlated to NES symptoms.

The nature of association between stress/anxiety and NES is relatively unknown. Although some studies have found elevated rates of anxiety disorders in those with NES (de Zwaan et al., 2006; Lundgren et al., 2008), others have indicated that increased anxiety may be most strongly associated with comorbid BED and NES, rather than NES itself. However, given the historical observations that nighttime eating is an indicator of psychological distress (e.g., Stunkard et al., 1955), and the mixed findings in the literature, it is apparent that much more research is needed in the area of anxiety comorbidity.

NES and Substance Abuse

The link between substance abuse and NES was noted by Stunkard et al. (1955), who observed that two out of 20 individuals in their initial

NES study woke in the night to consume alcohol. However, because most researchers have used drug and alcohol abuse as exclusionary criteria, little is known about the substance use patterns of persons with NES. Since 1955, only four published studies have examined NES and substance use (Lundgren et al., 2006; Lundgren et al., 2008; Rand et al., 1997; Striegel-Moore et al., 2008).

Rand et al. (1997) found no differences in substance abuse/dependence between those with NES and those without NES. Lundgren et al. (2008) compared rates of substance abuse within a non-obese sample with or without NES. Twenty-six percent of the participants with NES met lifetime criteria for a substance abuse or dependence disorder, which was significantly greater than the rates of non-NES participants. This corroborates an earlier study by Lundgren et al. (2006), in which people with NES reported higher rates of substance use disorders.

Striegel-Moore et al. (2008) briefly investigated lifetime use of marijuana, crack/cocaine, and alcohol in a national survey sample consisting of nearly 9,000 respondents ages 15 to 39 years. Within this sample, 2,068 reported night eating symptoms on a single 24-hour dietary recall. These participants were more likely to have a lifetime history of marijuana or crack/cocaine use, but less likely than non-night eaters to engage in binge drinking in the last year (five or more drinks in a day). When the night eaters were split according to discriminating factors, they fell into two categories: NES characterized by depression and NES characterized by late-night eating.

NES in Psychiatric Populations

Kruger, Shugar, and Cooke (1996) were the first to report rates of night eating behaviors in a sample of persons with bipolar disorder (BPD). In a study examining the rates of binge eating in a sample of 61 persons with BPD I or II, they found that 10 participants reported nighttime eating episodes 2 to 6 nights per week. The authors described the patterns of night eating in their sample, noting that these 10 participants reported awakening between 2:00 and 4:00 A.M. and eating indiscriminately, including the consumption of "unusual and inappropriate food combinations" (p. 49). They further noted that this eating pattern may be particularly significant in persons with BPD because mood switches are reported to occur in these early morning hours (cf. Bunney, Dennis, Goodwin, & Borge, 1972). Although this study did not attempt formally to diagnose NES, the findings provided support for the possible link between night eating patterns and BPD.

Providing further evidence of the link between NES and more serious psychopathology, Lundgren et al. (2006) found elevated rates of NES in an outpatient psychiatric clinic population of 399 adults. NES was diagnosed if participants had evening hyperphagia (one-third of total calories after evening meal) and/or nocturnal awakenings with food consumption three or more times per week. Forty-nine (12.3%) of the participants were diagnosed with NES, while an additional 28 were diagnosed with subthreshold NES. Furthermore, when analyses excluded 84 participants who were unable to be contacted for follow-up interviews, the prevalence of NES in this sample was 15.6%. Interestingly, the study did not reveal differences in rates of NES among various diagnostic subgroups, including mood, anxiety, personality, or psychotic disorders. However, a greater proportion of the NES subgroup was prescribed atypical antipsychotic medication when compared to those without NES. As mentioned previously, this study also found that current and remitted substance use disorders were more prevalent in persons with NES than those without NES.

As a follow-up, Lundgren, Rempfer, Brown, Goetz, and Hamera (2010) examined rates of NES in a sample of overweight and obese individuals with SMI who were enrolling in a group weight loss treatment program. In this study, SMI was defined in accordance with National Institute of Mental Health (NIMH, 1991) criteria (i.e., diagnosis of schizophrenia-spectrum or mood disorder, and functional impairment of 2 or more years). Given the varying criteria for NES reported in the literature, Lundgren et al. (2010) reported rates of NES associated with the various diagnostic criteria. Using a conservative estimate for NES, the authors reported a prevalence rate of 25.0% in this sample (≥ 50% evening hyperphagia and ≥ 3 nocturnal food ingestions/week). The authors note that this observed prevalence is greater than rates reported in nonpsychiatric obese samples. This study also examined BED and found that this sample of persons with SMI were more likely to experience NES than BED, with little comorbidity between the diagnoses. Lundgren et al. cited several issues that might explain the link between SMI and risk for NES, including stress, sleep disturbance, and medication effects.

Indeed, emerging evidence suggests the need to further examine the potential link between disturbed sleep patterns and NES in persons with mental illness. Various sleep disturbances are apparent among persons with schizophrenia and other serious mental illnesses (e.g., Cohrs, 2008).

Recently, a study by Palmese et al. (2011) reported high rates of NES in a sample of 175 persons with schizophrenia participating in a study for the treatment of insomnia. Forty-four percent of the participants met criteria for clinical insomnia. Those with severe insomnia had significantly higher rates of night eating than those with subthreshold or no insomnia. Rates of night eating in this schizophrenia sample increased as insomnia severity increased.

Although only a few studies have examined NES within psychiatric populations, the findings suggest a striking association between NES and serious mental illness. At present, it is unclear whether the observed rates of night eating in these populations may be related to psychopathology, medication effects, or both.

NES and Other Psychological Factors

Several researchers have included self-esteem measures as part of their assessment batteries in NES studies. The findings have consistently suggested that self-esteem is significantly lower in persons with NES. Gluck et al. (2001) found in their weight loss program sample of overweight persons, the participants with NES had significantly lower self-esteem than the participants with obesity and no night eating. In another study by Striegel-Moore et al. (2010), researchers found that participants with comorbid night eating and binge eating had significantly lower self-esteem than the participants with binge eating alone. This difference represented a moderate effect.

Given the association between childhood maltreatment and a variety of eating and weight concerns, Allison, Grilo, Masheb, and Stunkard (2007) examined the relationship between NES and childhood abuse and neglect. This study compared adults with NES ($N = 57$), adults with BED ($N = 176$), and a group of overweight/obese control participants ($N = 38$) on self-report measures of childhood abuse and neglect. Although reported rates of physical and sexual abuse were similar across all three groups, the NES and BED groups reported higher rates of emotional abuse and forms of neglect than the controls. Furthermore, these levels of abuse and neglect were associated with higher levels of depressive symptomatology. Although this cross-sectional study does not address causality, it suggests that there may be an association between NES and childhood adverse experiences, which is in need of further study.

Clinical Implications and Recommendations

The emerging literature on psychiatric comorbidity in NES highlights the need for increased assessment and treatment efforts in both weight loss and mental health settings.

Addressing Psychiatric Comorbidity within a Weight/Eating Setting

With the growing recognition of NES as a significant clinical condition in its own right, it is apparent that an increasing number of clinicians will recognize and treat it in weight loss and other health care settings. Existing literature suggests that, as a matter of standard care, mood and psychological distress should be evaluated in persons identified with NES. Clinicians should be particularly aware of possible co-occurrence of depression, anxiety, and substance use disorders. Furthermore, clinicians should recognize that persons with co-occuring NES and mood complaints may be more likely to view their eating patterns as distressing (e.g., de Zwaan et al., 2006). Indeed, NES symptoms (nocturnal eating in particular), may serve as a behavioral indicator of distress levels and/ or current life stressors (e.g., Stunkard et al., 1955; Colles et al., 2007).

Some, but certainly not all, persons with NES may present with a clinically significant mood or anxiety disorder that requires appropriate behavioral and/or pharmacological intervention. For instance, persons with NES who meet criteria for MDD should be evaluated for appropriate treatments for that condition, such as antidepressant medication and psychotherapy. The existing literature suggests, however, that a substantial proportion of persons with comorbid NES and depression/anxiety might exhibit only low to moderate levels of psychological complaints. In these situations, the specific treatment course will likely be tailored to individual concerns. Individualized functional analysis to determine the specific behaviors and symptoms of most concern may help identify the relative clinical focus on disordered eating versus psychological symptomatology. For some individuals with NES, their distress may be focused on concerns about disordered eating patterns, sleep disruption, and/or weight gain. In these instances, it may be clinically appropriate to focus treatment on the primary NES concerns (see Chapters 12 to 15, this volume, for further discussion of NES treatment options). Nonetheless, when comorbid psychological concerns are present, ongoing evaluation of the relevant symptom dimensions (e.g., anxiety, depression) will help providers evaluate the effectiveness of the NES treatment in ameliorating these complaints and/or determining whether further psychological intervention is warranted at any point.

In contrast, another likely clinical scenario is one in which a client/patient is relatively less concerned with the specific NES behaviors except to the extent that they reflect other stress-related or emotional concerns. In such cases, it may be appropriate to view the psychological distress as a primary focus of treatment, with attention to the eating patterns as a useful behavioral indicator of the psychological concerns such as stress, anxiety, or depression. Self-monitoring through daily mood and food recordings may help individuals recognize the patterns among night eating behavior and emotional status, and can also serve as treatment outcome data in this regard.

It is worth noting that several published treatment approaches for NES have logical implications for the accompanying psychological comorbidity. For instance, Pawlow, O'Neil, and Malcolm (2003) published data demonstrating that a brief relaxation training significantly reduced stress, anxiety, and depression levels in adults with NES. Furthermore, after a week, those who received relaxation training also demonstrated a trend toward less night eating. In addition, potential pharmacological treatments for NES have primarily targeted the neurotransmitter serotonin (e.g., O'Reardon et al., 2004), and have clear overlap with current treatments of choice for depression and anxiety symptoms. Further treatment research is needed that directly examines outcomes in terms of both NES symptomatology and the known psychological comorbidities.

Addressing NES within a Mental Health Setting

A related clinical consideration is the recognition that persons in mental health settings may exhibit high rates of unrecognized NES. Although no data have yet been published on the patterns of NES evaluation and treatment in mental health clinics, it is presumed that mental health clinicians are largely unaware of NES and thus are not identifying it in many affected individuals. There is but a nascent literature on the link between NES and serious psychiatric diagnoses, but the existing literature provides compelling evidence that a significant number of persons in mental health settings may be experiencing NES or subthreshold night eating behaviors (e.g., Lundgren et al., 2006; Lundgren et al., 2008). In particular, persons with psychotic disorders such as schizophrenia or schizoaffective disorder, and others who may be taking antipsychotic medications, appear to have particularly elevated rates of night eating behaviors. It is likely that individuals within the mental health system are largely unaware of NES and may not independently seek treatment, either out of stigma concerns or lack of awareness about the condition itself. Therefore, more formal screening efforts will assist in identifying individuals who might not otherwise seek treatment.

The integration of NES surveillance within the mental health system would align with contemporary efforts to better integrate medical and mental health systems of care. In recent years, there has been increasing attention to the high rates of obesity and related health concerns in mental health populations (e.g., Brown, Goetz, VanSciver, Sullivan, & Hamera, 2006; Daumit et al., 2011; Dixon, Postrado, Delahanty, Fischer, & Lehman, 1999). In fact, rates of overweight and obesity in persons with serious mental illness are at epidemic levels (Daumit et al., 2011). There is a push toward improved monitoring of physical health status of persons within mental health service settings (e.g., Parks & Radke, 2008). In this vein, evaluation and management of obesity risk factors, including NES and other eating concerns, are an important part of best practice in mental health settings. Mental health clinicians should be aware of the risk for NES in their client populations and include assessment of eating patterns and concerns as part of standard practice.

Certainly, much more research is needed in order to understand the mechanisms that underlie the observed comorbidities between psychiatric status and NES. However, the emerging literature suggests that primary sleep difficulties may be an important focus of clinical attention (e.g., Palmese et al., 2011). It is known that persons with various mental health conditions are at risk for sleep difficulties, and the link between NES and sleep continues to emerge (see Chapter 9 [Howell & Crow]). Thus, in addition to evaluating eating patterns, it is recommended that mental health clinicians consider the presence of primary sleep difficulties among clients. Although no published treatment studies exist for treating NES in a psychiatric population, the related weight loss literature demonstrates that factors such as medication status and metabolic changes can pose significant challenges with eating and weight interventions in this population (e.g., Daumit et al., 2011). Treatment approaches for NES within psychiatric populations will likely need to be adapted to the particular challenges of more serious psychopathology, such as accounting for any cognitive challenges. For instance, there are established difficulties with attention, memory, and problem-solving associated with many major mental illnesses (including schizophrenia, bipolar disorder, depression and anxiety; e.g., Rempfer, Hamera, Brown, & Bothwell, 2006). Furthermore, given the preliminary evidence that stress and relaxation training may benefit individuals with NES (Pawlow et al., 2003), similar interventions can be easily integrated within the mental health system, as stress-related concerns are of particular benefit to persons with existing mental health concerns (e.g., Hoffmann et al., 2005).

Areas for Future Research

Although psychopathology has been linked to NES since the first NES publication, the research directly investigating the two has been relatively slow to develop. In addition, there are problems with the existing literature that make it difficult to generalize the findings or draw firm conclusions. The first major issue in this and all other NES literature is the lack of agreed-upon diagnostic criteria. Even though many of the investigators use similar criteria, there is significant variability between studies, which could contribute to inconsistent findings. For instance, it appears that differentiating the NES symptoms of evening hyperphagia and nocturnal eating may reveal differences in mood or psychiatric comorbidities.

Several methodological issues also exist in the current NES and psychopathology literature. Many of the publications reviewed in this chapter were studies in which psychopathology was a small or cursory component of the original study's purpose. As a result, several studies investigated NES within the context of other disordered eating (e.g., BED and obesity), and these comorbidities are likely contributing to the reported patterns of psychopathology. For example, some of the most significant psychopathology findings were in people with comorbid BED and NES (Napolitano et al., 2001; Sassaroli et al., 2009). Although these findings are clinically relevant, as co-occurring BED and NES are relatively frequent, they artificially inflate the reported rates of psychopathology in NES. Also, many of the NES samples are collected from weight loss groups with obese participants. This is problematic, as persons with obesity may have higher psychological distress or psychopathology independent of any NES symptomatology. Several researchers have addressed this critique by investigating NES in non-obese samples (de Zwaan et al., 2006; Lundgren et al., 2008; Thompson & DeBate, 2010).

As previously suggested, many of the publications on NES and psychopathology seem to be extensions of existing projects that are focused on other research questions. As a result, several of the studies reviewed had current or past psychiatric diagnoses, such as major depressive disorder, substance abuse disorder, psychotic disorders, or bipolar disorder, as exclusion criteria. These criteria preclude the researchers from truly evaluating the role of psychopathology in NES. Similarly, the depth of psychiatric assessment warrants improvement. In many of the studies reviewed, psychopathology was assessed using a single, brief depression questionnaire. Future research would benefit by including the simultaneous assessment of multiple disorders using more complex diagnostic (e.g., SCID and Mini-International Neuropsychiatric Interview), depression, anxiety, and personality measures.

Similar to the aforementioned methodology and sampling issues, one future improvement of the NES and psychopathology literature would be to investigate the role of psychological factors from many angles. Specifically, there is a need for more studies, like Lundgren et al. (2010), in which NES is evaluated within people with primary psychiatric disorders, as opposed to evaluating psychiatric disorders within people primarily diagnosed with NES. This is important, as it would give a clearer assessment of the true rates of NES among persons with psychiatric disorders. In addition, NES appears to be a relatively unassessed condition within psychiatric populations, yet even subclinical NES symptoms may cause significant psychological distress (Colles et al., 2007; Striegel-Moore et al., 2010). Another suggested improvement of the literature would be to expand the research on previous and existing psychological disorders within persons with NES alone, as much of the previous research includes samples with several comorbid eating disorders.

Other sampling improvements of note include sample sizes and diversity. Although sample sizes have increased in the more recent NES literature, there continues to be a need for larger studies. In addition to small sample sizes, the majority of the studies reviewed in this chapter included predominately Caucasian, female samples, with only one study (Striegel-Moore et al., 2005) investigating NES and psychopathology in African American women. Therefore, another future direction is to explore NES and related psychopathology in more ethnically, culturally, and gender-diverse samples.

In reviewing the current literature on NES and psychological disorders, it is clear that NES can be an independent eating disorder. However, due to the mixed methodologies of much of the research, the etiology of NES and psychological disorders remains unclear. Some of the psychiatric comorbidity literature suggests that NES may be a function of (or attributed to) insomnia-related issues in psychiatric disorders such as schizophrenia (Cohrs, 2008) and depression (e.g., de Zwaan et al., 2006). A more precise understanding of night eating in persons with serious mental illness could refine treatment efforts, for instance, if effective treatment for NES should include specific insomnia interventions.

While the relationship among NES and depression has been repeatedly researched, much less is known regarding NES and other psychological disorders. Specifically, despite early observations of Stunkard et al. (1955), there is little research exploring the link between stress/anxiety and NES. In addition, much more research is needed on the association between NES and substance use disorders, serious mental illnesses, and other psychological factors such as personality dimensions/disorders. Finally, additional research is needed on effective treatments for comorbid NES and psychological disorders. Future directions should focus on identifying mechanisms for treatment effectiveness and investigating whether these mechanisms vary according to psychiatric comorbidities. Pawlow et al. (2003) found promising results for a relaxation intervention that affected both NES behaviors and psychological functioning. It is hoped that future research will more fully explore effective treatments in this domain.

References

Allison, K. C., Ahima, R. S., O'Reardon, J. P., Dinges, D. F., Sharma, V., Cummings, D. E., et al. (2005). Neuroendocrine profiles associated with energy intake, sleep, and stress in night eating syndrome. *Journal of Clinical Endocrinology and Metabolism, 90,* 6214–6217.

Allison, K. C., Grilo, C. M., Masheb, R. M., & Stunkard, A. J. (2007). High self-reported rates of neglect and emotional abuse by persons with binge eating disorder and night eating syndrome. *Behaviour Research and Therapy, 45,* 2874–2883.

Allison, K., Lundgren, J., O'Reardon, J. P., Geliebter, A., Gluck, M. E., Vinai, P., et al. (2010). Proposed diagnostic criteria for night eating syndrome. *International Journal of Eating Disorders, 43,* 241–247.

Birketvedt, G. S., Florholmen, J., Sundsfjord, J., Osterud, B., Dinges, D., Bilker, W., et al. (1999). Behavioral and neuroendocrine characteristics of the night-eating syndrome. *Journal of the American Medical Association, 282,* 657–663.

Boseck, J. J., Engel, S. G., Allison, K. C., Crosby, R. D., Mitchell, J. E., & de Zwaan, M. (2007). The application of ecological momentary assessment to the study of night eating. *International Journal of Eating Disorders, 40,* 271–276.

Brown, C., Goetz, J., VanSciver, A., Sullivan, D., & Hamera, E. (2006). A psychiatric rehabilitation approach to weight loss. *Psychiatric Rehabilitation Journal, 29,* 267–273.

Bunney, W. E., Dennis, M. L., Goodwin, F. K., & Borge, G. F. (1972). The "switch process" in manic-depressive illness. *Archives of General Psychiatry, 27,* 295–302.

Calugi, S., Grave, R. D., & Marchesini, G. (2009). Night eating syndrome in class II–III obesity: Metabolic and psychopathological features. *Internation Journal of Obesity, 33,* 899–904.

Cohrs, S. (2008). Sleep disturbances in patients with schizophrenia: Impact and effect of antipsychotics. *Central Nervous System Drugs, 22,* 939–962.

Colles, S. L., Dixon, J. B., & O'Brien, P. E. (2007). Night eating syndrome and nocturnal snacking: Association with obesity, binge eating, and psychological distress. *International Journal of Obesity, 31,* 1722–1730.

Daumit, G. L., Dalcin, A. T., Jerome, G. J., Young, D. R., Charleston, J., Crum, R. M., et al. (2011). A behavioral weight-loss intervention for persons with serious mental illness in psychiatric rehabilitation centers. *International Journal of Obesity, 35,* 1114–1123.

de Zwaan, M., Roerig, D. B., Crosby, R. D., Karaz, S., & Mitchell, J. E. (2006). Nighttime eating: A descriptive study. *International Journal of Eating Disorders, 39,* 224–232.

Dixon, L., Postrado, L., Delahanty, J., Fischer, P., & Lehman, A. (1999). The association of medical comorbidity in schizophrenia with poor physical and mental health. *Journal of Nervous and Mental Disease, 187,* 496–502.

Gluck, M. E., Geliebter, A., & Satoy, T. (2001). Night eating syndrome is associated with depression, low self-esteem, reduced daytime hunger, and less weight loss in obese outpatients. *Obesity Research, 9,* 264–267.

Hoffmann, V. P., Ahl, J., Meyers, A., Schuh, K. S., Shults, K. S., Collins, D. M., et al. (2005). Wellness intervention for patients with serious and persistent mental illness. *Journal of Clinical Psychiatry, 66,* 1576–1579.

Kruger, S., Shugar, G., & Cooke, R. G. (1996). Comorbidity of binge-eating disorder and the partial binge-eating syndrome with bipolar disorder. *International Journal of Eating Disorders, 19,* 45–52.

Kuldau, J. M., & Rand, C. S. W. (1986). The night eating syndrome and bulimia nervosa in the morbidly obese. *International Journal of Eating Disorders, 5,* 143–148.

Lundgren, J. D., Allison, K. C., Crow, S., O'Reardon, J. P., Berg, K. C., Galbraith, J., et al. (2006). Prevalence of the night eating syndrome in a psychiatric population. *American Journal of Psychiatry, 163,* 156–158.

Lundgren, J. D., Allison, K. C., O'Reardon, J. P., & Stunkard, A. J. (2008). A descriptive study of non-obese persons with night eating syndrome and a weight-matched comparison group. *Eating Behaviors, 9,* 343–351.

Lundgren, J. D., Rempfer, M. V., Brown, C. E., Goetz, J., & Hamera, E. (2010). The prevalence of night eating syndrome and binge eating disorder among overweight and obese individuals with serious mental illness. *Psychiatry Research, 175,* 233–236.

Napolitano, M. A., Head, S., Babyak, M. A., & Blumenthal, J. A. (2001). Binge-eating disorder and night eating syndrome: Psychological and behavioral characteristics. *International Journal of Eating Disorders, 30,* 193–203.

National Institute of Mental Health. (1991). *Task force report: Toward a national definition of severe and persistent mental illness.* Bethesda, MD: Author.

O'Reardon, J. P., Ringel, B. L., Dinges, D. F., Allison, K. C., Rogers, N. L., Martino, N. S., et al. (2004). Circadian eating and sleeping patterns in the night eating syndrome. *Obesity Research, 12,* 1789–1796.

Palmese, L., DeGeorge, P. C., Srihari, V. H., Wexler, B. E., Krystal, A. D., & Tek, C. (2011). Sleep patterns of individuals with schizophrenia. *Schizophrenia Bulletin, 37*(S1), 277.

Parks, J., & Radke, A. Q. (Eds.). (2008). *Obesity reduction and prevention strategies for individuals with serious mental illness.* Washington, DC: National Association of State Mental Health Program Directors, Medical Directors Council.

Pawlow, L. A., O'Neil, P. M., & Malcolm, R. J. (2003). Night eating syndrome: Effects of brief relaxation training on stress, mood, hunger, and eating patterns. *International Journal of Obesity, 27,* 970–978.

Powers, P. S., Perez, A., Boyd, F., & Rosemurgy, A. (1999). Eating pathology before and after bariatric surgery: A prospective study. *International Journal of Eating Disorders, 25,* 293–300.

Rand, C. S. W., & Kuldau, J. M. (1986). Eating patterns in normal-weight individuals: Bulimia, restrained eating, and the night eating syndrome. *International Journal of Eating Disorders, 5,* 75–84.

Rand, C. S. W., Macgregor, A. M. C., & Stunkard, A. J. (1997). The night eating syndrome in the general population and among postoperative obesity surgery patients. *International Journal of Eating Disorders, 22,* 65–69.

Rempfer, M., Hamera, E., Brown, C., & Bothwell, R. (2006). Learning proficiency on the Wisconsin Card Sorting Test in people with serious mental illness: What are the cognitive characteristics of good learners? *Schizophrenia Research, 87,* 316–322.

Sassaroli, S., Ruggiero, G. M., Vinai, P., Cardetti, S., Carpegna, G., Ferrato, N., et al. (2009). Daily and nightly anxiety among patients affected by night eating syndrome and binge-eating disorder. *Eating Disorders, 17,* 140–145.

Striegel-Moore, R. H., Dohm, F.-A., Hook, J. M., Schreiber, G. B., Crawford, P. B., & Daniels, S. R. (2005). Night eating syndrome in young adult women: Prevalence and correlates. *International Journal of Eating Disorders, 37,* 200–206.

Striegel-Moore, R. H., Franko, D. L., Thompson, D., Affenito, S., May, A., & Kraemer, H. C. (2008). Exploring the typology of night eating syndrome. *International Journal of Eating Disorders, 41,* 411–418.

Striegel-Moore, R. H., Rosselli, F., Wilson, G. T., Perrin, N., Harvey, K., & DeBar, L. (2010). Nocturnal eating: Association with binge eating, obesity, and psychological distress. *International Journal of Eating Disorders, 43,* 520–526.

Stunkard, A., Berkowitz, R., Wadden, T., Tanrikut, C., Reiss, E., & Young, L. (1996). Binge-eating disorder and the night-eating syndrome. *International Journal of Obesity, 20,* 1–6.

Stunkard, A. J., Grace, W. J., & Wolff, H. G. (1955). The night-eating syndrome. *American Journal of Medicine, 19,* 78–86.

Thompson, S. H., & DeBate, R. D. (2010). An exploratory study of the relationship between night eating syndrome and depression among college students. *Journal of College Student Psychotherapy, 24,* 39–48.

Vinai, P., Allison, K. C., Cardetti, S., Carpegna, G., Ferrato, N., Masante, D., et al. (2008). Psychopathology and treatment of night eating syndrome: A review. *Eating and Weight Disorders, 13,* 54–63.

Chapter 9

Nocturnal Eating
and Sleep Disorders

Michael J. Howell
Scott J. Crow

$\mathbf{S}$leep-related eating disorder (SRED) is characterized by a disruption of the nocturnal fast with episodes of feeding after an arousal from sleep. The nocturnal eating may result in adverse health consequences such as: weight gain, the consumption of inedible substances, insomnia, or sleep-related injury (American Academy of Sleep Medicine [AASM], 2005). The dysfunctional eating is associated with sedative hypnotic medications, in particular the benzodiazepine receptor agonists such as zolpidem, inducing varying degrees of diminished awareness, such as amnesia zolpidem (Morgenthaler & Silber, 2002; Schenck et al., 2005). SRED is recognized as a parasomnia (i.e., a behavioral disorder accompanying sleep) and is often associated with other sleep disorders such as sleepwalking and obstructive sleep apnea (AASM, 2005). Recently, compelling evidence suggests that many cases of nocturnal eating may be a nonmotor manifestation of restless legs syndrome (RLS) (Howell, Schenck, Larson, & Pusalavidyasagar, 2010; Provini et al., 2009).

This chapter first reviews the physiology that maintains the normal overnight fast and provide a historical description of sleep-related eating. The clinical characteristics of SRED are described, with a focus on the association with sedative hypnotic medications. Subsequently, we review the relationship between SRED and other sleep and eating disorders, in particular recent insights regarding the relationship between SRED and RLS. Although treatment trials are still in their infancy, we review the initial reports on therapies. Finally, we conclude by considering the relationship between SRED and night eating syndrome (NES). See Table 9.1 for terms and definitions used in this chapter.

Normal Metabolic Physiology during Sleep

Under normal human physiological conditions, nighttime is characterized by a prolonged period of fasting associated with sleep. Energy homeostasis is maintained through the sleep period by alterations in metabolism and appetite modulation (see Table 9.2). This stands in contrast to fasting during sedentary wakefulness, which demonstrates a progressive hypoglycemia over 12 hours (Van Cauter, Polonsky, & Scheen, 1997).

Sleep and circadian-related changes in glucose utilization and tolerance helps maintain stable energy stores. First, the diminished motor activity of sleep decreases peripheral metabolism. Second, brain metabolism of glucose is reduced during sleep, particularly non-rapid-eye-movement (NREM) sleep (Boyle et al., 1994; Maquet et al., 1990). Third, insulin is rapidly disposed of during sleep, resulting in more available glucose (Van Cauter et al., 1991). Fourth, growth hormone is secreted with sleep onset, stimulating hepatic gluconeogenesis and inhibiting glucose uptake

TABLE 9.1. Terms and Definitions

Night eating	Eating after the evening meal and prior to final awakening
Evening hyperphagia	Excessive eating after the evening meal and prior to falling asleep
Nocturnal eating	Eating that occurs after an arousal from sleep prior to final awakening
Restless legs syndrome	Motor restlessness that interferes with sleep onset and maintenance
Psychophysiological insomnia	A state of central nervous system hypervigilance that interferes with sleep onset and maintenance

TABLE 9.2. Processes That Maintain Energy Homeostasis during Sleep

Decreased glucose utilization	Impaired glucose tolerance	Appetite suppression
• Decreased motor activity • Decreased cerebral glucose activity (NREM sleep)	• Growth hormone secretion at sleep onset • Increased insulin disposal • Cortisol secretion during second half of sleep period	• Increased leptin (satiety hormone)

(Holl, Hartman, Veldhuis, Taylor, & Thorner, 1991; Van Cauter & Spiegel, 1999). This relationship allows anabolic processes to occur during periods of musculoskeletal and cerebral quiescence. Finally, cortisol secretion near the end of the sleep period stimulates gluconeogenesis, promotes lipolysis, and mobilizes amino acids and ketones (Van Cauter & Spiegel, 1999).

Sleep changes in hormone secretion promote satiety and suppress appetite. In particular, leptin, a peptide hormone secreted by adipocytes, inhibits hunger centers in the hypothalamus. Leptin peaks soon after sleep onset, helping to suppress feeding behavior (Simon, Gronfier, Schlienger, & Brandenberger, 1998). Conversely, the hormone ghrelin, (a hunger signal) has increased levels during sleep in humans (Dzaja et al., 2004). Presumably, therefore, during sleep there is a balance between increased ghrelin and increased leptin activity that does not promote eating.

Definition of SRED

The normal sleep-related fast is lost with nocturnal eating. SRED is characterized by recurrent episodes of nocturnal eating after an arousal with adverse consequences. The episodes are described as occurring in an involuntary, compulsive, or "out of control" manner. Often, patients describe an inability to return to sleep without eating, and in this regard SRED resembles other sleep-related compulsions such as RLS. In the setting of sedative hypnotic medications, the patient often cannot be awakened and thus SRED resembles somnambulism. Adverse consequences include: weight gain, consumption of peculiar combinations of food or inedible substances, dangerous food preparation behavior, sleep-related injury, dental caries, hyperglycemia in diabetic patients, and painful abdominal distention (AASM, 2005; Schenck, Hurwitz, Bundlie, & Mahowald, 1991; Winkelman, 1998).

Historical Background of SRED

Prior to the publication of the 1991 article that defined SRED (Schenck et al., 1991), there were several reports of dysfunctional nocturnal eating in relation to other sleep disorders. In fact, the original description of RLS in 1960 by Ekbom noted frequent compulsive nocturnal eating in association with a motor restlessness that impaired sleep (Ekbom, 1960). In 1981, eating during a sleepwalking episode was described in a 35-year-old woman with schizoaffective disorder (Nadel, 1981). This case was also the first description of unconscious nocturnal eating in association with psychotropic medications. Subsequently, a series of three sleep-related eating cases was published in 1990 (Whyte, 1990). All three patients described eating unpalatable foods such as raw bacon, often with subsequent amnesia, and polysomnography (PSG) studies demonstrated disorders of arousal from NREM sleep.

In 1991 a series of 19 patients with nocturnal eating seen over 5 years was reported (Schenck et al., 1991). This condition was named SRED, and PSG studies demonstrated evidence of an arousal disorder, leading to its classification as a parasomnia in the *International Classification of Sleep Disorders* (AASM, 2005).

Importantly, nocturnal eating is frequently noted among patients with NES, originally reported in 1955 by Stunkard et al. among a group of obese patients (Stunkard, Grace, & Wolff, 1955). SRED and NES share many similarities, represent a spectrum of abnormal nocturnal eating behavior, and may be best explained as similar phenomena interpreted differently by separate clinical fields with distinct patient populations. Investigations have suggested that NES is a circadian delay in meal timing that results in evening hyperphagia, nocturnal eating, and morning anorexia (Stunkard, Allison, Lundgren, & O'Reardon, 2009). NES is currently diagnosed if 25% of food intake is consumed after the evening meal and/or at least two episodes of nocturnal eating per week with clinical consequences. SRED has historically been distinguished from NES by amnestic eating alone, without evening hyperphagia. However, recent changes in the definition of SRED (AASM, 2005) have expanded SRED to include nonamnestic eating, increasing the overlap between these two conditions. One potentially distinctive feature of SRED is its close association with RLS (see later section on SRED and RLS). For further consideration of the relationship between SRED and NES please see the final section below.

Epidemiology of SRED

Epidemiological studies suggest that nocturnal eating (both dysfunctional and nondysfunctional) and SRED (dysfunctional nocturnal eating alone) are common, particularly among patients with other sleep disorders. The most striking relationship is between RLS and SRED. In a survey of 53 patients with RLS who presented to a sleep disorder center, 66% had frequent nocturnal eating and 45% had SRED (Howell et al., 2010). These findings are similar to a survey of 100 patients with RLS who demonstrated a 33% prevalence of SRED (Provini et al., 2009). These and other reports suggest a fundamental relationship between RLS and nocturnal eating (see section on RLS and SRED below). SRED is also frequently associated with other parasomnias. Three studies have reported comorbid sleepwalking in 48 to 65% of patients with SRED (Lam, Fong, Yu, Li, & Wing, 2009; Schenck et al., 1991; Winkelman, 1998). Sleepwalking without eating may precede SRED, and once nocturnal eating develops, it often becomes the predominant sleepwalking behavior (Schenck et al., 1991). The majority (60–83%) of reported cases are female (Schenck et al., 1991; Vetrugno et al., 2006; Winkelman, 1998).

Amnestic SRED is often related to psychotropic medications, in particular sedative hypnotics. These cases are often characterized by prolonged and dramatic sleepwalking with eating events (Dolder & Nelson, 2008). More recently SRED has been implicated with use of the benzodiazepine receptor agonists, in particular zolpidem (Morgenthaler & Silber, 2002; Schenck et al., 2005) (see section on SRED and benzodiazepine receptor agonists below).

Psychiatric comorbidities are frequently reported in the setting of patients with dysfunctional nocturnal eating. In the original 1991 case series, 47% of SRED patients (9/19) had an Axis I disorder and many had daytime anxiety about the possibility of choking or starting fires (Schenck et al., 1991). A more recent report noted that 40% (14/35) of patients with nocturnal eating met criteria for depressed mood (Vetrugno et al., 2006); a separate study noted that patients with SRED endorsed more symptoms of depression and dissociation than those without SRED (Winkelman, Herzog, & Fava, 1999).

SRED has also been noted among eating disorder groups. A self-administered questionnaire determined prevalence rates of 17% in an inpatient eating disorder group, 9% in an outpatient eating disorder group, and 5% among a group of college students (Winkelman et al., 1999). This later finding is similar to a survey of 1,235 general psychiatry patients, which noted a 4% lifetime prevalence of SRED and a 2.4% 1-year prevalence (Lam, Fong, Ho, Yu, & Wing, 2008).

SRED is associated with weight gain and obesity; however, a causal relationship has not been established. In the original 1991 case series nearly half of all patients fulfilled established criteria for being overweight (Schenck et al., 1991), and in a follow-up report 44% of patients claimed that greater than 20% of their excess weight was related to nocturnal eating (Schenck & Mahowald, 1994).

Clinical Characteristics of SRED

SRED is a relentless, chronic condition. In the original description, more than half (58%) described nocturnal eating at least once a night (Schenck et al., 1991). In another study the majority of patients described a long history of involuntary nocturnal eating (mean duration 16 years), and nearly all reported eating on a nightly basis (Winkelman, 1998). A substantial proportion (23%) describe eating more than five times per night (Vetrugno et al., 2006).

SRED is characterized by consumption of high-calorie foods, sometimes by dangerous preparation, and by the occasional ingestion of nonfood substances. The most commonly consumed nocturnal foods are higher in carbohydrates and fats than daytime ingestions. Interestingly, hunger is notably absent, with patients often describing instead a compulsion to eat so that sleep may be reinitiated (Vetrugno et al., 2006; Winkelman, 1998). Unconscious food preparation has resulted in injuries such as drinking excessively hot liquids, choking, and lacerations. Furthermore, inedible and toxic substances have been consumed such as: egg shells, coffee grounds, sunflower shells, buttered cigarettes, glue, and cleaning solutions. Finally, patients with food allergies have ingested substances that during the daytime they take extreme precautions to avoid (Schenck, 2006; Schenck & Mahowald, 1994; Winkelman, 1998).

Various medical consequences can occur from repeated nocturnal eating. Weight gain is commonly reported, and SRED may precipitate or aggravate diabetes mellitus, hyperlipidemia, hypercholesterolemia, hypertension, and OSA (Schenck, 2006; Schenck & Mahowald, 1994; Winkelman, 1998). Patients with nocturnal eating are at increased risk for dental caries, as oral hygiene practices rarely follow feeding episodes

(Schenck & Mahowald, 1994). Furthermore, patients will often fall back asleep with an oral food bolus, which is combined with a circadian decline in salivary flow. Finally, failure to exhibit control over nocturnal eating can be associated with secondary depressive disorders (Winkelman, 1998).

PSG is used to characterize SRED with commonly consumed nocturnal food made available at bedside in order to facilitate eating behavior. If a patient eats during the PSG study, the concomitant sleep–wake state is then identified and the technologist can assess level of awareness during the event and subsequently the patient's morning recall. Similar to sleepwalking, SRED most commonly arises out of NREM sleep. One study documented that 44 of 45 feeding episodes in 26 patients arose from NREM sleep. Furthermore, elevated periodic limb movements and rhythmic masticatory muscle activity (RMMA) associated with arousal from NREM sleep have been reported in the majority of SRED cases studied with PSG (Schenck & Mahowald, 1994; Vetrugno et al., 2006).

Very limited early reports suggest that SRED may have a genetic predisposition. In one case a 31-year-old female with SRED reported that her dizygotic twin sister and father were also affected (De Ocampo, Foldvary, Dinner, & Golish, 2002). Another study described that 26% (6/23) of patients with SRED claimed to have a first-degree relative with nocturnal eating behavior (Winkelman, 1998). Conversely, in a separate report only 6% (2/36) of subjects described similar behaviors in family members (Vetrugno et al., 2006). Clearly, additional research is needed to determine whether dysfunctional nocturnal eating is an inherited trait.

SRED and Benzodiazepine Receptor Agonists

Many of the early reports suggested that amnestic nocturnal eating was frequently associated with sedating psychotropic medications (see Table 9.3 for a list of medications commonly associated with SRED). In fact, the first case study of amnestic nocturnal eating in 1981 was associated with a combination of chlorpromazine, amitriptyline, and methyprylon (Nadel, 1981). Subsequently, SRED has been reported induced with triazolam, lithium, olanzapine, risperidone, zopiclone, and zaleplon (Lam, Fong, Ho, Yu, & Wing, 2008; Lu & Shen, 2004; Molina & Joshi, 2010; Paquet, Strul, Servais, Pelc, & Fossion, 2002; Schenck & Mahowald, 1994) as well as zolpidem extended-release formulation (Chiang & Krystal, 2008; Najjar, 2007).

The majority of drug cases are related to zolpidem, a benzodiazepine

TABLE 9.3. Medications Associated with SRED

• Zolpidem—immediate release	• Triazolam
• Zolpidem—sustained release	• Midazolam
• Zopiclone	• Risperidone
• Zaleplon	• Olanzapine

receptor agonist (BRA). The first reported case of amnestic nocturnal eating related to zolpidem use was described in member of the armed services in 1999 (Harazin & Berigan, 1999). A series of zolpidem-associated SRED followed in 2002. Five middle-age patients were described, two of whom already had intermittent episodes of conscious nocturnal eating prior to starting zolpidem. All five patients were on various neuropsychiatric agents, and interestingly all had a history of RLS. Soon after initiating zolpidem each patient described amnestic nocturnal eating that stopped with discontinuation (Morgenthaler & Silber, 2002).

Further reports have strengthened the relationship between zolpidem and SRED. In a series of 1,235 patients at an outpatient psychiatry clinic the combination of zolpidem and antidepressants posed the greatest risk for SRED. In another report of 29 sleepwalkers where a high usage of BRA for sleep was noted (86%), 65.5% of patients described sleep-related eating behavior (Lam et al., 2009). More recently, eight patients reported that nocturnal eating began on average 40 days after starting zolpidem (Valiensi, Cristiano, Martinez, Reisin, & Alvarez, 2010). The vast majority of reports note improvement if not outright resolution once the agents are discontinued (Dang, Garg, & Rataboli, 2009; Harazin & Berigan, 1999; Morgenthaler & Silber, 2002; Sansone & Sansone, 2008; Valiensi et al., 2010; Wing, Lam, Li, Zhang, & Yu, 2010).

The spectrum of feeding behavior is diverse in drug-induced SRED. A typical case report described a 51-year-old female with RLS who noted empty food packages the mornings after she started taking zolpidem. She later discerned that she had been eating sandwiches on several occasions (Sansone & Sansone, 2008). A more alarming example included prolonged amnestic behavior in a 45-year-old male. After 10 days of treatment, he was missing on two occasions after going to bed. Subsequently it was discovered that after driving his car more than 2 kilometers he had climbed into his place of business through the shutter and ate chocolate and other carbohydrate-rich snacks (Dang et al., 2008).

Uncontrollable nocturnal eating is often reported after patients ingest greater than the maximum recommended dose of zolpidem (10 mg) (Schenck et al., 2005; Tsai, Tsai, & Huang, 2007). Often this occurs when, in a desperate attempt to initiate sleep, patients escalate their dose without a new prescription (Schenck et al., 2005). Recently a cross-sectional pilot study of 125 psychiatric patients on hypnosedatives evaluated the risk factors for complex sleep behaviors such as amnestic sleep eating. Multiple regression analysis showed that a higher dose of zolpidem was the only significant predictor of complex sleep behaviors. Furthermore, none of the subjects that demonstrated complex sleep behaviors took a dose of less than 10 mg (Hwang, Ni, Chen, Lin, & Liao, 2010).

BRAs enhance gamma-aminobutyric acid (GABA) activity at central GABA-A receptors, resulting in hypnotic phenomena such as sleep and amnesia. It has been suggested that the complex behavior noted with some BRAs is in part related to increasing binding affinity and that zolpidem has the highest binding affinity among the BRAs (Dolder & Nelson, 2008; Yun & Ji, 2010).

Investigators have utilized functional neuroimaging to explore the neuropharmacological mechanisms of drug-induced SRED. A case of zolpidem-induced SRED was studied with fluorodeoxyglucose–positron emission tomography (FDG-PET) during sleep on and off zolpidem but did not demonstrate significant differences in brain metabolism (Hoque & Chesson, 2009). Interestingly these findings are consistent with a larger FDG-PET study that did not demonstrate metabolic differences during sleep in 12 normal volunteers studied on and off zolpidem (Gillin et al., 1996). Further functional imaging studies are needed to better explain the underlying mechanisms associated with dysfunctional nocturnal eating.

Because hypnotic agents suppress executive function it may be that zolpidem, by itself, does not activate SRED but instead disinhibits the behavior in a patient population at risk for nocturnal feeding. Patients with RLS demonstrate a greater tendency toward nocturnal eating (Howell et al., 2010; Provini et al., 2009), and a substantial number of BRA-associated amnestic nocturnal eating cases have been reported in patients with RLS (Chiang & Krystal, 2008; Howell et al., 2010; Morgenthaler & Silber, 2002; Provini et al., 2009; Sanofi-Aventis, 2006) (see section below on RLS and SRED).

SRED and Amnesia

Impaired consciousness as a defining criterion for SRED has evolved since complete or at least partial unconsciousness was necessary for diagnosis. In the original series of SRED cases, 84% (32/38) patients claimed an impairment in awareness (Schenck et al., 1991). In another case series, 91% (21/23) of patients had incomplete consciousness and/or amnesia for the behavior (Winkelman, 1998). Conversely, a subsequent report noted full awareness in all 26 patients after episodes of nocturnal eating in a sleep laboratory. However, the authors did not report whether the subjects typically had full awareness during nocturnal eating at home (Vetrugno et al., 2006). This is an important distinction, as the level of consciousness may be different in a sleep laboratory compared to a more familiar sleeping environment. Also, in SRED, awareness will vary night to night and sometimes between episodes of the same night (Winkelman, 2006b). Currently, reduced awareness and subsequent amnesia is not a required diagnostic criterion for SRED in the *International Classification of Sleep Disorders* (AASM, 2005).

The discrepancy in consciousness among SRED reports may be best explained by the use of sedating medications and comorbid sleepwalking disorders (Vetrugno et al., 2006). The first case reports of amnestic nocturnal eating were associated with sedative psychotropic medications as well as other parasomnias (Nadel, 1981; Schenck & Mahowald, 1994; Whyte, 1990). Moreover, the majority of patients in the original series were taking hypnotic medication or had a previous history of sleepwalking (Schenck et al., 1991). However, in a community survey of 92 subjects who admitted to nocturnal eating only 18% reported at least partial unawareness, and none of those who were fully aware had a history of sleepwalking. Conversely, if subjects did have a sleepwalking history they were far more likely (73%) to be at least partially unaware of the behavior (de Zwaan, Roerig, Crosby, Karaz, & Mitchell, 2006). Moreover, it is expected that many parasomnia patients would be on sedative hypnotic medications, as these agents are often the treatment of choice for sleepwalking disorders. More definitively, all 26 patients with full consciousness during nocturnal eating episodes in a sleep laboratory were drug free and only one had a history of sleepwalking (Vetrugno et al., 2006).

SRED and RLS

A critical review of both the SRED and RLS literature suggests an intimate, possibly causal, relationship between these conditions. This conclusion is based on similarities in epidemiology, polysomnographic phenomena, clinical course, and treatment response. The evidence is especially compelling in cases of medication-induced SRED where the mistreatment of RLS as psychophysiological insomnia (PI) is plausible, and, based on recent investigations, amnestic eating is the expected result. Here we present the data supporting such a link with a summary conclusion at the end of the section.

RLS is a disorder affecting approximately 8 to 10% of the population and thus a common cause of sleep initiation and maintenance failure (Allen et al., 2005; AASM, 2005; Berger, Luedemann, Trenkwalder, John, & Kessler, 2004). Further, while RLS is distinct from, it is commonly confused with PI. Thus it may be expected that many patients with RLS will be mistakenly treated with therapies designed to treat PI, including agents such as benzodiazepine receptor agonists.

Like SRED, and unlike sleepwalking, RLS has a higher prevalence in women (AASM, 2005; Berger et al., 2004; Ohayon, Guilleminault, & Priest, 1999). Furthermore, medication-induced SRED is also more common in women (Hwang et al., 2010; Schenck et al., 2005).

Similar to RLS (Paulus, Dowling, Rijsman, Stiasny-Kolster, & Trenkwalder, 2007), several features of SRED suggest an underlying dopamine dysfunction. First, dopamine mediates impulsive behaviors such as motor restlessness, smoking, and binge eating (Bello & Hajnal, 2010; Paulus et al., 2007). Second, a PSG study of 35 patients with SRED demonstrated that 77% had PSG confirmation of wakeful RLS and periodic limb movement during sleep (Vetrugno et al., 2006). Third, RMMA and bruxism, dopaminergic phenomena (Lavigne, Kato, Kolta, & Sessle, 2003; Vetrugno et al., 2006) associated with RLS (Lavigne & Montplaisir, 1994), are commonly seen in SRED (Schenck & Mahowald, 1994; Vetrugno et al., 2006). In the original SRED case series prominent repetitive chewing movements were described during NREM sleep and after arousals (Schenck & Mahowald, 1994). Recently, RMMA was found in 29 of 35 patients diagnosed with SRED during their PSG evaluations (Vetrugno et al., 2006).

Recently, two investigations demonstrated a high prevalence of both SRED and nondysfunctional nocturnal eating in patients with RLS. A community survey of 100 patients with RLS reveals a high prevalence of SRED in RLS (33%) compared to normal population controls (1%) (Provini et al., 2009). The authors pondered whether the compulsive nocturnal eating was related to underlying RLS brain pathology or whether nocturnal eating was merely "killing time," as previously suggested (Manni, Ratti, & Tartara, 1997). This question was addressed in another study of 80 patients with either RLS or PI who presented to sleep disorders center noted. This report noted that 66% of patients with RLS described either nondysfunctional nocturnal eating (21%) or SRED (45%). Conversely, no patients with PI described nocturnal eating alone and only 7% met criteria for SRED. This study suggests that nocturnal eating in RLS is not merely "killing time," as patients with PI were more likely to have prolonged (> 5 minutes) nightly awakenings (85%), compared to patients with RLS (30%) (Howell et al., 2010).

Like nondysfunctional nocturnal eating (a nonpathological variation of SRED), RLS also has a mild form that does not interfere with sleep onset (Satija & Ondo, 2008). Moreover, RLS is often a difficult condition to diagnose because current symptomatic criteria fail to identify many cases, and atypical variants may go unrecognized during routine clinical evaluation (Allen, 2007). Thus it may be expected that among the SRED clinical population there exist many cases of mild or atypical RLS.

A recent case helps illustrate the intimate relationship between SRED and RLS. A 74-year-old woman presented 20 years ago with history of uncontrollable RLS and SRED. Both the nocturnal eating and RLS were well controlled with various combinations of alpazolam, acetaminophen/codeine, and carbidopa/levodopa. Subsequently, ropinerole was added to fully control symptoms. Then, with the eruption of a right lower extremity zoster, the patient had a relapse of both RLS (bilateral symptoms) as well as nocturnal eating. Compellingly, the RLS and SRED resolved in parallel with the resolution of the skin lesions. Medications were not adjusted in the period immediately prior to, during, or after the zoster event (Mahowald, Cramer Bornemann, & Schenck, 2010). While the underlying mechanism in this case is unknown, iron-related proteins (iron is a catalyst in dopamine metabolism) are noted to change in the setting of herpetic infections (Maffettone et al., 2008).

Intriguingly, the nocturnal feeding behavior of SRED closely resembles the motor activity of RLS. RLS is characterized by an underlying feeling (often poorly described) of discomfort in the lower extremities that compels the patient to move. Movement relieves the discomfort, and sleep is unable to be reinitiated until this urge is addressed (Walters, 1995). In SRED, patients state that, after an awakening from sleep, they have a compulsion to eat (often without hunger) that interferes with sleep maintenance. Subsequently, once food is ingested the feeling abates and sleep may be reinitiated (AASM, 2005; Provini et al., 2009; Provini et al., 2010; Schenck & Mahowald, 1994).

Compulsive nocturnal eating is not unexpected, as patients with RLS often describe other nonmotor comorbidities such as: mood and anxiety disorders, nicotine addiction (Lee et al., 2008; Picchietti & Winkelman, 2005; Winkelman, Finn, & Young, 2006), as well as other nocturnal compulsions that interfere with sleep, such as sleep-related smoking (Provini et al., 2010). It has even been suggested that the name itself be changed from RLS to Ekbom's syndrome to recognize the various nonmotor manifestations of this condition (International Restless Legs Syndrome Study Group, 2010). Recently, six cases of nocturnal eating and nocturnal smoking were reported. Five of the six cases either presented with or were noted to have RLS. Patients claimed that they would wake up and be unable to return to sleep without eating and/or smoking. In a follow-up study that investigated the prevalence of sleep-related smoking, RLS patients demonstrated an increased prevalence (12%) compared to matched controls (2%). Interestingly, among RLS patients with nocturnal smoking SRED was common (83%), and both phenomena often began simultaneously (Provini et al., 2010). Further patients with nonmotor manifestations of RLS have more severe motor restlessness as measured by the International RLS Rating Scale (Provini et al., 2010). These findings suggest that nonmotor manifestations of RLS often arise in concert and are a marker of more severe disease.

It has been suggested that nocturnal eating and other nonmotor manifestations of RLS may be caused by dopaminergic agents, as these agents are known to trigger daytime impulsive behaviors such as gambling (Driver-Dunckley et al., 2007; Giladi, Weitzman, Schreiber, Shabtai, & Peretz, 2007; Nirenberg & Waters, 2006, 2010; Tippmann-Peikert, Park, Boeve, Shepard, & Silber, 2007). However, dopamine agents suppress feeding behavior in animal models (Martin-Iverson & Dourish, 1988), and recent reports suggest that dopaminergic agents are not the cause of the nocturnal eating. In a survey of 33 patients with SRED and RLS, 10 patients reported that nocturnal eating emerged prior to or concomitant with motor restlessness, and none reported that nocturnal eating emerged after the start of dopaminergic therapy. Also, RLS patients with SRED were not significantly more likely to use dopaminergic drugs compared to RLS patients without SRED. In fact, subjects whose nocturnal eating symptoms were under control were more likely to be on these agents than subjects who continued to have nocturnal eating (Provini et al., 2009). Furthermore, a double-blind treatment trial of pramipexole for SRED demonstrated improved sleep and reduced nighttime activity. Admittedly, nocturnal ingestions were not reduced in this small study (Provini et al., 2005). Among our series of patients with RLS, some early prospective data indicate that dopaminergic treatment results in a reduction (not an exacerbation) of nocturnal eating. Of the eight RLS patients with nocturnal eating who had not yet been exposed to dopaminergic medications five had resolution and three had improvement of nocturnal eating with dopaminergic therapy. Consistent with other reports, nocturnal eating symptoms demonstrated a clinical response in parallel to motor RLS symptoms (Howell et al., 2010). Finally, treatment with dopaminergic agents appears to improve other nonmotor manifestations of RLS. In particular, all patients who reported a remission of nocturnal smoking had been treated with dopaminergic agonists (Provini et al., 2010).

Importantly, a substantial number of zolpidem-induced SRED cases occur in the setting of RLS (Chiang & Krystal, 2008; Mahowald et al., 2010; Morgenthaler & Silber, 2002; Sansone & Sansone, 2008; Yun & Ji, 2010). As mentioned above, RLS is a condition distinct from, but often clinically mistaken for, PI. It is notable that SRED, sleepwalking, and other complex sleep behaviors are rare (1% or less) in zolpidem-treated PI patients when RLS has been carefully excluded (Ganzoni, Santoni, Chevillard, Sebille, & Mathy, 1995; Holm & Goa, 2000; Roth, Roehrs, & Vogel, 1995; Roth, Soubrane, Titeux, Walsh, & Zoladult Study Group, 2006; Sauvanet et al., 1988). In one compelling case of zolpidem-induced SRED with RLS, both motor restlessness and amnestic nocturnal eating resolved once zolpidem was stopped and RLS therapy began. The same authors subsequently reviewed 10 other cases and noted that in all eight cases of zolpidem-induced SRED in which RLS was considered, RLS was confirmed (Yun & Ji, 2010). However, in a study of 19 patients with zolpidem-induced complex sleep behaviors, screening for RLS was notably absent (Hwang et al., 2010). Thus the mistreatment of RLS as PI may be a crucial underlying step in the pathogenesis of many amnestic SRED cases.

In conclusion, the following lines of evidence suggest that SRED may be a nonmotor manifestation of RLS and that mistreatment of RLS as PI is a crucial step in the pathogenesis of drug-induced SRED cases:

1. RLS has frequently been described in cases of medication and non-medication-induced SRED.
2. Nocturnal eating is common in patients with RLS (including the original 1960 description by Ekbom).
3. SRED is common in patients with RLS.
4. The nocturnal eating in RLS is not merely "killing time," as patients with other causes of fragmented sleep, such as PI, have more awakenings yet rarely break the nighttime fast.
5. The compulsive nature of nocturnal eating in SRED is similar

in character to the motor and other nonmotor manifestations of RLS.

6. PSG studies demonstrate PLMs, RMMA, and bruxism in SRED. These phenomena are frequently noted in RLS and, like RLS, are associated with dopaminergic dysfunction.

7. The nocturnal eating and motor restlessness of RLS frequently arise, intensify, and subside in parallel.

8. In several reports the underlying sleep fragmentation of drug-induced SRED was not caused by PI, but instead RLS, a common condition that is easily confused with (and treated as) PI.

9. The rise of amnestic SRED parallels the rise of BRA use.

10. The CNS actions of sedative–hypnotic medications (suppression of memory and judgement) unleash predisposed behaviors, which in the case of RLS include inappropriate and amnestic ambulation with eating behavior.

11. Conversely, the incidence of SRED is rarely noted when patients with underlying motor restlessness are rigorously excluded from hypnotic treatment.

12. Finally, dopaminergic agonist treatments for RLS appear to improve rather than exacerbate nocturnal eating and SRED.

Treatment of SRED

The first goal in treating SRED is to eliminate implicated medications (see Table 9.3) and correct comorbid sleep disorders, especially RLS. The majority of patients with drug-induced SRED note improvement if not outright resolution of nocturnal eating behavior after inducing agents are discontinued (Chiang & Krystal, 2008; Dang et al., 2008; Harazin & Berigan, 1999; Morgenthaler & Silber, 2002; Sansone & Sansone, 2008; Schenck et al., 2005; Tsai et al., 2007; Valiensi et al., 2010; Wing et al., 2010). Rarely, patients who do not have nocturnal eating prior to exposure will have persisting episodes after cessation. A subject's dysfunctional nocturnal eating can be controlled by treating comorbid RLS (see section SRED and RLS above). Dopaminergics, opiods, and benzodiazepines are agents typically employed in the treatment of RLS (see Table 9.4). Interestingly, SRED comorbid with sleepwalking can also be effectively treated with these agents. In one case series, eight sleepwalking patients with SRED were effectively treated with bromocriptine and/or clonazepam (Schenck, Hurwitz, O'Connor, & Mahowald, 1993). Finally, in both reported cases of SRED with

TABLE 9.4. Treatments for Nocturnal Eating and SRED

Medication class	Agent	Authors and year	Study design	Primary diagnosis (no. of subjects)	Results (responders/total subjects)[a]
Dopaminergics	Carbidopa/ levodopa	Schenck et al. (1993)	Case series	SRED (12)	(10/12); temporary remission in 2/12.
	Bromocriptine	Schenck et al. (1993)	Case series	SRED (3)	(2/3); temporary remission in 1/3.
	Pramipexole	Provini et al. (2005)	Pilot double blind, placebo, crossover	SRED (11)	Decreased nocturnal activity as measured by actigraphy, no change in number of awakenings or ingestions
Antiseizure	Topiramate	Winkelman (2003)	Open-label trial	SRED (2); NES (2)	(4/4); mean weight loss of 11.1 kg over 8.5 months
	Topiramate	Martinez-Salio et al. (2007)	Case report	SRED (1)	(1/1); 2-year follow-up
	Topiramate	Schenck et al. (2006)	Case series	SRED (17)	(12/17); mean weight loss of 9.2 kg among responders after 1.8 years
	Topiramate	Winkelman (2006)	Open-label trial	SRED (25)	(17/25); mean weight loss of 11.1 kg over mean 11.6 months; 21/25 adverse events and 7/17 responders discontinued after 1 year

[a] Responders defined as elimination of nocturnal eating or diminished nocturnal eating with other clinical improvement such as weight loss.

obstructive sleep apnea, continuous positive airway pressure eliminated both the sleep-disordered breathing and the nocturnal eating (Schenck & Mahowald, 1994).

At this time two classes of pharmacotherapies have been studied in SRED and appear to be potentially effective in the treatment of dysfunctional nocturnal eating. In particular, dopaminergics and the antiseizure medication topiramate have both demonstrated preliminary yet promising results. However, research on the therapy of SRED is still in its infancy, and further investigations, in particular large randomized controlled trials, are necessary.

Dopaminergic agents are effective treating SRED even in the absence of motor restlessness. The original case series noted that either bedtime levodopa or bromocriptine was effective in eliminating nocturnal eating (Schenck et al., 1993). Recently pramipexole, a dopamine agonist, was investigated in a small double-blind, placebo-controlled crossover trial. Pramipexole was well tolerated in all patients, including those without diagnosed RLS or PLMD. On pramipexole, improved sleep and reduced nighttime activity was documented with actigraphy. There was no improvement in the number or duration of awakenings (Provini et al., 2005). The main side effects of dopamine agonist include sedation, orthostasis, and impulsive behaviors.

Early reports indicate that the antiseizure medication topiramate may be an effective therapy. An open-label trial of topiramate in four patients with nocturnal eating demonstrated positive results. The agent was well tolerated, reports of nocturnal eating were diminished, and weight loss (mean of 11.1 kg) was noted in all four individuals over 8.5 months (Winkelman, 2003). More recently, a 28-year-old obese male had a 10-year history of nocturnal eating episodes that were eliminated with topiramate. It was also reported that the agent was well tolerated over a 2-year follow-up (Martinez-Salio, Soler-Algarra, Calvo-Garcia, & Sanchez-Martin, 2007). In another case series, 12 of 17 patients with SRED treated with topiramate responded to treatment. The agent was well tolerated, and over 1.8 years there was a mean weight loss of 9.2 kg among the treatment responders (Schenck & Mahowald, 2006). Another review of 25 SRED patients on topiramate reported that 68% of patients with SRED responded to treatment. Furthermore, over 1 year, 28% of patients lost more than 10% of their body weight. Adverse events were high, however, and 41% of patients discontinued the medication (Winkelman, 2006a). The main side effects of topiramate include weight loss, paresthesias, renal calculus, cognitive dysfunction, and orthostasis.

Serotonergic therapies have efficacy for nocturnal eating in cases of NES (reviewed in Patel, O'Reardon, & Cristancho, Chapter 12).

Clinical Conclusion

SRED occurs when there is a break in the sleep-related fast. Clinical evaluation should attempt to identify comorbid sleep disorders and to eliminate inducing agents. In particular RLS, PLMD, sleepwalking, and OSA are reversible conditions and commonly associated with nocturnal eating. SRED is associated with psychotropic medication, most notably the BRA zolpidem. PSG with a seizure montage is often necessary to identify and treat the comorbid sleep disorders.

At this time, two types of pharmacotherapies (the antiseizure medication topiramate and dopaminergic agents) have been studied and appear to be potentially effective in SRED.

SRED and NES

Dysfunctional eating during the main sleep period has been categorized as either NES or SRED. These reversible conditions represent a unique opportunity in the struggle against obesity; however, ideal therapies will not arise until the correlations between these two conditions are better understood.

There are some notable similarities and distinctions between NES and SRED (see Table 9.5). Both share a chronic course, familial associations, comorbid neuropsychiatric disease, and are frequently associated with weight gain and obesity. They differ in level of consciousness and control noted during feeding, as well as the inappropriate timing of associated food intake (evening hyperphagia) (Howell, Schenck, & Crow, 2009).

It is notable that, in comparison to the extensive investigations of NES, our understanding of SRED is still in its infancy. For example, many SRED reports fail to comment on the presence or absence of evening hyperphagia, suggesting that many of these patients may be better characterized as having NES. We have noted that individual patients will demonstrate overlap between these conditions, which can confound treatment.

Distinguishing these conditions historically have been their purported pathophysiological mechanisms. The evening hyperphagia and

TABLE 9.5. Comparison of SRED and NES

	SRED	NES
Original description	Schenck et al. (1991)	Stunkard et al. (1955)
Field of origin	Sleep medicine	Eating disorders
Patient population	Sleep disorders	Obesity
Clinical characteristics		
Evening hyperphagia	Uncertain	Yes
Nocturnal eating	Yes	Yes
Morning anorexia	Uncertain	Yes
Amnesia	Yes[a]	No
Purported mechanism	Breakdown in the nocturnal fast	Circadian delay in the timing of food intake
Associated disorders		
RLS	Yes	Uncertain
Sleepwalking	Yes	Uncertain
Obstructive sleep apnea	Yes	Uncertain
Eating disorders	Uncertain	Yes
Pharmacological treatments	Dopaminergics; topiramate	Sertraline

[a] Usually in association with sedative–hypnotic medication.

nocturnal eating of NES has been attributed to an abnormality in the circadian timing of caloric intake relative to sleep, while SRED has been characterized as a breakdown in nocturnal fasting mechanisms (Howell et al., 2009). Of course these explanations are not mutually exclusive, and one could suggest that the circadian delay of feeding may in fact be the process leading to both sleep disruption and a breakdown in the nocturnal fast. In this regard the RLS findings in SRED cases noted above may in fact be complementary to the circadian delay hypothesis of NES. RLS symptoms, both motor and nonmotor, have circadian fluctuations that reach a symptomatic crescendo during the late evening in parallel with the abnormal nighttime feeding in NES and SRED (Allen, 2007).

Conversely, one study suggests that RLS symptoms may in fact distinguish these pathologies, as NES was rare in patients with RLS. This investigation of 100 patients with RLS and controls surveyed subjects for both SRED and NES (Provini et al., 2009). SRED was noted in 33% of patients, similar to another report of 45% (Howell et al., 2010). However, only 3% of patients with RLS met criteria for NES (Provini et al., 2009). Importantly, this study utilized a 1999 definition of NES (Birketvedt, Florholmen, Sundsfjord, et al., 1999), likely excluding patients with NES under the revised criteria (Allison et al., 2010).

One notable study (Rogers et al., 2006) investigated NES patients with PSG and demonstrated an increased number of awakenings and reduced sleep duration, suggesting an underlying sleep-disrupting process. No comment was made regarding the presence or absence of RLS or periodic limb movements, a PSG finding often correlated with RLS. Further data on the incidence of RLS in patients with NES are lacking. However, an investigation of motor restlessness in NES would be intriguing because RLS symptoms typically progress in the early to late evening, similar to evening hyperphagia.

The patient's primary presenting symptoms may explain the divergence of these similar conditions into different clinical fields, for it would be expected that patients who are predominantly affected by sleep initiation and maintenance difficulty (with nocturnal eating) would present to a sleep clinician. Conversely, patients whose predominant concern is excessive eating prior to sleep (with some sleep disruption) would more likely arrive at an eating disorder clinic. This range of clinical presentation suggests that evening hyperphagia and nocturnal eating may in fact be situated on opposite poles of a potentially unifying disorder.

Clearly, further investigations are needed in patients with abnormal nocturnal eating. Ecological momentary assessment (EMA), where a portable electronic device periodicially surveys appetite, food intake, sleep perception, as well as other symptoms, is an elegant method of evaluating circadian phenomena. EMA has been used by NES investigators (Boseck et al., 2007) and would be ideal for considering whether patients with SRED have evening hyperphagia and morning anorexia, or whether patients with NES have motor restlessness of RLS.

A critical review of the literature suggests that SRED may be better classified as dysfunctional nocturnal eating upon the NES spectrum. At this point the only nocturnal eating that is undisputably characterized as SRED is unconscious nocturnal eating, which, as noted above, rarely occurs outside of the setting of sedative hypnotic medications. In review, patients with RLS have an urge to ambulate as well as eat and can be frequently misdiagnosed and treated for insomnia. In these cases amnestic nocturnal eating is then the expected manifestation of treatment with sedative hypnotic agents, which inhibit executive function and impair memory. Thus it is plausible that the only "pure SRED" cases are in fact adverse events related to medication misapplications.

Ultimately, integration between sleep and eating disorder medicine is of paramount importance to better unravel pathophysiological mechanisms and reverse the contribution of nighttime eating to weight gain. Collaboration will either unify these currently disparate disorders or with greater insight demonstrate fundamentally distinct pathologies. Regardless, engagement between investigators will help us reach the ultimate goal of identifying effective therapy for all patients.

References

Allison, K. C., Lundgren, J. D., O'Reardon, J. P., Geliebter, A., Gluck, M. E., Vinai, P., et al. (2010). Proposed diagnostic criteria for night eating syndrome. *International Journal of Eating Disorders, 43*(3), 241–247.

Allen, R. P. (2007). Controversies and challenges in defining the etiology and pathophysiology of restless legs syndrome. *American Journal of Medicine, 120*(1, Suppl. 1), S13–S21.

Allen, R. P., Walters, A. S., Montplaisir, J., Hening, W., Myers, A., Bell, T. J., et al. (2005). Restless legs syndrome prevalence and impact: REST general population study. *Archives of Internal Medicine, 165*(11), 1286–1292.

American Academy of Sleep Medicine. (2005). *International classification of sleep disorders: Diagnostic and coding manual* (2nd ed.). Westchester, IL: Author.

Bello, N. T., & Hajnal, A. (2010). Dopamine and binge eating behaviors. *Pharmacology, Biochemistry, and Behavior, 97*(1), 25–33.

Berger, K., Luedemann, J., Trenkwalder, C., John, U., & Kessler, C. (2004). Sex and the risk of restless legs syndrome in the general population. *Archives of Internal Medicine, 164*(2), 196–202.

Birketvedt, G., Florholmen, J., & Sundsfjord, J., et al. (1999). Behavioral and neuroendocrine characteristics of the night-eating syndrome. *Journal of the American Medical Association, 282*, 657–666.

Boseck, J. J., Engel, S. G., Allison, K. C., Crosby, R. D., Mitchell, J. E., & de Zwaan, M. (2007). The application of ecological momentary assessment to the study of night eating. *International Journal of Eating Disorders, 40*(3), 271–276.

Boyle, P. J., Scott, J. C., Krentz, A. J., Nagy, R. J., Comstock, E., & Hoffman, C. (1994). Diminished brain glucose metabolism is a significant determinant for falling rates of systemic glucose utilization during sleep in normal humans. *The Journal of Clinical Investigation, 93*(2), 529–535.

Chiang, A., & Krystal, A. (2008). Report of two cases where sleep-related eating behavior occurred with the extended-release formulation but not the immediate-release formulation of a sedative–hypnotic agent. *Journal of Clinical Sleep Medicine, 4*(2), 155–156.

Dang, A., Garg, G., & Rataboli, P. V. (2009). Zolpidem induced nocturnal sleep-related eating disorder (NSRED) in a male patient. *International Journal of Eating Disorders, 42*(4), 385–386.

De Ocampo, J., Foldvary, N., Dinner, D. S., & Golish, J. (2002). Sleep-related eating disorder in fraternal twins. *Sleep Medicine, 3*(6), 525–526.

de Zwaan, M., Roerig, D. B., Crosby, R. D., Karaz, S., & Mitchell, J. E. (2006). Nighttime eating: A descriptive study. *International Journal of Eating Disorders, 39*(3), 224–232.

Dolder, C. R., & Nelson, M. H. (2008). Hypnosedative-induced complex behaviours: Incidence, mechanisms and management. *CNS Drugs, 22*(12), 1021–1036.

Driver-Dunckley, E. D., Noble, B. N., Hentz, J. G., Evidente, V. G., Caviness, J. N., Parish, J., et al. (2007). Gambling and increased sexual desire with dopaminergic medications in restless legs syndrome. *Clinical Neuropharmacology, 30*(5), 249–255.

Dzaja, A., Dalal, M. A., Himmerich, H., Uhr, M., Pollmacher, T., & Schuld, A. (2004). Sleep enhances nocturnal plasma ghrelin levels in healthy subjects. *American Journal of Physiology, Endocrinology, and Metabolism, 286*(6), E963–E967.

Ekbom, K. A. (1960). Restless legs syndrome. *Neurology, 10,* 868–873.

Ganzoni, E., Santoni, J. P., Chevillard, V., Sebille, M., & Mathy, B. (1995). Zolpidem in insomnia: A 3-year post-marketing surveillance study in Switzerland. *Journal of International Medical Research, 23*(1), 61–73.

Giladi, N., Weitzman, N., Schreiber, S., Shabtai, H., & Peretz, C. (2007). New onset heightened interest or drive for gambling, shopping, eating, or sexual activity in patients with Parkinson's disease: The role of dopamine agonist treatment and age at motor symptoms onset. *Journal of Psychopharmacology, 21*(5), 501–506.

Gillin, J. C., Buchsbaum, M. S., Valladares-Neto, D. C., Hong, C. C., Hazlett, E., Langer, S. Z., et al. (1996). Effects of zolpidem on local cerebral glucose metabolism during non-REM sleep in normal volunteers: A positron emission tomography study. *Neuropsychopharmacology, 15*(3), 302–313.

Harazin, J., & Berigan, T. R. (1999). Zolpidem tartrate and somnambulism. *Military Medicine, 164*(9), 669–670.

Holl, R. W., Hartman, M. L., Veldhuis, J. D., Taylor, W. M., & Thorner, M. O. (1991). Thirty-second sampling of plasma growth hormone in man: Correlation with sleep stages. *Journal of Clinical Endocrinology and Metabolism, 72*(4), 854–861.

Holm, K. J., & Goa, K. L. (2000). Zolpidem: An update of its pharmacology, therapeutic efficacy, and tolerability in the treatment of insomnia. *Drugs, 59*(4), 865–889.

Hoque, R., & Chesson, A. L., Jr. (2009). Zolpidem-induced sleepwalking, sleep-related eating disorder, and sleep-driving: Fluorine-18-flourodeoxyglucose positron emission tomography analysis, and a literature review of other unexpected clinical effects of zolpidem. *Journal of Clinical Sleep Medicine, 5*(5), 471–476.

Howell, M. J., Schenck, C. H., & Crow, S. J. (2009). A review of nighttime eating disorders. *Sleep Medicine Reviews, 13*(1), 23–34.

Howell, M. J., Schenck, C. H., Larson, S., & Pusalavidyasagar, S. (2010). Nocturnal eating and sleep-related eating disorder (SRED) are common among patients with restless legs syndrome. *Sleep, 33,* A227.

Hwang, T. J., Ni, H. C., Chen, H. C., Lin, Y. T., & Liao, S. C. (2010). Risk predictors for hypnosedative-related complex sleep behaviors: A retrospective, cross-sectional pilot study. *Journal of Clinical Psychiatry, 71*(10), 1331–1335.

International Restless Legs Syndrome Study Group. (2010, June). *Restless legs syndrome, or Ekbom's syndrome.* Unpublished roundtable discussion, SLEEP Conference, San Antonio, TX.

Lam, S. P., Fong, S. Y., Ho, C. K., Yu, M. W., & Wing, Y. K. (2008). Parasomnia among psychiatric outpatients: A clinical, epidemiologic, cross-sectional study. *Journal of Clinical Psychiatry, 69*(9), 1374–1382.

Lam, S. P., Fong, S. Y., Yu, M. W., Li, S. X., & Wing, Y. K. (2009). Sleepwalking in psychiatric patients: Comparison of childhood and adult onset. *Australian and New Zealand Journal of Psychiatry, 43*(5), 426–430.

Lavigne, G. J., Kato, T., Kolta, A., & Sessle, B. J. (2003). Neurobiological mechanisms involved in sleep bruxism. *Critical Reviews in Oral Biology and Medicine, 14*(1), 30–46.

Lavigne, G. J., & Montplaisir, J. Y. (1994). Restless legs syndrome and sleep bruxism: Prevalence and association among Canadians. *Sleep, 17*(8), 739–743.

Lee, H. B., Hening, W. A., Allen, R. P., Kalaydjian, A. E., Earley, C. J., Eaton, W. W., et al. (2008). Restless legs syndrome is associated with DSM-IV major depressive disorder and panic disorder in the community. *Journal of Neuropsychiatry and Clinical Neurosciences, 20*(1), 101–105.

Lu, M. L., & Shen, W. W. (2004). Sleep-related eating disorder induced by risperidone. *Journal of Clinical Psychiatry, 65*(2), 273–274.

Maffettone, C., De Martino, L., Irace, C., Santamaria, R., Pagnini, U., Iovane, G., et al. (2008). Expression of iron-related proteins during infection by bovine herpes virus type-1. *Journal of Cellular Biochemistry, 104*(1), 213–223.

Mahowald, M. W., Cramer Bornemann, M. A., & Schenck, C. H. (2010). A case of reversible restless legs syndrome (RLS) and sleep-related eating disorder relapse triggered by acute right leg herpes zoster infection: Literature review of spinal cord and peripheral nervous system contributions to RLS. *Sleep Medicine, 11*(6), 583–585.

Manni, R., Ratti, M. T., & Tartara, A. (1997). Nocturnal eating: Prevalence and features in 120 insomniac referrals. *Sleep, 20*(9), 734–738.

Maquet, P., Dive, D., Salmon, E., Sadzot, B., Franco, G., Poirrier, R., et al. (1990). Cerebral glucose utilization during sleep–wake cycle in man determined by positron emission tomography and [18F]2-fluoro-2-deoxy-D-glucose method. *Brain Research, 513*(1), 136–143.

Martinez-Salio, A., Soler-Algarra, S., Calvo-Garcia, I., & Sanchez-Martin, M. (2007). Nocturnal sleep-related eating disorder that responds to topiramate. [Sindrome de ingesta nocturna relacionada con el sueno con respuesta al topiramato] *Revista De Neurologia, 45*(5), 276–279.

Martin-Iverson, M. T., & Dourish, C. T. (1988). Role of dopamine D-1 and D-2 receptor subtypes in mediating dopamine agonist effects on food consumption in rats. *Psychopharmacology, 96*(3), 370–374.

Molina, S. M., & Joshi, K. G. (2010). A case of zaleplon-induced amnestic sleep-related eating disorder. *Journal of Clinical Psychiatry, 71*(2), 210–211.

Morgenthaler, T. I., & Silber, M. H. (2002). Amnestic sleep-related eating disorder associated with zolpidem. *Sleep Medicine, 3*(4), 323–327.

Nadel, C. (1981). Somnambulism, bed-time medication and over-eating. *The British Journal of Psychiatry, 139,* 79.

Najjar, M. (2007). Zolpidem and amnestic sleep-related eating disorder. *Journal of Clinical Sleep Medicine, 3*(6), 637–638.

Nirenberg, M. J., & Waters, C. (2006). Compulsive eating and weight gain related to dopamine agonist use. *Movement Disorders, 21*(4), 524–529.

Nirenberg, M. J., & Waters, C. (2010). Nocturnal eating in restless legs syndrome. *Movement Disorders, 25*(1), 126–127.

Ohayon, M. M., Guilleminault, C., & Priest, R. G. (1999). Night terrors, sleep-walking, and confusional arousals in the general population: Their frequency and relationship to other sleep and mental disorders. *Journal of Clinical Psychiatry, 60*(4), 268–276; quiz 277.

Paquet, V., Strul, J., Servais, L., Pelc, I., & Fossion, P. (2002). Sleep-related eating disorder induced by olanzapine. *Journal of Clinical Psychiatry, 63*(7), 597.

Paulus, W., Dowling, P., Rijsman, R., Stiasny-Kolster, K., & Trenkwalder, C. (2007). Update of the pathophysiology of the restless legs syndrome. *Movement Disorders, 22*(Suppl. 18), S431–S439.

Picchietti, D., & Winkelman, J. W. (2005). Restless legs syndrome, periodic limb movements in sleep, and depression. *Sleep, 28*(7), 891–898.

Provini, F., Albani, F., Vetrugno, R., Vignatelli, L., Lombardi, C., Plazzi, G., et al. (2005). A pilot double-blind placebo-controlled trial of low-dose pramipexole in sleep-related eating disorder. *European Journal of Neurology, 12*(6), 432–436.

Provini, F., Antelmi, E., Vignatelli, L., Zaniboni, A., Naldi, G., Calandra-Buonaura, G., et al. (2009). Association of restless legs syndrome with nocturnal eating: A case–control study. *Movement Disorders, 24*(6), 871–877.

Provini, F., Antelmi, E., Vignatelli, L., Zaniboni, A., Naldi, G., Calandra-Buonaura, G., et al. (2010). Increased prevalence of nocturnal smoking in restless legs syndrome (RLS). *Sleep Medicine, 11*(2), 218–220.

Rogers, N. L., Dinges, D. F., Allison, K. C., Maislin, G., Martino, N., O'Reardon, J. P., et al. (2006). Assessment of sleep in women with night eating syndrome. *Sleep, 29*(6), 814–819.

Roth, T., Roehrs, T., & Vogel, G. (1995). Zolpidem in the treatment of transient insomnia: A double-blind, randomized comparison with placebo. *Sleep, 18*(4), 246–251.

Roth, T., Soubrane, C., Titeux, L., Walsh, J. K., & Zoladult Study Group. (2006). Efficacy and safety of zolpidem-MR: A double-blind, placebo-controlled study in adults with primary insomnia. *Sleep Medicine, 7*(5), 397–406.

Sanofi-Aventis. (2006). *Sanofi-Aventis 2005 financial report.*

Sansone, R. A., & Sansone, L. A. (2008). Zolpidem, somnambulism, and nocturnal eating. *General Hospital Psychiatry, 30*(1), 90–91.

Satija, P., & Ondo, W. G. (2008). Restless legs syndrome: Pathophysiology, diagnosis, and treatment. *CNS Drugs, 22*(6), 497–518.

Sauvanet, J. P., Maarek, L., Roger, M., Renaudin, J., Louvel, E., & Orofiamma, B. (1988). Open long-term trials with zolpidem in insomnia. In S. Z. Langer,

J. P. Sauvanet, & P. L. Morselli (Eds.), *Imidozopyridines in sleep disorders* (pp. 339–349). New York: Raven Press.

Schenck, C. H. (2006). *Paradox lost: Midnight in the battleground of sleep and dreams* (1st ed.). Minneapolis: Extreme-Nights, LLC.

Schenck, C. H., Connoy, D. A., Castellanos, M., Johnson, B., Wills, L., Cramer-Bornemann, M. A., et al. (2005). Zolpidem-induced sleep-related eating disorder (SRED) in 19 patients. *Sleep, 28*(Suppl.), a259.

Schenck, C. H., Hurwitz, T. D., Bundlie, S. R., & Mahowald, M. W. (1991). Sleep-related eating disorders: Polysomnographic correlates of a heterogeneous syndrome distinct from daytime eating disorders. *Sleep, 14*(5), 419–431.

Schenck, C. H., Hurwitz, T. D., O'Connor, K. A., & Mahowald, M. W. (1993). Additional categories of sleep-related eating disorders and the current status of treatment. *Sleep, 16*(5), 457–466.

Schenck, C. H., & Mahowald, M. W. (1994). Review of nocturnal sleep-related eating disorders. *International Journal of Eating Disorders, 15*(4), 343–356.

Schenck, C. H., & Mahowald, M. W. (2006). Topiramate therapy of sleep-related eating disorder (SRED). *Sleep, 29*, a268.

Simon, C., Gronfier, C., Schlienger, J. L., & Brandenberger, G. (1998). Circadian and ultradian variations of leptin in normal man under continuous enteral nutrition: Relationship to sleep and body temperature. *Journal of Clinical Endocrinology and Metabolism, 83*(6), 1893–1899.

Stunkard, A. J., Allison, K. C., Lundgren, J. D., & O'Reardon, J. P. (2009). A biobehavioural model of the night eating syndrome. *Obesity Reviews, 10*(Suppl. 2), 69–77.

Stunkard, A. J., Grace, W. J., & Wolff, H. G. (1955). The night-eating syndrome: A pattern of food intake among certain obese patients. *The American Journal of Medicine, 19*(1), 78–86.

Tippmann-Peikert, M., Park, J. G., Boeve, B. F., Shepard, J. W., & Silber, M. H. (2007). Pathologic gambling in patients with restless legs syndrome treated with dopaminergic agonists. *Neurology, 68*(4), 301–303.

Tsai, M. J., Tsai, Y. H., & Huang, Y. B. (2007). Compulsive activity and antero-grade amnesia after zolpidem use. *Clinical Toxicology, 45*(2), 179–181.

Valiensi, S. M., Cristiano, E., Martinez, O. A., Reisin, R. C., & Alvarez, F. (2010). Sleep-related eating disorders as a side effect of zolpidem. [Sindrome de ingesta nocturna como efecto colateral del zolpidem] *Medicina, 70*(3), 223–226.

Van Cauter, E., & Spiegel, K. (1999). Circadian and sleep control of endocrine secretions. In F. W. Turek & P. C. Zee (Eds.), *Monograph on "Neurobiology of Sleep and Circadian Rhythms"* (pp. 397–425). New York: Marcel Dekker.

Van Cauter, E., Blackman, J. D., Roland, D., Spire, J. P., Refetoff, S., & Polonsky, K. S. (1991). Modulation of glucose regulation and insulin secretion by circadian rhythmicity and sleep. *Journal of Clinical Investigation, 88*(3), 934–942.

Van Cauter, E., Polonsky, K. S., & Scheen, A. J. (1997). Roles of circadian rhythmicity and sleep in human glucose regulation. *Endocrine Reviews, 18*(5), 716–738.

Vetrugno, R., Manconi, M., Ferini-Strambi, L., Provini, F., Plazzi, G., & Montagna, P. (2006). Nocturnal eating: Sleep-related eating disorder or night eating syndrome? A videopolysomnographic study. *Sleep, 29*(7), 949–954.

Walters, A. S. (1995). Toward a better definition of the restless legs syndrome. the international restless legs syndrome study group. *Movement Disorders, 10*(5), 634–642.

Whyte, J. K. N. (1990). Somnambulistic eating: A report of three cases. *International Journal of Eating Disorders, 9,* 577–581.

Wing, Y. K., Lam, S. P., Li, S. X., Zhang, J., & Yu, M. W. (2010). Sleep-related eating disorder and zolpidem: An open interventional cohort study. *Journal of Clinical Psychiatry, 71*(5), 653–656.

Winkelman, J. W. (1998). Clinical and polysomnographic features of sleep-related eating disorder. *Journal of Clinical Psychiatry, 59*(1), 14–19.

Winkelman, J. W. (2003). Treatment of nocturnal eating syndrome and sleep-related eating disorder with topiramate. *Sleep Medicine, 4*(3), 243–246.

Winkelman, J. W. (2006a). Efficacy and tolerability of open-label topiramate in the treatment of sleep-related eating disorder: A retrospective case series. *Journal of Clinical Psychiatry, 67*(11), 1729–1734.

Winkelman, J. W. (2006b). Sleep-related eating disorder and night eating syndrome: Sleep disorders, eating disorders, or both? *Sleep, 29*(7), 876–877.

Winkelman, J. W., Finn, L., & Young, T. (2006). Prevalence and correlates of restless legs syndrome symptoms in the Wisconsin sleep cohort. *Sleep Medicine, 7*(7), 545–552.

Winkelman, J. W., Herzog, D. B., & Fava, M. (1999). The prevalence of sleep-related eating disorder in psychiatric and non-psychiatric populations. *Psychological Medicine, 29*(6), 1461–1466.

Yun, C. H., & Ji, K. H. (2010). Zolpidem-induced sleep-related eating disorder. *Journal of the Neurological Sciences, 288*(1–2), 200–201.

PART IV

ASSESSMENT

Chapter 10

Conceptual Issues Related to the Assessment of Eating Behavior, Mood, and Sleep in Night Eating Syndrome

Drew A. Anderson
Scott G. Engel
Ross D. Crosby

Night eating syndrome (NES) has three core problem areas: eating, mood, and sleep (Stunkard & Allison, 2003). An accurate assessment of all three areas is critical for diagnosis and treatment of this disorder. This chapter will broadly review current assessment practices of these areas in the context of NES, including strengths and weaknesses as well as areas of diagnostic concern.

Assessment of Eating in NES

The primary behavioral feature of NES is a circadian delay in the pattern of food intake, manifested by either evening hyperphagia (defined as the consumption of at least 25% of daily caloric intake after the evening meal) or regular (defined as at least two per week) nocturnal awakenings with food ingestions (Allison, Lundgren, O'Reardon, et al., 2010). The assessment of eating behavior relating to NES represents a particular challenge in that two separate aspects of eating must be evaluated: the quantity and the timing of food intake. The following sections discuss several approaches to assessing eating behavior along with the relative strengths and limitations of each approach.

Self-Report Measures of NES

Some research investigating NES has been based primarily on self-report instruments (e.g., de Zwaan, Roerig, Crosby, Karaz, & Mitchell, 2006). The most frequently used self-report measure of NES is the Night Eating Questionnaire (NEQ; Allison, Lundgren, et al., 2008). The NEQ was developed at the University of Pennsylvania as a self-rating screening instrument for NES. The items and responses have been revised several times; however, six core items have been present throughout the revisions: morning hunger, time of first meal, percentage of caloric intake after the evening meal, initial insomnia, frequency of awakenings, and frequency of nocturnal eating episodes. The psychometric properties of the NEQ have been established across several studies (Allison, Lundgren, et al., 2008; Allison, Engel, et al., 2008). The primary advantages of self-report measures such as the NEQ are convenience and ease of administration. As such, the NEQ is an ideal measure for initial screening of NES. However, the NES has limited utility for the assessment of eating behavior for several reasons. First, as with all measures of self-report, the NES is susceptible to retrospective recall biases that may limit the accurate assessment of both the quantity and timing of food ingestion. Second, respondents may not have the knowledge to make an accurate judgment about the amount of kilocalories consumed across various time intervals. Third, self-report measures do not provide prompts or follow-up questions that may clarify the questions and obtain more accurate responses.

Interview-Based Diagnostic Assessments of NES

There is currently only one unpublished semistructured diagnostic interview that has been used specifically to assess NES, the Night Eating Syndrome History and Inventory (NESHI; reported in de Zwaan et al., 2006). The NESHI assesses detailed characteristics of night eating, including age of onset, level of control, foods eaten, activities during awakenings, and family history. Unfortunately, the psychometric properties of this interview have not been established. Semistructured interviews are generally considered to be the gold standard for diagnostic assessment.

One disadvantage of a semistructured interview is the time and resources needed to administer it, including staff and training time. A recent paper proposing diagnostic criteria for NES (Allison, Lundgren, O'Reardon, et al., 2010) noted that the field would benefit from the development of a diagnostic interview for NES that would be similar to the Structured Diagnostic Interview for DSM-IV (SCID). However, as valuable as a NES semistructured interview would be for diagnostic purposes, such an interview would likely have more limited utility as a precise measure of eating behavior for many of the same reasons noted above for self-report measures. Recollections of eating behaviors by respondents may be influenced by retrospective recall biases. Furthermore, respondents may have limited knowledge about the kilocalorie content of the foods they eat, making judgments about the quantity of food ingested suspect.

Food Diary Assessment of Eating Behavior

A number of studies have used food diaries to assess eating behavior in the context of NES (Pawlow, O'Neill, & Malcolm, 2003; Lundgren, Allison, O'Reardon, & Stunkard, 2008; O'Reardon, Ringel, et al., 2004). These diaries can provide reasonably reliable measures of both the quantity and timing of food ingestion, particularly if respondents complete diary recordings immediately after eating. However, the assessment of eating behavior with food diaries is not without its limitations. Respondents typically require extensive training on how to record eating episodes accurately. Furthermore, the conversion of diary recordings into kilocalories consumed can be time intensive. The accuracy of food diaries is reduced if respondents do not complete ratings immediately after eating. When diaries are completed using paper and pencil, there is no easy way to determine when they were completed. Finally, food diaries often underestimate the amount of food that is typically consumed by participants, due to either underreporting (i.e., failure to record what is eaten) or undereating (i.e., voluntary food restriction during the assessment period) (Monnier et al., 2001).

Interviewer-Administered Assessment of Eating Behavior

One of the most accurate methods for gathering detailed nutrient information on foods consumed over a 24-hour period is with an interviewer-administered assessment such as the Nutritional Data System for

Research (NDS-R; Schakel, Sievert, & Buzzard, 1988). The NDS-R is a computer-based, interviewer-administered assessment that allows for nutrient intake calculation of foods eaten over a 24-hour interval. The NDS-R is considered by many to be the gold standard method of food intake assessment (Feskanich, Sielaff, Chong, & Buzzard, 1999). Caloric intake as determined by NDS-R has been shown to correlate with data from doubly-labeled water, supporting the validity of the assessment (Raymond, Neumeyer, Warren, Lee, & Peterson, 2003). Although we are not aware of any NES studies using the NDS-R, it has been used successfully with research on samples of overweight and obese individuals, including those with binge eating disorder (Raymond et al., 2003; Ebbeling et al., 2004; Engel et al., 2009). While interviewer-administered assessments of eating like the NDS-R have a number of advantages, they depend on the accuracy of the information provided by the participants. As such, they are susceptible to the same threats of underreporting that were described above for food diaries. The validity of these interviewer-administered assessments may be improved by coupling them with other assessment strategies, such as ecological momentary assessment (Engel et al., 2009), which is described below.

Ecological Momentary Assessment of Eating Behavior

Ecological momentary assessment (EMA) is an intensive "real-time" data collection strategy in the participant's natural environment. EMA has been recommended for the study of eating disorders (Smyth et al., 2001), and at least one study has used EMA to measure mood and behavior in participants with NES (Boseck et al., 2007). EMA is designed to circumvent many of the limitations of self-report data (e.g., retrospective recall bias) and laboratory methods (e.g., limited external validity) by having participants report immediate or very recent events that have occurred in their natural environment. EMA may be useful as a way of measuring the timing of eating events, but has limited utility for the assessment of the quantity of food consumed unless coupled with other assessment strategies, such as the NDS-R (see Engel et al., 2009). Another possible limitation of EMA for the study of NES is that participants may be reluctant to complete recordings during the night. In the EMA study reported by Boseck and colleagues (2007), the 14 participants completed only 71 EMA recordings during the night eating episodes, compared to 118 morning recordings reporting night eating episodes the previous night.

Activity-Monitoring Assessment of Eating Behavior

The timing of eating behaviors may also be measured by activity monitors. Birketvedt and colleagues (1999) conducted a behavioral observation study of NES using motion sensors coupled with food diaries to record food consumption across a 24-hour interval. Likewise, O'Reardon and colleagues (O'Reardon, Ringel, et al., 2004) used a similar methodology to compare eating behavior in obese participants with NES and controls. The advantage of the activity-monitoring strategy is that it provides precise records of the onset and duration of activity. However, neither the nature of that activity (e.g., eating vs. going to the bathroom) nor the amount of food ingested can be determined using activity monitoring alone. As such, activity monitoring is most effective for the study of NES when coupled with other assessment strategies such as food diaries or interviewer-administered nutritional assessments such as the NDS-R.

Feeding Laboratory Assessment of Eating Behavior

Feeding laboratories provide a standardized, controlled environment in which to study eating behaviors. This approach has been used to study individuals with anorexia nervosa, bulimia nervosa, and binge-eating disorder (see Mitchell, Crow, Peterson, Wonderlich, & Crosby, 1998, for a review). In addition, at least two feeding laboratory NES studies have been conducted to date. Birketvedt and colleagues (1999) compared the neuroendrocrine characteristics (e.g., melatonin, leptin, cortisol) of participants with NES to controls in a 24-hour feeding laboratory paradigm. Rogers and colleagues (2006) compared the sleeping and eating patterns of 15 women with NES and 14 controls in a feeding laboratory over a 3-day period. Feeding laboratories provide an ideal environment in which to evaluate contextual variables (e.g., amount of food presented) as well as a reliable way to evaluate the effects of pharmacological and psychotherapeutic interventions on eating behaviors. The primary limitation of feeding laboratory assessment is in terms of external validity; laboratory settings are by definition not naturalistic, and it is impossible to replicate or even approximate the natural environment in which eating typically occurs. As such, feeding laboratory studies may provide useful information that can validate, suggest, or challenge established clinical observations about NES. However, it is essential that findings from feeding laboratory studies be validated using one of more of the other assessment strategies described.

Conclusions

Each of the assessment strategies described above has certain strengths as well as significant limitations. Researchers should be aware of these and take them into consideration when designing NES studies. The ideal assessment strategy for measuring eating behavior may well be coupling two or methods, thereby building on the strengths of each approach.

NES and Mood

On numerous occasions NES has been discussed as having a significant mood-related component. As noted previously, Stunkard and Allison (2003) stated that NES "appears to be a unique combination of an eating disorder, a sleep disorder, and a mood disorder" (p. 7). Indeed, two of the key features of the disorder, namely disturbed sleep and eating patterns, are also commonly disturbed in mood disorders. Also, a number of studies have found that NES frequently co-occurs with depression.

Before discussing some of the research related to mood and NES we briefly review some of the common approaches to measuring mood and disturbances of mood that researchers studying NES may employ. Consistent with the previous section on the assessment of eating in NES, the measurement of mood in NES patients is also commonly done using one or more of the following approaches: self-report questionnaires, interviews, and/or ecological momentary assessment (EMA). Each of these approaches is briefly discussed below.

Self-Report Questionnaires and the Assessment of Mood in NES

Far and away the most frequently used mood-related measure is the Beck Depression Inventory (BDI; Beck, Ward, Mendelson, Mock, & Erbaugh, 1961). The BDI was developed to assess behavioral aspects of depression. In its original form the BDI is a 21-item self-report questionnaire that is relatively quick and easy to administer and score. The psychometric properties of the BDI have been thoroughly tested and typically can be described as good to excellent. Not only can the total score of the BDI be used as an index of depression level in those with NES, but it is relatively common practice for clinicians to check patients' responses to the item that taps suicidality. In addition to the BDI a number of other self-report questionnaires are commonly used to assess mood disturbances and would be appropriate for individuals with NES (e.g., Zung Self-Rating Depression Scale [Zung, 1965], Internal State Scale [Bauer et al., 1991]).

Interview Assessment of Mood in NES

In clinical practice two interviews are most commonly administered to assess mood and mood disturbance: the Hamilton Rating Scale for Depression (Ham-D; Hamilton, 1960) and the Structured Clinical Interview for DSM-IV Disorders (SCID-I; First, Spitzer, Gibbon, Williams, & Benjamin, 1996). The Ham-D characterizes the severity of depressive symptoms of patients and is to be administered by trained assessors. The psychometric properties of the Ham-D have been reported numerous times, and the instrument generally demonstrates good to excellent indices of reliability and validity (e.g., Hamilton, 1960; Bech et al., 1975). While the Ham-D provides information regarding the severity of mood disturbance, it was not designed as a diagnostic tool for mood disorders. The SCID-I is an assessor-administered diagnostic interview. In addition to the other Axis I disorders, mood disorders are assessed with the SCID-I. When used in psychiatric samples the psychometric properties of the SCID-I are generally reported to be from fair to excellent (Williams et al., 1992).

EMA and the Assessment of Mood in NES

As with the assessment of eating, one final assessment method worthy of mention is EMA. EMA involves the use of small electronic devices that are carried by participants in their natural environment (Stone & Shiffman, 1994). These electronic devices gather data from participants while they go about their everyday routine. While most self-report questionnaire or interview measures provide data on participants' mood over the course of a relatively longer period of time, EMA allows for the measurement of momentary mood states. This may be particularly relevant to NES given that relatively transient affective states may play a causal role in the behavior of interest (Boseck et al., 2007).

Current Mood-Related Literature and NES

de Zwaan and colleagues (2006) found that approximately 56% of their sample of night eaters reported meeting criteria for major depressive disorder in their lifetime. In addition, nearly 70% of their sample met criteria for any affective disorder. Besides diagnoses of mood disorders, the literature suggests that daily mood is also impaired in patients with NES. In support of this notion, Stunkard's original 1955 description of NES included increasing negative mood throughout the day, which peaks during the evening or night, as an optional criterion for the disorder. Consistent with this, Birketvedt and colleagues (1999) demonstrated that the mood of patients with NES was generally lower than control participants, and that patients with NES experienced more negative affect in the evening when compared to control participants, as reported through visual analogue mood scales kept in logs throughout the day. In general, momentary negative mood states appeared to be more common in the NES group than the control group.

In a more intensive assessment of momentary affect Boseck and colleagues (2007) gathered momentary ratings of mood from self-reported night eaters using EMA. Participants carried palmtop computers and provided ratings of momentary mood multiple times from when they woke up to the time they went to bed each day. In this study participants reported lower mood in the morning than at any other time of day, which contrasts the earlier findings obtained through more conventional means of assessment. Future studies should seek to clarify these conflicting findings.

Another possible indication that NES may have a significant mood component can be seen in the treatment literature for NES. While initial efforts to treat NES were psychodynamic in nature and focused on stress reduction (Stunkard, 1976), more recent treatment literature has largely been pharmacological in nature (Miyaoka et al., 2003; O'Reardon et al., 2006; O'Reardon, Stunkard, & Allison, 2004; Stunkard et al., 2006). Importantly, these studies have employed selective serotonin reuptake inhibitors (SSRIs), which are indicated for mood disorders. In addition, cognitive-behavioral therapy (CBT), which was initially developed for use in mood disorders (Beck, Rush, Shaw, & Emery, 1979) has been used successfully in patients with NES (Allison, Lundgren, Moore, O'Reardon, & Stunkard, 2010).

One interesting and relevant finding is that the improvements seen in NES appear to occur, at least for the most part, independent of improvements in mood. In the previously mentioned O'Readon and colleagues (2006) study NES patients were treated with the SSRI sertraline. Of the 17 participants who were treated with sertraline, seven achieved remission of their core night eating symptoms. Importantly, the correlation between improvement in depression and NES symptoms was relatively low ($r = 0.28$, $p = .40$). These data provide some support for the idea that the depression and NES symptoms occurred somewhat independently and responded to SSRI treatment differentially.

In 2008 Striegel-Moore and colleagues reported on the typology of NES. Interestingly, they found that two of the four groups comprising individuals with NES had significant depression associated with their condition. Of the 1,771 participants with NES in the study, 626 were categorized in a group of patients who were characterized by considerable depression. Of these depressed NES participants, 296 were called "depressed evening eaters" and 330 were considered "depressed late-night eaters." It is interesting that a significant proportion of NES patients were grouped based on their levels of mood disturbance. However, a counterpoint is also relevant: nearly two-thirds of these patients were placed in two "nondepressed" groups, suggesting that impaired mood is not present in the majority of NES patients.

Conclusion

Data currently suggest that a large percentage of NES patients have co-occurring mood disorders (e.g., de Zwaan et al., 2006), and that it should be regularly assessed in this population. Furthermore, treatments that have been effective for NES have also been effective treatments for depression (CBT and SSRIs). These findings have led experts in the field to speculate that mood may be a key component of NES (Stunkard & Allison, 2003). However, two key findings in the literature support the notion that disordered mood is not a necessary component of NES: (1) a considerable percentage of NES patients do not appear to meet criteria for any mood disorder in their lifetime or to cluster in a "currently depressed" group, and (2) NES and mood symptoms appear to respond to treatment relatively independently to each other.

Assessment of Sleep-Related Issues in NES

Assessment of Insomnia

Insomnia has been considered to be a core criterion of NES since its first description (Allison et al., 2008; Allison, Lundgren, O'Reardon, Geliebter, Gluck, et al., 2010; de Zwann et al., 2006; Stunkard, Grace, & Wolff, 1955; Vinai et al., 2008), and it has been suggested that NES could be classifed as an insomnia-related disorder (Allison, O'Reardon, Geliebter, et al., 2010). Thus the assessment of insomnia is an important consideration in the diagnosis of NES.

Insomnia is particularly relevant to two of the proposed criteria for NES (Allison, O'Reardon, Geliebter, et al., 2010). First, one of the daily patterns of eating that fulfills the criteria of "a significantly increased intake in the evening and/or nighttime" is at least two nocturnal awakenings per week with ingestions of food. In this case it is not the insomnia per se that is primarily of concern; rather, it is the nocturnal eating that is of concern, and the awakenings merely allow the possibility for eating to occur. It is important to note that many individuals do not wake up specifically to eat, however. For example, de Zwann and colleagues (2006) found that less than 20% of a sample of persons with nighttime eating problems reported that they woke up primarily to eat, and the authors suggested some of their participants ate simply as a way to "kill time" while awake, a pattern has been found by others (Manni, Ratti, & Tartara, 1997). Also, Birketvedt and colleagues (1999) found that only half of all nighttime awakenings in persons with NES were associated with food intake. Thus many of the awakenings in individuals with NES may not involve food or eating, and the function of nocturnal eating may differ among individuals. Likewise, awakenings within a given individual may occur for different reasons at different times. At this point it is unclear whether differentiating episodes where an individual awakens specifically to eat from those where an individual eats simply because he or she is awake will make any clinical or theoretical significance to the diagnosis and treatment of NES. The proposed criteria for NES do include a criterion related to the presence of a belief that one must eat in order to initiate or return to sleep (Allison, Lundgren, O'Reardon, et al., 2010), but there is currently no criterion related to the reason or reasons for awakening. Until this issue is investigated further, we recommend that assessors document the functions of, and reasons for, awakenings.

The second NES criterion related to insomnia requires that sleep onset and/or sleep maintenance insomnia be present four or more nights per week. This criterion is one of five diagnostic signs and symptoms, three of which must be present for a diagnosis of NES (Allison, Lundgren, O'Reardon, et al., 2010). In this case the focus of the criterion is on the insomnia itself. However, there are some potential problems with the assessment of this criterion. First, insomnia has been defined inconsistently in the medical literature, with the term being used to define both a simple symptom of sleeplessness as well as a more severe and complex disorder (Manber & Ong, 2010; Roth, 2007). It is not clear how the term is being used in either the NES literature or proposed criteria. Also, insomnia is a common disorder, with symptoms of sleeplessness affecting up to 30–50% of the population and roughly 10% meeting the more stringent criteria involving distress or impairment (Roth, 2007; Schutte-Rodin, Broch, Buysse, Dorsey, & Sateia, 2008). Having such a common criterion as part of the diagnosis might artificially inflate the numbers of individuals meeting criteria for NES. On the other hand, requiring more stringent definitions for insomnia may necessitate more detailed assessments than is desirable, given that a strict diagnosis of insomnia does not appear to have been used in studies of NES. Current guidelines from the American Academy of Sleep Medicine (AASM) recommend that a full assessment of insomnia should contain, at a minimum, an evaluation to identify comorbid disorders and medication use, a self-report measure of sleepiness, and a 2-week sleep log to document patterns of sleeping (Schutte-Rodin et al., 2008), which do not appear to be common in the NES literature.

Assessment Measures of Insomnia

Clinical Interview

A careful patient history via clinical interview is the foundation of a good assessment of insomnia (Doghramji & Cologne, 2010; Sateia, Doghramji, Hauri, & Morin, 2000; Schutte-Rodin et al., 2008). While no one interview has been found to be the best, guidelines exist to assist with conducting a thorough and systematic sleep history (Doghramji & Cologne, 2010; Edinger & Carney, 2008; Sateia et al., 2000; Schutte-Rodin et al., 2008).

Polysomnography

While polysomnography is considered to be the gold standard for evaluating many sleep-related disorders (Kushida et al., 2005), it is not recommended for the routine evaluation of chronic insomnia (Germain & Moul, 2010; Martin & Ancoli-Israel, 2002; Schutte-Rodin et al., 2008), although some have argued that it provides useful information (Jacobs, Reynolds, Kupfer, Lovin, & Ehrenpreis, 1988). Shortcomings include that fact that it: (1) is expensive and time consuming, (2) does not adequately capture the subjective complaints that are part of the definition of insomnia, and (3) may be difficult to reproduce normal sleep in a laboratory or clinic setting (Martin & Ancoli-Israel, 2002).

Actigraphy

Actigraphy has been increasingly used in the assessment of insomnia (Morgenthaler et al., 2007). It has the advantages of being much less expensive than polysomnography and may be used at home. Its routine use is somewhat controversial, however; it has been recommended as an assessment tool for insomnia by some practice guidelines of the AASM (Morgenthaler et al., 2007) but not by other practice guidelines of the same organization (Schutte-Rodin et al., 2008). It also has some limitations; a recent review concluded that while actigraphy has reasonable sensitivity to detect differences between clinical groups of individuals with insomnia and controls, it generally overestimates sleep time because of its inability to detect the motionless wakefulness that is common in insomnia (Sadeh, 2011).

Self-Report Questionnaires

Self-report questionnaires are the most common method for assessing insomnia (Germain & Moul, 2010), and a number of such measures have been developed to assess insomnia and related behaviors. Many of them have good reliability and validity, but it is beyond the scope of this chapter to discuss all of them in detail. Interested readers can review these measures elsewhere (e.g., Devine, Hakim, & Green, 2005; Germain & Moul, 2010; Moul, Hall, Pilkonis, & Buysse, 2004; Sateia et al., 2000; Vernon, Dugar, Revicki, Treglia, & Buysse, 2010).

Sleep Diaries

Sleep diaries have been widely used in studies of NES (e.g., Lundgren et al., 2008; O'Reardon, Ringel, et al., 2004; Rogers et al., 2006) and have been validated in persons with NES (O'Reardon, Ringel, et al., 2004). One week of monitoring appears to be the norm in the NES literature, but AASM guidelines suggest 2 weeks (Schutte-Rodin et al., 2008). Assessors should consider extending the assessment period to conform with current guidelines.

In summary, a number of methodologies are available to clinicians who wish to assess insomnia to aid in the diagnosis of NES. However, it does not appear that the assessment of insomnia as related to NES is typically as thorough as is recommended by sleep medicine specialists (Schutte-Rodin et al., 2008). Future research should use more precise definitions and more thorough assessments to improve the reliability and validity of the NES criteria related to insomnia.

Differential Diagnosis of NES versus Sleep-Related Eating Disorder

NES must be distinguished from sleep-related eating disorder (SRED), the disorder it most resembles (Allison, Lundgren, O'Reardon, et al., 2010). Several characteristics related to eating and sleep can help the assessor make an accurate diagnosis.

One of the principal distinguishing characteristics between these disorders is the level of awareness during eating episodes. Individuals with NES are typically described as being aware of their nocturnal eating episodes and having good recall of them, while those with SRED are often described as having only partial or no awareness during such episodes (Allison, Lundgren, O'Reardon, et al., 2010; Howell, Schenck, & Crow, 2009; O'Reardon, Ringel, et al., 2004). The assessment of awareness in the NES literature has been criticized as being too vague, however, and some episodes of eating in SRED can occur with partial or full awareness (Howell et al., 2009; Vertrungo et al., 2006) (see Chapter 9 [Howell & Crow]). Thus there can be some diagnostic confusion between these disorders on this point. The use of other criteria listed in this section may clarify the diagnosis when patient reports of level of consciousness during eating are vague or otherwise questionable.

Another difference between the disorders relates to the foods eaten during nocturnal eating episodes. Individuals with NES typically eat foods similar to those eaten during the daytime, while individuals with SRED have been found to eat foods not typically ingested during the daytime, including some bizarre food items (Howell et al., 2009). Thus individuals reporting eating more bizarre food items should be suspected of having SRED, not NES.

An additional differentiating factor concerns the timing of eating in these patients. It is well established that individuals with NES have a circadian shift in their pattern of eating, with evening hyperphagia after dinner and before bedtime extremely common (Allison, Lundgren, O'Reardon, et al., 2010). Conversely, it has been suggested that this pattern of eating is not seen in SRED, with problematic eating episodes in individuals with this disorder occurring only after bedtime (Schenck, 2006). While this observation needs to be validated by formal research (Schenck, 2006), it still may be a useful heuristic for differential diagnosis.

Conclusion

Sleep disturbance is a key feature of NES, and there are many methods available to assess the sleep-related problems typically found as part of the disorder. Questions remain, however, about the level of methodological rigor required to document sleep disturbance in the context of NES. Nevertheless, researchers and clinicians should strive to use guidelines from sleep-related organizations such as the AASM to help guide their assessment process.

Discussion

There are well-established guidelines and procedures for assessing eating, mood, and sleep. Current practice for the assessment of these domains in the context of NES is generally good, although there is some room for improvement. Assessors are encouraged to follow the literature in each of these domains to keep up with changing assessment measures and procedures.

References

Allison, K. C., Engel, S. G., Crosby, R. D., deZwaan, M., O'Reardon, J. P., Wonderlich, S. A., et al. (2008). Evaluation of diagnostic criteria for night eating syndrome using item response theory analysis. *Eating Behaviors, 9,* 398–407.

Allison, K. C., Lundgren, J. D., Moore, R. H., O'Reardon, J. P. & Stunkard, A. J. (2010). Cognitive behavior therapy for night eating syndrome: A pilot study. *American Journal of Psychotherapy, 64,* 91–107.

Allison, K. C., Lundgren, J. D., O'Reardon, J. P., Geliebter, A., Gluck, M. E., Vinai, P., et al. (2010). Proposed diagnostic criteria for night eating syndrome. *International Journal of Eating Disorders, 43,* 241–247.

Allison, K. C., Lundgren, J. D., O'Reardon, J. P, Martino, N. S., Sarwer, D. B., Wadden, T. A., et al. (2008). The Night Eating Questionnaire (NEQ): Psychometric properties of a measure of severity of the night eating syndrome. *Eating Behaviors, 9,* 62–72.

Bauer, M. S., Crits-Christoph, P., Ball, W. A., Jacobsen, O., Vitger, J., Bulwig, T. G., et al. (1991). Independent assessment of manic and depressive symptoms by self-rating: Scales characteristics and implications for the study of mania. *Archives of General Psychiatry, 48,* 807–812.

Bech, P., Gram, L. F., Dein, E., Jacobsen, O., Vitger, J., Bulwig, T. G., et al. (1975). Quantitative rating of depressive states: Correlation between clinical assessment, Beck's self-rating scale, and Hamilton's objective rating scale. *Acta Psychiatrica Scandinavica, 71,* 315–317.

Beck, A. T., Rush, A. J., Shaw, B. F., & Emery, G. (1979). *Cognitive therapy of depression*. New York: Guilford Press.

Beck, A. T., Ward, C. H., Mendelson, M., Mock, J., & Erbaugh, J. (1961). An inventory for measuring depression. *Archives of General Psychiatry, 4*, 53–63.

Birketvedt, G., Florholmen, J., Sundsfjord, J., Osterud, B., Dinges, D., Bilker, W., et al. (1999). Behavioral and neuroendocrine characteristics of night eating syndrome. *Journal of the American Medical Association, 282*, 657–663.

Boseck, J. J., Engel, S. G., Allison, K. C., Crosby, R. D., Mitchell, J. E., & de Zwaan, M. (2007). The application of ecological momentary assessment to the study of night eating. *International Journal of Eating Disorders, 40*, 271–276.

Devine, E. B., Hakim, Z., & Green, J. (2005). A systematic review of patient-reported outcome instruments measuring sleep dysfunction in adults. *Pharmacoeconomics, 23*, 889–912.

de Zwaan, M., Roerig, D. B., Crosby, R. D., Karaz, S., & Mitchell, J. E. (2006). Nighttime eating: A descriptive study. *International Journal of Eating Disorders, 39*, 224–232.

Doghramji, K., & Cologne, S. E. (2010). History taking in insomnia. In M. J. Sateia & D. J. Buysse (Eds.), *Insomnia: Diagnosis and treatment* (pp. 84–88). London: Informa Healthcare.

Ebbeling, C. B., Sinclair, K. B., Pereira, M. A., Garcia-Lago, E., Feldman, H. A. & Ludwig, D. S. (2004). Compensation for energy intake from fast food among overweight and lean adolescents. *Journal of the American Medical Association, 291*, 2828–2833.

Edinger, J. D., & Carney, C. E. (2008). *Overcoming insomnia: A cognitive-behavioral therapy approach therapist guide*. New York: Oxford University Press.

Engel, S. G., Kahler, K. A., Lystad, C. M., Crosby, R. D., Simonich, H. K., Wonderlich, S. A., et al. (2009). Eating behavior in obese BED, obese non-BED and non-obese control subjects: A naturalistic study. *Behaviour Research and Therapy, 47*, 897–900.

Feskanich, D., Sielaff, B. H., Chong, K., & Buzzard, L. M. (1999). Computerized collection and analysis of dietary intake information. *Computer Methods Programs in Biomedicine, 30*, 47–57.

First, M. B., Spitzer, R. L., Gibbon, M., Williams, J. B. W., & Benjamin, L. (1996). *Structured Clinical Interview for DSM-IV Disorders—Patient edition (with psychotic screen, version 2.0)*. New York: Biometrics Research Department, New York State Psychiatric Institute.

Germain, A., & Moul, D. E. (2010). Evaluation instruments and methodology. In M. J. Sateia & D. J. Buysse (Eds.), *Insomnia: Diagnosis and treatment* (pp. 89–97). London: Informa Healthcare.

Hamilton, M. (1960). A rating scale for depression. *Journal of Neurology, Neurosurgery, and Psychiatry, 23*, 56–62.

Howell, M. J., Schenck, C. H., & Crow, S. J. (2009). A review of nighttime eating disorders. *Sleep Medicine Reviews, 13*, 23–34.

Jacobs, E. A., Reynolds, C. F. I., Kupfer, D. J., Lovin, P. A., & Ehrenpreis, A. B.

(1988). The role of polysomnography in the differential diagnosis of chronic insomnia. *American Journal of Psychiatry, 145,* 346–349.

Kushida, C. A., Littner, M. R., Morgenthaler, T., Alessi, C. A., Bailey, D., Coleman, J., et al. (2005). Practice parameters for the indications for polysomnography and related procedures: An update for 2005. *Sleep, 28,* 499–521.

Lundgren, J. D., Allison, K. C., O'Reardon, J. P., & Stunkard, A. J. (2008). A descriptive study of non-obese persons with night eating syndrome and a weight-matched comparison group. *Eating Behaviors, 9,* 343–351.

Manber, R., & Ong, J. C. (2010). Clinical assessment of insomnia: Primary insomnias. In M. J. Sateia & D. J. Buysse (Eds.), *Insomnia: Diagnosis and treatment* (pp. 113–125). London: Informa Healthcare.

Manni, R., Ratti, M. T., & Tartara, A. (1997). Nocturnal eating: Prevalence and features in 120 insomniac referrals. *Sleep, 20,* 734–738.

Martin, J. L., & Ancoli-Israel, S. (2002). Assessment and diagnosis of insomnia in non-pharmacological intervention studies. *Sleep Medicine Reviews, 6,* 379–406.

Mitchell, J. E., Crow, S., Peterson, C., Wonderlich, S., & Crosby, R. D. (1998). Feeding laboratory studies in patients with eating disorders. *International Journal of Eating Disorders, 24,* 115–124.

Miyaoka, T., Yasukawa, R., Tsubouchi, K., Miura, S., Shimizu, Y., Sukegawa, T., et al. (2003). Successful treatment of nocturnal eating/drinking syndrome with selective serotonin reuptake inhibitors. *International Clinical Psychopharmacology, 18,* 175–177.

Monnier, L., Colette, C., Percheron, C., Pham, T. C., Sauvanet, J. P., Ledevehat, C., et al. (2001). Dietary assessment in current clinical practice: How to conciliate rapidity, simplicity, and reliability. *Diabetes and Metabolism, 27,* 388–395.

Morgenthaler, T., Alessi, C., Friedman, L., Owens, J., Kapur, V., Boehlecke, B., et al. (2007). Practice parameters for the use of actigraphy in the assessment of sleep and sleep disorders: An update for 2007. *Sleep, 30,* 519–529.

Moul, D. E., Hall, M., Pilkonis, P. A., & Buysse, D. J. (2004). Self-report measures of insomnia in adults: Rationales, choices, and needs. *Sleep Medicine Reviews, 8,* 177–198.

O'Reardon, J. P., Allison, K. C., Martino, N. S., Lundgren, J. D., Heo, M., & Stunkard, A. J. (2006). A randomized placebo-controlled trial of sertraline in the treatment of the night eating syndrome. *American Journal of Psychiatry, 164,* 893–898.

O'Reardon, J. P., Ringel, B. L., Dinges, D. F., Allison, K. C., Rogers, N. L., Martino, N. S., et al. (2004). Circadian eating and sleeping patterns in the night eating syndrome. *Obesity Research, 12,* 1789–1796.

O'Reardon, J. P., Stunkard, A. J., & Allison, K. C. (2004). A clinical trial of sertraline in the treatment of night eating syndrome. *International Journal of Eating Disorders, 35,* 16–26.

Pawlow, L. A., O'Neill, P. M., & Malcolm, R. J. (2003). Night eating syndrome: Effects of brief relaxation training on stress, mood, hunger and eating patterns. *International Journal of Obesity and Related Metabolic Disorders, 27,* 970–978.

Raymond, N. C., Neumeyer, B., Warren, C. S., Lee, S. S., & Peterson, C. B. (2003). Energy intake patterns in obese women with binge eating disorder. *Obesity Research, 11,* 869–879.

Rogers, N. L., Dinges, D. F., Allison, K. C., Maislin, G., Martino, N., O'Reardon, J. P., et al. (2006). Assessment of sleep in women with night eating syndrome. *Sleep, 29,* 814–819.

Roth, T. (2007). Insomnia: Definition, prevalence, etiology, and consequences. *Journal of Clinical Sleep Medicine, 15*(Suppl. 5), S7–S10.

Sadeh, A. (2011). The role and validity of actigraphy in sleep medicine: An update. *Sleep Medicine Reviews, 15,* 259–267.

Sateia, M. J., Doghramji, K., Hauri, P. J., & Morin, C. M. (2000). Evaluation of chronic insomnia: An American Academy of Sleep Medicine review. *Sleep, 23,* 243–308.

Schakel, S. F., Sievert, Y. A., & Buzzard, I. M. (1988). Sources of data for developing and maintaining a nutrient database. *Journal of the American Dietetic Association, 88,* 1268–1271.

Schenck, C. H. (2006). A study of circadian eating and sleeping patterns in night eating syndrome (NES) points the way to future studies on NES and sleep-related eating disorder. *Sleep Medicine, 7,* 653–656.

Schutte-Rodin, S., Broch, L., Buysse, D., Dorsey, C., & Sateia, M., (2008). Clinical guideline for the evaluation and management of chronic insomnia in adults. *Journal of Clinical Sleep Medicine, 4,* 487–504.

Smyth, J., Wonderlich, S., Crosby, R. D., Miltenberger, R., Mitchell, J., & Rorty, M. (2001). The use of ecological momentary assessment approaches in eating disorder research. *International Journal of Eating Disorders, 30,* 83–95.

Stone, A. A., & Shiffman, S. (1994). Ecological momentary assessment (EMA) in behavioral medicine. *Annals of Behavioral Medicine, 16,* 199–202.

Striegel-Moore, R. H., Franko, D. L., Thompson, D., Affenito, S., May, A., & Kraemer, H. C. (2008). Exploring the typology of night eating syndrome. *International Journal of Eating Disorders, 41,* 411–418.

Stunkard, A. J. (1976). *The pain of obesity.* Palo Alto, CA: Bull.

Stunkard, A. J., & Allison, K. C. (2003). Two forms of disordered eating in obesity: Binge eating and night eating. *International Journal of Obesity, 27,* 1–12.

Stunkard, A. J., Allison, K. C., Lundgren, J. D., Martino, N. S., Heo, M., Eremad, B., et al. (2006). A paradigm for facilitating pharmacotherapy at a distance: Sertraline treatment of the night eating syndrome. *Journal of Clinical Psychiatry, 67,* 1558–1572.

Stunkard, A., Grace, W. J., & Wolff, H. G. (1955). The night-eating syndrome: A pattern of food intake among certain obese patients. *American Journal of Medicine, 19,* 78–86.

Vernon, M. K., Dugar, A., Revicki, D., Treglia, M., & Buysse, D. (2010). Measurement of non-restorative sleep in insomnia: A review of the literature. *Sleep Medicine Reviews, 14,* 205–212.

Vertrungo, R., Manconi, M., Ferini-Strambi, L., Provini, F., Plazzi, G., & Montagna, P. (2006). Nocturnal eating: Sleep-related eating disorder or night eating syndrome? A videopolysomnographic study. *Sleep, 29,* 949–954.

Vinai, P., Allison, K. C., Cardetti, S., Carpegna, G., Ferrato, N., Masante, D., et al. (2008). Psychopathology and treatment of night eating syndrome: A review. *Eating and Weight Disorders, 13,* 54–63.

Williams, J. W., Gibbon, M., First, M. B., Spitzer, R. L., Davies, M., Borus, J., et al. (1992). The Structured Clinical Interview for DSM-III-R (SCID), II: Multisite test–retest reliability. *Archives of General Psychiatry, 49,* 630–636.

Zung, W. W. K. (1965). A self-rating depression scale. *Archives of General Psychiatry, 12,* 63–70.

Chapter 11

Assessment Instruments for Night Eating Syndrome

Jennifer D. Lundgren
Kelly C. Allison
Piergiuseppe Vinai
Marci E. Gluck

Several instruments are available for assessing the symptoms and associated features of night eating syndrome (NES). These range from brief self-report tools that quantify symptom severity to longer, semistructured clinical interviews designed to establish a NES diagnosis and aid in treatment planning. Three self-report instruments have been developed for the assessment of NES: the Night Eating Questionnaire (NEQ; Allison et al., 2008), the Night Eating Symptom Scale (NESS; O'Reardon, Stunkard, & Allison, 2004), and the Night Eating Diagnostic Questionnaire (NEDQ; Morrow, Gluck, Flancbaum, Lorence, & Geliebter, 2008; Gluck, Geliebter, & Satov, 2001). The first two (NEQ and NESS) are similar, with the main distinction being their function; the NEQ assesses symptoms over an unspecified duration and is meant to screen for NES symptoms broadly, while the NESS assesses symptoms over the previous 7 days, and is meant to be used to monitor progress in treatment. Both are reviewed in detail below. The NEDQ, as its name implies, is a self-report diagnostic questionnaire. It differs significantly from the NEQ and NESS in that it is used to establish a diagnosis of NES, rather than an assessment of the individual's symptom severity, independent of a NES diagnosis. It too is reviewed in more detail below.

In addition to these self-report instruments, two clinical interviews are available that assess night eating behavior: the Night Eating Syndrome History and Inventory (NESHI) and a portion of the Eating Disorder Examination (EDE; Fairburn, Cooper, & O'Connor, 2008). The NESHI is a semistructured clinical interview that is used to establish a diagnosis of NES in addition to gathering information on NES symptom severity, distress due to night eating behavior and its impact on functioning, as well as the history of one's night eating behavior and precipitating factors. The NEQ is embedded in the interview so that a quantitative NES symptom severity score can be obtained. The NESHI has recently been revised to incorporate NES research diagnostic criteria (Allison, Lundgren, O'Reardon, Geliebter, et al., 2010). Its description and use, as well as the full interview, are included below.

Finally, several other assessment methods are available to understand more fully the sleep, mood, and eating patterns of individuals with NES. These include prospective food records, dietary recalls, actigraphy, polysomnography, and mood assessments such as the Beck Depression Inventory-II (Beck, 1996). See Chapter 10 (Anderson, Engel, & Crosby) for a review of these tools.

Self-Report Assessments

NEQ and NESS

The NEQ (Allison et al., 2008) is a 14-item, self-report instrument that assesses the behavioral and psychological symptoms of NES. Specifically, the NEQ assesses morning hunger and timing of first food consumption (two items), food cravings and control over eating behavior both before bedtime (two items) and during nighttime awakenings (two items), percent of food consumed after dinner (one item), initial insomnia (one item), frequency of nocturnal awakenings and ingestion of food (three items), mood disturbance (two items), and awareness of nocturnal eating episodes (one item, included to differentiate a diagnosis of sleep-related eating disorder from NES, but not included in the total score). Each item is rated on a Likert-type scale and scores can range from 0 to 52. The NEQ and its scoring instructions are included in the Allison and colleagues (2008) validation paper.

The NEQ is not designed to diagnose NES (although a diagnosis can be approximated), but rather is intended to help clinicians and researchers (1) screen for NES so that more comprehensive assessments (e.g., the NESHI) can confirm a diagnosis, and (2) assess changes in symptom severity across time (e.g., as a measure of symptom stability or treatment outcome).

The psychometric properties of the NEQ have been assessed in three separate samples: 1,980 individuals from 76 countries who completed the NEQ online, 81 outpatients diagnosed with NES who were enrolled in a comprehensive assessment study of NES, and 194 bariatric surgery candidates (all published in Allison et al., 2008). The NEQ has also been administered to psychiatric outpatients (Lundgren, Allison, Crow, Berg, Galbraith, et al., 2006), obese individuals with serious mental illness (Lundgren, Rempfer, Brown, Goetz, & Hamera, et al., 2010), and individuals diagnosed with eating disorders (Lundgren et al., 2008; Lundgren et al., 2011). With the exception of descriptive data on NEQ scores in these populations (see Table 11.1), no psychometric data with these samples have been published. Readers are encouraged to review Chapters 7 (Latzer & Tzischinsky) and 8 (Rempfer & Murphy) for discussions of the comorbidity between NES and other psychiatric and eating disorders.

In the sample of 1,980 Internet participants (representing the United States and 75 additional countries), the NEQ was found to have a four-factor structure: (1) nocturnal ingestions, (2) evening hyperphagia, (3) morning anorexia, and (4) mood/sleep. This factor structure reflects both early and contemporary conceptualizations of NES and its associated features (Stunkard, Grace, & Wolf, 1955; Allison, Lundgren, O'Reardon, Geliebter, Gluck, et al., 2010). Confirmatory factor analysis, for which the four factors were considered to be part of a single higher-order factor, was supported, and hence a single NEQ score is most often reported in the literature. In this diverse sample, which included many participants who likely completed the NEQ while browsing the website for information about NES, the average score was 33.1 ± 7.5 (range 2–49 points).

In the second validation sample (81 adult outpatient research participants diagnosed with NES), the convergent validity of the NEQ was examined. The NEQ correlated significantly with the percent of total daily food intake consumed after the evening meal (measured with 7-day prospective food records), frequency of nocturnal ingestions of food (measured with 7-day prospective food records), the EDE Dietary Restraint, Eating Concern, and Shape Concern subscales, as well as the EDE global score, the Pittsburg Sleep Quality Index, the Perceived Stress Scale, and the Beck Depression Inventory. The NEQ did not correlate significantly with morning hunger ratings or subscales of the Three Factor Eating Questionnaire (Eating Inventory). The mean NEQ score in

TABLE 11.1. Normative NEQ Data for Different Populations

Population	Mean (SD) NEQ score
1,980 individuals from 76 countries who completed the NEQ online (Allison et al., 2008)	33.1 (7.5)
81 outpatient research participants diagnosed with NES; all body mass index ranges (Allison et al., 2008)	
Total sample	32.4 (6.8)
Nonobese NES (*n* = 14)	36.0 (6.8)
Overweight NES (*n* = 26)	33.1 (4.3)
Obese NES (*n* = 41)	31.1 (7.2)
194 bariatric surgery candidates (Allison et al., 2008)	
Surgery candidates diagnosed with NES (*n* = 19)	26.2 (8.1)
Surgery candidates not diagnosed with NES (*n* = 175)	16.0 (6.3)
399 psychiatric outpatients (Lundgren et al., 2006)	21.1 (10.0)
68 overweight/obese individuals with serious mental illness enrolled in an outpatient behavioral weight loss program (Lundgren et al., 2010)	19.0 (7.3)
31 females enrolled in an outpatient treatment for bulimia nervosa (Lundgren, Shapiro, & Bulik, 2008)	20.1 (6.6)
68 inpatients seeking treatment for eating disorders (Lundgren et al., 2011)	
Total sample	21.2 (8.6)
Patients diagnosed with anorexia nervosa (*n* = 32)	16.6 (7.5)
Patients diagnosed with bulimia nervosa (*n* = 32)	25.7 (7.9)

this sample was 32.4 ± 6.8 (range 12–45 points). Interestingly, non-obese individuals scored significantly higher than obese individuals on both the NEQ total score and the Nocturnal Ingestion factor.

Finally, Allison and colleagues (2008) examined the positive predictive value and the discriminant validity of the NEQ in 194 individuals seeking evaluation as candidates for bariatric surgery. The positive predictive value, or the number of cases who screened positive on the NEQ and whose diagnosis was later confirmed with interview, increased with higher NEQ values. For example, at a cut score of 25 points (out of a possible 52), the NEQ had a positive predictive value of only 40.7%, meaning that nearly 60% of cases who screened positive were not positive upon interview. At a NEQ cut score of 30 or higher, however, the positive predictive value increased to 72.7%, indicating that, for bariatric surgery candidates, scores of 30 or higher were more indicative of an actual NES diagnosis. Nonetheless, diagnostic confirmation with a more comprehensive clinical interview, as well as sleep and dietary records is suggested (see Chapter 10 [Anderson, Engel, & Crosby] of this volume for a review).

There are some limitations to the design and use of the NEQ. First, the items do not assess the absolute frequency of nocturnal ingestions per week, so that diagnostic criteria cannot be fully assessed. In addition, the proposed diagnostic criteria for NES (Allison, Lundgren, O'Reardon, Geliebter, et al., 2010) state that persons need to exhibit evening hyperphagia (consumption of at least 25% of daily caloric intake after the evening meal) *and/or* nocturnal ingestions twice per week. On the NEQ, responders who only endorse evening hyperphagia do not have the opportunity to score above 30 points, and usually do not even score above 25 points, and thus would not be identified successfully if only the cut scores were used. We have found it helpful to look specifically at the evening hyperphagia item (#5) in addition to the total NEQ score, to reduce the number of false negatives.

The NEQ has been translated into several languages, with several validation studies underway. Harb and colleagues published a Brazilian translation of the NEQ in Portuguese (Harb, Cuamo, & Hidalgo, 2008), while Vinai and colleagues have published an Italian version (Vinai, 2011). Other translations in the process of validation include Spanish (Moize, personal communication), French (Drapeau, personal communication), Hebrew (Latzer et al., personal communication), Korean (in Allison, Stunkard, & Their, 2004, as translated into Korean), and Greek (Karekla, personal communication). Because many of these translations have not yet been published, readers are encouraged to contact the editors of this book for copies or contact information for those individuals who prepared the translations.

The NESS was originally published in a form identical to that of the NEQ except for the focus on symptoms in the previous week (O'Reardon et al., 2004). As such, it is a better tool for tracking symptom change on a frequent basis, for example during treatment. Since its original publication, it has been revised by the research group at the University of Pennsylvania to track the specific number of awakenings and nocturnal ingestions experienced each week. Furthermore, the awareness question was omitted, with the reasoning that, once established at baseline, the level of awareness over eating episodes would likely not vary significantly with the worsening or improvements in symptoms.

In summary, the NEQ is a brief NES symptom scale designed to (1) screen for NES and (2) assess symptom change over time, while the NESS is designed to assess specific symptom levels during the previous week, ideal for use to track progress in an intervention. A copy of the NEQ, along with its instructions for use and scoring, are available in the Allison and colleagues (2008) publication. Of note, in addition to its publication in the Allison paper, it is included in the Weight and Lifestyle Inventory (WALI; Wadden & Foster, 2006) as part of a comprehensive assessment of factors involved in the development, maintenance, and treatment of obesity. The NESS and its scoring key are included in Figures 11.1a and 11.1b.

Directions: Refer to your experiences in the past week. Please give ONE answer for each question.

1. How hungry were you in the morning during the past week?

0	1	2	3	4
Not at all	A little	Somewhat	Moderately	Very

2. When did you usually eat for the first time each day?

0	1	2	3	4
Before 9:00 A.M.	9:01 A.M. to 12:00 P.M.	12:01 to 3:00 P.M.	3:01 to 6:00 P.M.	6:01 P.M. or later

3. Did you have cravings or urges to eat snacks after supper, but before bedtime this week?

0	1	2	3	4
None at all	A little	Somewhat	Very much so	Extremely so

4. How much control do you have over your eating between supper and bedtime?

0	1	2	3	4
None at all	A Little	Somewhat	Very much	Complete

5. How much of your daily food intake did you consume *after* suppertime?

0	1	2	3	4
0% (none)	1–24% (up to a quarter)	25–49% (between a quarter and a half)	50–74% (more than half)	75–100% (almost all)

6. How often did you have trouble getting to sleep this week?

0	1	2	3	4
Never	1–2 times	3–4 times	5–6 times	Every night

7. How many times *total* did you get up in the middle of the night *in the past week*?

_____ # times whole week

8. When you got up in the middle of the night, how many times *total* did you snack *in the past week*?

_____ # times whole week

9. Did you have cravings or urges to eat snacks when you woke up at night this week?

0	1	2	3	4
None at all	A little	Somewhat	Very much so	Extremely so

10. **When you were up at night this week, how much did you need to eat in order to get back to sleep?**

0	1	2	3	4	Check here
Not at all	A little	Somewhat	Very much so	Extremely so	_____

if you did
not get up

11. **How much control do you have over your eating while you are up at night?**

0	1	2	3	4	Check here
Not at all	A little	Some	Very much	Complete	_____

if you did
not get up

12. **Were you feeling blue or down in the dumps this week?**

0	1	2	3	4
Not at all	A little	Somewhat	Very much so	Extremely so

13. **When you were feeling blue, was your mood lower in the:**

0	1	2	3	4	Check here if you
Early morning	Late morning	Afternoon	Early evening	Late evening/ nighttime	did not feel blue at all

FIGURE 11.1a. Night Eating Symptom Scale (NESS). Developed by Kelly C. Allison, Albert J. Stunkard, and John P. O'Reardon. Copyright 2011 by the University of Pennsylvania. For commercial usage, please contact the Center for Technology Transfer of the University of Pennsylvania.

- Step 1: Reverse-score items 1, 4, and 11.
- Step 2: Recode items 7 and 8. A response of 0 = 0 points, 1–2 times = 1 point, 3–4 times = 2 points, 5–6 times = 3 points, and 7+ times = 4 points.
- Step 3: Sum all items for the total score.

FIGURE 11.1b. Night Eating Symptom Scale (NESS) scoring.

Night Eating Diagnostic Questionnaire

The first version of the NEDQ was developed in 2001 by Marci Gluck and Allan Geliebter at the New York Obesity Research Center (Gluck et al., 2001). NEDQ has 21 questions and takes about 10 to 15 minutes to complete. It was designed to assess NES based on the criteria set forth by Stunkard and colleagues in 1999 (Birketvedt, Florholmen, Sundsfjord, Osterud, Dinges, et al., 1999). More recently, the questionnaire was revised to include questions that would diagnose NES based on the recently proposed diagnostic criteria (Allison, Lundgren, O'Reardon, Geliebter, et al., 2010). One of the unique aspects of this questionnaire is that it assesses morning anorexia and also includes an objective measure of the number of days in which patients eat breakfast and experience sleep difficulties and/or wake up in the night to eat. In addition, evening hyperphagia is assessed based both on the criteria of 25% of daily food intake after the evening meal, as stated by the most recent criteria for NES (Allison, Lundgren, O'Reardon, Geliebter, et al., 2010), and on 25% of daily food intake after 7:00 P.M., as stated by previous criteria (Stunkard et al., 1996). Although the scoring is based on the new criteria, because the hour of evening meal differs cross-culturally (Adami, Meneghelli, & Scopinaro, 1997), it might be useful to assess a variety of symptomatology and be able to report that information in published papers as the diagnostic criteria for NES continue to evolve. Lastly, the authors created an experimental hierarchical scoring method to assess mild, moderate, and full-syndrome night eaters. A validation study of the NEDQ is currently being conducted by Allan Geliebter at the New York Obesity Research Center. The NEDQ and its scoring key are included in Figures 11.2a and 11.2b. Citation and information for use are included below the questionnaire.

Directions: Please answer the following questions carefully and be sure to answer each question. Thank you for your participation.

1. What time do you usually go to bed in the evening (turn out the lights in order to go to sleep)? _____ P.M.

2. What time do you usually get out of bed in the morning? _____ A.M.

3. On most days, do you experience loss of appetite in the morning?   ☐ No ☐ Yes

4. How often do you typically eat breakfast (after your final _____ times/week morning awakening)?

5. What time do you usually have the first meal of the day? _____ A.M./P.M. (please circle)

6. How much food do you generally eat after 7:00 P.M. as a (0–100) _____% percentage (%) from 0 to 100? (Please be specific, for example, 15%.)

7. What time do you usually have your evening meal? _____ P.M.

8. How much food do you generally eat after your evening meal as a percentage (%) from 0 to 100? (Please be specific, for example, 15%.)   (0–100) _____%

8a. For how long have you been consuming at least this much

_____ years

after your evening meal?   _____ months

9. On most days, do you have a strong urge to eat between dinner and sleep onset
and/or during the night?   □ No □ Yes

10. Do you have trouble falling asleep at night?   □ No □ Yes

10a. If YES, how many times each week?   _____ times/week

11. Do you have trouble staying asleep at night?   □ No □ Yes

11a. If YES, how many times each week?   _____ times/week

11b. If YES, how many times each week do you get out of bed during these
awakenings?   _____ times/week

12. How many times each week do you awake from sleep during the night to use the
bathroom?   _____ times/week   □ None

13. Do you awake from sleep during the night and eat food?   □ No □ Yes

IF NO, SKIP TO QUESTION 14.

13a. If yes, how many times per week?   _____ times/week

13b. For how long have you been getting up at this frequency to eat?

_____ years
_____ months

13c. Do you believe you need to eat in order to fall back to sleep when
you wake up at night?   □ No □ Yes

13d. How aware are you of your eating during the night?   □ Not at all
□ Somewhat
□ Extremely

13e. How often do you recall your eating during the night the next day?
□ Never
□ Sometimes
□ Always

14. Would you consider yourself a night eater?   □ No □ Yes
IF NO, SKIP TO QUESTION 15.
IF YES (please answer the following questions):

14a. IF YES, how upset are you about your night eating?   □ Not at all
□ Somewhat
□ Extremely

14b. IF YES, how much has your eating at night impaired your functioning and/or
interfered with your daily life?   □ Not at all
□ Somewhat
□ Extremely

14c. For how long have you been experiencing this night eating behavior?

□ Less than 3 months
□ 3–6 months
□ 6–12 months
□ More than 1 year

FIGURE 11.2a. (*continued on next page*)

15. Do you have sleep apnea?   □ No □ Yes
                                                               □ Don't know
16. Do you work an evening or night shift?   □ No □ Yes
   16a. IF YES, is it: □ Evening
                                                               □ Night
                                                               □ Rotating
   16b. IF YES, for how long have you been working this shift? _____ years
                                                                _____ months
17. Have you been feeling depressed or down nearly every day?   □ No □ Yes
18. In general, when you are feeling depressed or down, is your mood lower in the:
                                                               □ Morning
                                                               □ Afternoon
                                                               □ Evening/nighttime
                                                               □ Not applicable
19. Are you currently dieting to lose weight?   □ No □ Yes
   19a. IF YES, how much weight have you lost in the past 3 months? _____ lb.
20. What is your current height and weight (without clothing or shoes)?
                                                               _____Height (in.)
                                                               _____Weight (lb.)
21. Please take a moment to review your responses. Have you answered
    each question completely?   □ No □ Yes

FIGURE 11.2a. Night Eating Diagnositc Questionnaire (NEDQ).

To be diagnosed with NES, the individual must have the following:

I. The daily pattern of eating demonstrates a significantly increased intake in the
   evening and/or nighttime, as manifested by one or both of the following:
   A. At least 25% of food intake is consumed after the evening meal
      Q 8 ≥ 25% and Q 8a ≥ 3 months
   B. At least two episodes of nocturnal eating per week
      Q 13 = yes AND Q 13a ≥ 2 d/wk AND Q 13b ≥ 3 months
II. Awareness and recall of evening and nocturnal eating episodes are present.
    Q 13d = somewhat or extremely and/or Q 13e = sometimes or always
III. The clinical picture is characterized by *at least three* of the following features:
    A. Lack of desire to eat in the morning and/or breakfast is omitted on four or more
       mornings per week
       Q3 = yes OR Q4 ≤ 3 times/week
    B. Presence of a strong urge to eat between dinner and sleep onset and/or during
       the night
       Q 9 = yes
    C. Sleep onset and/or sleep maintenance insomnia are present four or more
       nights per week
       Q 10 or Q 11 = Yes and Q 10a or Q 11a ≥ 4 times/week
    D. Presence of a belief that one must eat in order to initiate or return to sleep
       Q 13c = Yes
    E. Mood is frequently depressed and/or mood worsens in the evening
       Q 17 = yes OR Q 18 = evening/nighttime

IV. The disorder is associated with significant distress and/or impairment in functioning.
Q 14a OR Q 14 b = somewhat or extremely
V. The disordered pattern of eating has been maintained for a minimum of 3 months.
14c = 3–6 months OR 6–12 months OR more than 1 year
VI. The disorder is not secondary to substance abuse or dependence, medical disorder, medication, or another psychiatric disorder: This cannot be assessed using the questionnaire but should be noted.

Standard Scoring Based on Above
Dichotomous
1. **Non-NE** = *normal* (does not meet criteria category below)
2. **NES** = *full-syndrome night eater* has 1 criterion from I **plus** ≥ 3 of 5 qualifiers from criteria III **plus** IV and V

Experimental Scoring
Hierarchical
1. **Non-NE** = *normal* (does not meet any criteria category below)
2. **N** = *mild night eater* has 1 criteria from I (but does not meet criteria NE or NES)
3. **NE** = *moderate night eater* has 1 criteria from I **plus** ≥ 3 of 5 qualifiers from criteria III (but does not meet criteria for NES)
4. **NES** = *full-syndrome night eater* has ≥ 1 from I **plus** ≥ 3 of 5 qualifiers from criteria III **plus** IV and V

FIGURE 11.2b. Night Eating Diagnostic Questionnaire (NEDQ) scoring.

Interview Assessments

Only two clinical interviews assess night eating behavior: the NESHI and a portion of the EDE. These are reviewed below.

Eating Disorder Examination

The EDE is the gold-standard clinical interview for the assessment of disordered eating behavior (Black & Wilson, 1996). It yields four quantitative subscales (Weight Concern, Shape Concern, Eating Concern, Dietary Restraint) and a Global Scale. The most recent version of the EDE (Fairburn, Cooper, & O'Connor, 2008; version 16.0) includes three questions on evening and nocturnal eating behavior in the "Pattern of Eating" section. Interviewers can obtain the frequency of evening snacks and nocturnal eating, defined as an episode of eating after the person has been to sleep, during the previous 28 days. In addition, a rating of one's awareness during nocturnal eating episodes is obtained for anyone who reports nocturnal eating behavior during the previous 28 days.

Two recent reports have suggested that night eating behavior is quite common among individuals diagnosed with eating disorders (Lundgren et al., 2008; Lundgren et al., 2011). Given the frequency with which night eating has been noted in these samples, clinicians and researchers are encouraged to report on the night eating questions when using the EDE in eating disorder assessment and treatment studies.

Night Eating Syndrome History and Inventory

The NESHI, originally developed by Kelly Allison, Albert Stunkard, and John O'Reardon at the University of Pennsylvania, is a semistructured clinical interview for the assessment and diagnosis of NES during the previous 28 days. To date it has not been published, and the version included in this chapter has been updated to reflect the recently proposed research diagnostic criteria for NES (Allison, Lundgren, O'Reardon, Geliebter, et al., 2010). The NESHI follows the NEQ content closely, because the NEQ questions are embedded in it, and an NEQ score is attainable from it. It differs substantially from the NEQ, however, in that it is clinician administered and there are several additional open-ended questions aimed to gather details about the individual's night eating and associated behaviors.

Perhaps the most difficult aspect of NES to assess is the concept of evening hyperphagia. We have found through our clinical and research assessment experience that persons overestimate the percentage of food consumed after the evening meal. One example of this comes from a study where we recruited participants based on the criteria of consuming half of daily intake after dinner. After completing food journals for a week, the average intake after dinner was calculated at 35%, not 50% (O'Reardon et al., 2004). We have also found that patients often have trouble weighting how much they have eaten in their previous meals, and then they overvalue the amount eaten at night. This may also be influenced by their belief that the evening or night is the period of time that is problematic, which may cause them to inflate their estimate of intake during this period. Whatever the reason, it is important to highlight the typical daily pattern of eating before estimating the percent of intake consumed after dinner. Thus the NESHI includes prompts for descriptions of food intake throughout a typical 24-hour period before determining whether evening hyperphagia is present.

When administering the NESHI, it is important for the clinician to use the follow-up questions to confirm or disconfirm the participant's verbal response to questions and to assign a response to numbered (and scored) items based on all information available, not just participant initial self-report. This version of the NESHI also includes several questions to assess impairment and distress associated with NES, compensatory

Overview: The NESHI was developed by Allison, Lundgren, O'Reardon, and Stunkard. It is a comprehensive semistructured clinical interview developed to assess the degree of and severity of NES symptoms and to establish a diagnosis of NES based on research diagnostic criteria (see Allison et al., 2010). The Night Eating Questionnaire (NEQ; Allison et al., 2008) is embedded in the NESHI (numbered items), and instructions for calculating the NEQ score are included in the interview. In addition, the NESHI includes a checklist to determine the patient's NEQ diagnosis (none, subthreshold, full threshold).

Patient name: _____ Date of interview: _____

Male: _____ Female: _____ Ethnicity: _____ Age: _____

Height: _____ Current weight: _____ Current BMI: _____

Section 1: Current Symptoms
Please answer the following questions according to your behavior during the past 4 weeks (28 days).
- What time do you typically get up each day?
1. How hungry are you usually in the morning?

0	1	2	3	4
Not at all	A little	Somewhat	Moderately	Very

2. When do you usually eat for the first time?

0	1	2	3	4
Before 9:00 A.M.	9:01 A.M. to 12:00 P.M.	12:01 to 3:00 P.M.	3:01 to 6:00 P.M.	6:01 P.M. or later

Estimate with the patient how many days per week he or she has experienced a lack of desire to eat in the morning or has omitted breakfast (Criterion III A): _____
For each possible eating episode ask how often that meal or snack is typically eaten (# days per week), what time it is usually consumed, and what types of food and how much are usually eaten.

Meal/snack	# Days/wk	Time	What and how much?
Breakfast			
Morning snack			
Lunch			
Afternoon snack			
Dinner			

3. Do you have cravings or urges to eat snacks after supper, but before bedtime? (Criterion III B)

0	1	2	3	4
None at all	A little	Somewhat	Very much so	Extremely so

FIGURE 11.3. (*continued*)

4. **How much control do you have over your eating between supper and bedtime?**

0	1	2	3	4
None at all	A Little	Somewhat	Very much	Complete

- When do you usually go to bed?
- Do you have any problems falling asleep? How long does it usually take (as long as 30 minutes)?

5. **How often do you have trouble getting to sleep? (Criterion III C)**

0	1	2	3	4
Never	Sometimes	About half the time	Usually	Always

6. **How often do you get up at least once in the middle of the night? (Criterion III C)**

0	1	2	3	4
Never	Less than once a week	About once a week	More than once a week	Every night

Criterion III C: Estimate with the patient how many nights per week he or she has difficulty falling asleep or maintaining sleep: _____

***** If answered "never," skip down to calculate percentage of food eaten after the evening meal and complete remaining interview questions. ****************

7. **Do you have cravings or urges to eat snacks when you wake up at night? (Criterion III B)**

0	1	2	3	4
None at all	A little	Somewhat	Very much so	Extremely so

8. **Do you need to eat in order to get back to sleep when you awake at night? (Criterion III D)**

0	1	2	3	4
None at all	A little	Somewhat	Very much so	Extremely so

9. **When you get up in the middle of the night, how often do you snack?**

0	1	2	3	4
Never	Sometimes	About half	Usually	Always

* If > "never," how many episodes of nocturnal eating do you experience per week? **(Criterion I B): _____**

Meal/ snack	# episodes /wk	Typical times?	What and how much?
Nocturnal ingestion			

- When you snack in the middle of the night, how aware are you of your eating? (Circle one; if "Not at all" or "A little," may be sleep-related eating disorder.) **(Criterion II)**
  Not at all   A little   Somewhat   Very much so   Completely

FIGURE 11.3. (*continued*)

10. How much control do you have over your eating while you are up at night?

0	1	2	3	4
None at all	A Little	Some	Very much	Complete

Based on the amount eaten during meals and snacks during the day, evening, and night, estimate with the patient what proportion of his or her total daily intake he or she consumes *after* the evening meal (this includes snacks before bedtime and nocturnal ingestions) :   % (Criterion I A)

11. How much of your daily food intake do you consume *after* suppertime?

0	1	2	3	4
0%	1–25%	26–50%	51–75%	76–100%

12. Are you currently feeling blue or down in the dumps? (Criterion III E)

0	1	2	3	4
Not at all	A little	Somewhat	Very much so	Extremely

13. When you are feeling blue, is your mood lower in the (circle one): (Criterion III E)

0	1	2	3	4	0
Early morning	Late morning	Afternoon	Early evening	Late evening/ nighttime	Mood does not change during the day

If the core features of NES (eating ≥ 25% of intake after evening meal and/or nocturnal ingestions ≥ 2 times per week) are present, rate the following (if not, stop interview here):

Section 2: Distress and Compensation
Criterion IV: Distress/Impairment in Functioning:
Answers must be reported at 3 or 4.

A. Is your night eating upsetting to you?

0	1	2	3	4
Not at all	A little	Somewhat	Very much so	Extremely

B. Have you felt any shame because of your night eating?

0	1	2	3	4
None	A little	Somewhat	Very much	Extreme

C. Have you felt guilty because of night eating?

0	1	2	3	4
None	A little	Somewhat	Very much	Extreme

D. How much has your night eating affected your life?

0	1	2	3	4
Not at all	A little	Somewhat	Very much so	Extremely

Assessment of Compensatory Behaviors:
A. Have you ever done or used the following during a time when (or shortly after) you were night eating?
   1) Make yourself vomit: Yes   No
   2) Laxatives: Yes   No

FIGURE 11.3. (*continued*)

3) Diuretics (water pills):	Yes	No
4) Diet pills (over the counter or prescription):	Yes	No
5) Exercise more than 2 hours per day:	Yes	No
6) Fast or not eat (for 24 hours or more):	Yes	No
7) Other methods—please indicate below:	Yes	No

B. If yes to any purgative method, how often? _____

Section 3: History and Course
Background:
A. At what age did you begin night eating? _____ **(Criterion V)**
B. How much did you weigh when you began night eating (to assess if normal weight or overweight at onset)? _____
C. How often did you diet before your night eating began?
    1. never
    2. once every couple of years
    3. once or twice a year
    4. once every 3 months or more
D. Before you began night eating, did you (circle all that apply; **Criterion IV**):
    1. stay up late at night regularly
    2. work a night shift; if yes, when/how long? _____
    3. endure a stressful event; if yes, identify: _____
    4. experience a medical condition that would account for night eating behavior
    5. begin medication/substance that would account for night eating behavior
E. Does anyone else in your family have symptoms of night eating?
_____

F. What strategies, medications, or supplements have you tried to stop night eating, and were they successful (e.g., sleeping pills, melatonin, SSRIs)?
    1. _____
    2. _____
    3. _____
G. What factors have influenced your night eating:
    1. Is it the same on weekdays and weekends? Y N
_____
    2. When you sleep at a hotel or away from home, do you still eat this way? Y N
_____
3. Do your symptoms differ during times of stress? Y N
_____

Section 4: Diagnosis
NES Diagnosis (check criteria based on NESHI interview and other corroborating clinical evidence [e.g., food record]):
_____ I. The daily pattern of eating demonstrates a significantly increased intake in the evening and/or nighttime, as manifested by *one or both* of the following:
    _____ A. At least 25% of food intake is consumed after the evening meal
    _____ B. At least two episodes of nocturnal eating per week
_____ II. Awareness and recall of evening and nocturnal eating episodes are present.
_____ III. The clinical picture is characterized by *at least three* of the following features are scored as a 3 or 4 on the appropriate items:
    _____ A. Lack of desire to eat in the morning and/or breakfast is omitted on four or more mornings per week

FIGURE 11.3. (*continued*)

_____ B. Presence of a strong urge to eat between dinner and sleep onset
and/or during the night
_____ C. Sleep onset and/or sleep maintenance insomnia are present four
or more nights per week
_____ D. Presence of a belief that one must eat in order to initiate or return
to sleep
_____ E. Mood is frequently depressed and/or mood worsens in the
evening
_____ IV. The disorder is associated with significant distress and/or impairment in
functioning (at least two of the features in this section are rated at a 3 or 4).
_____ V. The disordered pattern of eating has been maintained for at least 3 months.
_____ VI. The disorder is not secondary to substance abuse or dependence, medical
disorder, medication, or another psychiatric disorder.

Directions for scoring the NEQ: (1) Reverse-score items 1, 4, and 10. (2) Sum all
numbered items.
NEQ score after interview: _____
NES Diagnosis (circle): None_____ Subthreshold _____ Full threshold _____

FIGURE 11.3. Night Eating Syndrome History and Inventory (NESHI).
Copyright by the University of Pennsylvania. For commercial usage, please
contact the Center for Technology Transfer of the University of Pennsylvania.

behaviors in response to night eating behavior, background factors that
may have contributed to the onset of NES, and a checklist for establishing a diagnosis based on the interview. In Figure 11.3 we have included
the NESHI and its instructions for use.

Assessment in Clinical Contexts

As we have reviewed in this chapter, there are both brief and comprehensive instruments available for assessing NES and its associated features. Table 11.2 presents a side-by-side comparison of their features and
intended uses.

When beginning treatment with individuals with NES, we suggest that
a clinician begin by administering the NESHI (Figure 11.3). This allows
the clinician to determine the current pattern of night eating (both evening
hyperphagia and nocturnal ingestions of food), as well as the associated
mood, sleep, and hunger features. From this interview, the clinicians should
have a good sense of the potential etiology of NES for the individual, the
current factors that may serve to maintain the night eating behavior, previous treatment attempts, and several areas to target during treatment. (See
Chapters 13 and 14 [Allison] for a detailed review of cognitive-behavioral
therapy for NES; see also Chapter 12 [Patel, O'Reardon, and Cristancho]

TABLE 11.2. Comparison of NES Assessment Instruments

Instrument name	Assessment type	Assessment length/ administration time	Purpose of assessment instrument
NEQ	Self-report	14 items; 5–10 minutes	Symptom assessment, treatment outcome
NESS	Self-report	13 items; 5–10 minutes	Symptom assessment over past week, treatment outcome
NEDQ	Self-report	21 items; 10–15 minutes	Diagnosis
NESHI	Semistructured clinical interview	Several items, both open ended and Likert-type; 45–60 minutes	Diagnosis, history, symptom assessment
EDE	Structured clinical interview	3 items included in larger assessment; 5 minutes for night eating questions, 45–60 minutes for full assessment	Night eating behavior frequency and awareness; treatment outcome

Note. NEQ, Night Eating Questionnaire (Allison et al., 2008); NESS, Night Eating Symptom Scale; NEDS, Night Eating Diagnostic Questionnaire (Gluck, Geliebter, & Satov, 2001); NESHI, Night Eating Syndrome History and Inventory; EDE, Eating Disorder Examination (Fairburn, Cooper, & O'Connor, 2008).

for a review of pharmacological treatment for NES, and Chapter 15 [Pawlow] for a review of other approaches for the treatment of NES.)

If the patient notes compensatory behaviors, especially for individuals with a history of anorexia nervosa or bulimia nervosa, we suggest that the clinician also administer the EDE to get a better sense of their body-image concerns and general disordered eating behaviors. For obese individuals without additional eating-disordered and compensatory behaviors, an additional assessment tool such as the WALI (Wadden & Foster, 2006) would provide valuable information, especially if the patient planned to attempt weight loss as part of the treatment for NES.

Once treatment has begun, the NEQ is ideal for assessing symptom severity and change in symptoms over time. For more frequent symptoms assessment (e.g., weekly symptom monitoring), the NESS would be more appropriate. The NESS has been used successfully in both psychotherapeutic (Allison, Lundgren, O'Reardon, Moore, & Stunkard, 2010) and pharmacological treatments for NES (O'Reardon et al., 2004; O'Reardon et al., 2006; Stunkard et al., 2006).

In addition to the assessment resources reviewed in this chapter, clinicians are also encouraged to use daily food records to assess change in eating patterns, including the frequency and size of breakfast, evening hyperphagia, and nocturnal ingestions of food. Actigraphy and polysomnography can be helpful in ruling out sleep disorders and parasomnias (e.g., SRED and others are reviewed in Chapter 9 [Howell and Crow]), but may be of limited practicality in some clinical settings.

Areas for Future Research

The assessment of NES has developed significantly since Stunkard first observed the night eating patterns of "Ms. M." described in Chapter 2. Fortunately, there are both self-report and clinical interviews available for use in both clinical and research settings. Despite these advances in the assessment of NES, much work needs to be done.

First, psychometric studies are needed to replicate the Allison and colleagues (2008) validation study of the NEQ. In particular, given the high rates of NES in psychiatric and eating-disordered populations (Lundgren et al., 2006; Lundgren, Shapiro, & Bulik, 2008; Lundgren et al., 2010), the NEQ and NEDQ need to be validated in these samples. Based on the experience of the authors, this can be a challenging task. For example, the many executive functioning deficits noted among persons with schizophrenia (Zayat, Rempfer, Gajewski, & Brown, 2011) could affect the reliability of patient responses. The authors are not aware of any published papers that have assessed test–retest reliability of the NEQ or NEDQ in any sample, let alone a psychiatric sample.

Similarly, additional work needs to be done to develop and validate night eating assessment tools appropriate for children and adolescents. Although rare in children and young adults, night eating behavior has been documented (Streigel-Moore et al., 2004). In a recent study (Gallant, Lundgren, Allison, Stunkard, Lambert, et al., in press), children ages 8 to 10 completed the French NEQ, and their mother also responded to a subset of NEQ questions. Interestingly, there were substantial differences in child compared to mother report on the questions related to sleep disturbance, and minor discrepancies in the ratings for evening hyperphagia, nocturnal ingestions of food, and morning anorexia.

Finally, we recommend that researchers explore additional modes of assessment (e.g., real-time, *in vivo* self-monitoring) so as to better understand the functional relationship between night eating behavior and sleep and to help differentiate NES from other eating disorders, such as binge-eating disorder.

References

Adami, G. E., Meneghelli, A., & Scopinaro, N. (1997). Night eating syndrome in individuals with Mediterranean eating-style. *Eating and Weight Disorders: Studies on Anorexia, Bulimia, and Obesity, 2,* 203–206.

Allison, K. C., Lundgren, J. D., O'Reardon, J. P., Geliebter, A., Gluck, M., Vinai, P., et al. (2010). Proposed diagnostic criteria for night eating syndrome. *International Journal of Eating Disorders, 43,* 241–247.

Allison, K. C., Lundgren, J. D., O'Reardon, J. P., Moore, R. H., Stunkard, A. J. (2010). Cognitive behavior therapy for night eating syndrome: A pilot study. *American Journal of Psychotherapy, 64,* 94–106.

Allison, K. C., Lundgren, J. D., O'Reardon, J. P., Sarwer, D. B., Wadden, T. A., & Stunkard, A. J. (2008). The night eating questionnaire (NEQ): Psychometric properties of a screening tool for the diagnosis of night eating syndrome. *Eating Behaviors, 9,* 62–72.

Allison, K. C., Stunkard, A. J., & Their, S. L. (2004). *Overcoming the night eating syndrome: A step-by-step guide to breaking the cycle.* Oakland, CA: New Harbinger.

Beck, A. T. (1996). *The Beck Depression Inventory II.* San Antonio: Harcourt Brace.

Birketvedt, G., Florholmen, J., Sundsfjord, J., Osterud, B., Dinges, D., Bilker, W., et al. (1999). Behavioral and neuroendocrine characteristics of the night-eating syndrome. *Journal of the American Medical Association, 282,* 657–663.

Black, C. M. D., & Wilson, G. T. (1996). Assessment of eating disorders: Interview versus questionnaire. *International Journal of Eating Disorders, 20,* 43–50.

Fairburn, C. G., Cooper, Z., & O'Connor, M. E. (2008). Eating Disorder Examination (Edition 16.0D). In C. G. Fairburn (Ed.), *Cognitive behavior therapy and eating disorders* (pp. 265–308). New York: Guilford Press.

Gallant, A. R., Lundren, J. D., Allison, K. C., Stunkard, A. J., Lambert, M. O'Loughlin, J., et al. (in press). Validity of the night eating questionnaire in children. *International Journal of Eating Disorders.*

Gluck, M. E., Geliebter, A., & Satov, T. (2001). Night eating syndrome is associated with depression, low self-esteem, reduced daytime hunger, and less weight loss in obese outpatients. *Obesity Research, 9,* 264–267.

Harb, A. B., Caumo, W., & Hidalgo, M. P. (2008). Translation and adaptation of the Brazilian version of the Night Eating Questionnaire. *Cadernos de Saúde Pública, 24*(6), 1368–1376.

Lundgren, J. D., Allison, K. C., Crow, S., Berg, K. C., Galbraith, J., Martino, N. S., et al. (2006). Prevalence of the night eating syndrome in a psychiatric population. *American Journal of Psychiatry, 163*(1), 156–158.

Lundgren, J. D., McCune, A., Spresser, C. D., Harkins, P., Zolton, L., & Mandal, K. K. (2011). Night eating patterns of individuals with eating disorders: Implications for conceptualizing the night eating syndrome. *Psychiatry Research, 186*(1), 103–108.

Lundgren, J. D., Rempfer, M. V., Brown, C. E., Goetz, J., & Hamera, E. (2010).

The prevalence of night eating syndrome and binge-eating disorder among overweight and obese individuals with serious mental illness. *Psychiatry Research, 175,* 233–236.

Lundgren, J. D., Shapiro, J. R., & Bulik, C. (2008). Night eating patterns of patients with bulimia nervosa: A preliminary report. *Eating and Weight Disorders: Studies on Anorexia, Bulimia, and Obesity, 13*(4), 171–175.

Morrow, J., Gluck, M. E., Flancbaum, L., Lorence, M., & Geliebter, A. (2008). Night eating syndrome and weight loss after Ru-en-Y gastric bypass surgery. *Eating and Weight Disorders: Studies on Anorexia, Bulimia, and Obesity, 13*(4), e96–e99.

O'Reardon, J. P., Allison, K. C., Martino, N. S., Lundgren, J. D., Heo, M., & Stunkard, A. J. (2006). A randomized placebo-controlled trial of sertraline in the treatment of the night eating syndrome. *American Journal of Psychiatry, 163,* 893–898.

O'Reardon, J. P., Stunkard, A. J., & Allison, K. C. (2004). A clinical trial of sertraline in the treatment of night eating syndrome. *International Journal of Eating Disorders 35,* 16–26.

Striegel-Moore, R. H., Thompson, D., Franko, D. L., Barton, B., Affenito, S., Schreiber, G. B., et al. (2004). Definition of night eating in adolescent girls. *Obesity Research, 12,* 1311–1321.

Stunkard, A. J., Berkowitz, R., Wadden, T., Tanrikut, C., Reiss, E., & Young, L. (1996). Binge eating disorder and the night eating syndrome. *International Journal of Obesity and Related Metabolic Disorders, 20*(1), 1–6.

Stunkard, A. J., Allison, K. C., Lundgren, J. D., Martino, N. S., Heo, M., Etemad, B., et al. (2006). A paradigm for facilitating pharmacotherapy research at a distance: Treatment of the night eating syndrome. *Journal of Clinical Psychiatry 67,* 1568–1572.

Stunkard, A. J., Grace, W. J., Wolff, H. G. (1955). The night eating syndrome: A pattern of food intake among certain obese patients. *American Journal of Medicine, 19,* 78–86.

Vinai, P. (Ed.). (2011). *Pathways to obesity and main roads to recovery.* New York: Nova.

Wadden, T. A., & Foster, G. D. (2006). The Weight and Lifestyle Inventory (WALI). *Obesity, 14*(Suppl. 2), S99–S118.

Zayat, E., Rempfer, M., Gajewski, B., & Brown, C. E. (2011). Patterns of association between performance in a natural environment and measures of executive function in people with schizophrenia. *Psychiatry Research, 187*(1–2), 1–5.

PART V

TREATMENT

Chapter 12

Pharmacological Treatment of Night Eating Syndrome

Kajal R. Patel
John P. O'Reardon
Mario A. Cristancho

Night eating syndrome (NES) was initially described by Stunkard, Grace, and Wolff in 1955. One would expect given the evolution of more than five decades since its first elucidation, that extensive research on etiology and pharmacological treatment of NES would have been completed. To the contrary, only in last decade has the literature on NES started to expand and with it our understanding of this novel eating disorder. In fact, the First International Symposium of NES expert investigators took place just in 2008 and produced consensus provisional diagnostic criteria (Allison et al., 2010). The purpose of this chapter is to review the limited available literature to guide the pharmacological treatment of NES.

Recognition of NES and Target Symptoms

The diagnosis of NES is frequently missed due to lack of clinician awareness as well as patients' apparent aversion to volunteer symptoms due to embarrassment. It is therefore important to screen individuals actively for this disorder in clinical settings, including primary care medical practice.

NES is characterized by morning anorexia, evening hyperphagia, insomnia (both initial and middle), and nighttime awakenings that are frequently accompanied by food ingestion (Birketvedt et al., 1999). Individuals with NES are clearly distressed by the symptoms and its consequences such as weight gain and mood symptoms. Associated mood symptoms include depressed mood with sometimes diurnal variation (i.e., worse in the evening; Birketvedt et al., 1999; Stunkard et al., 1955). Other important clinical features include a perceived loss of control over night eating episodes and fatigue in the daytime, which is likely secondary to sleep deprivation. The consensus set of diagnostic criteria for NES will help to standardize the diagnosis and serve both research and clinical purposes. NES's diagnostic criteria, clinical characteristics, and differential diagnosis are discussed in more detail in Chapter 1 (Lundgren, Allison, & Stunkard) and earlier sections of this volume.

Pharmacotherapy of NES

Pathophysiology of NES

It is believed that alteration of neuroendocrine circadian rhythms is a core feature of this eating disorder. NES is fundamentally characterized by dissociation between eating and sleep rhythms with a delay in food intake but not in the onset and offset, timewise, of sleep rhythm (O'Reardon, Ringel, et al., 2004). Serotonergic neurons of the dorsal raphe nucleus have modulatory inputs to the suprachiasmatic nucleus (SCN), which maintains circadian rhythms (O'Reardon, Peshek, & Allison, 2005). Furthermore, studies on subjects with NES have shown that serotonin transporter (SERT) binding is increased in the midbrain (Lundgren et al., 2008).

Thus a plausible serotonergic hypothesis of the etiology of NES is a that a relative deficiency of synaptic serotonin in serotonergic nuclei in the midbrain due to hyperactivity of the serotonin transporter SERT leads to downstream dysregulation of sleep and food intake circadian rhythms in the SCN in the hypothalamus (Stunkard, Allison, Lundgren, & O'Reardon, 2009). The cause of the fundamental SERT hyperactivity is unknown. Based on these observations, it has been hypothesized that increasing postsynaptic serotonergic activity by blockade of the serotonin reuptake transporter by means of selective serotonin reuptake inhibitors (SSRIs) should be efficacious in treating NES (Stunkard et al., 2009).

Selective Serotonin Reuptake Inhibitors

Evidence of the beneficial role of SSRIs in the treatment of NES includes case reports, case series, open-label clinical trials, and one randomized placebo-controlled trial.

Case Reports

A positive role of serotoninergic agents in the treatment of NES was initially reported by Spaggiari et al. (1994). They treated seven patients with NES with *d*-fenfluramine (a serotonin releaser) and reported benefit. Later, Friedman, Even, Dardennes, and Guelfi (2002) reported the successful treatment of NES with 14 sessions of phototherapy in a 51-year-old obese female patient. Phototherapy is known to have a serotonergic basis biologically. The use of serotonergic agents in NES was further investigated by Miyaoka et al. (2003) who treated four female patients with night eating and clinical characteristics of NES. Three of these subjects responded robustly to paroxetine (20–40 mg/day) with resolution of NES symptoms within 2 weeks. The fourth subject had a similar response to a low dosage of fluvoxamine (25 mg/day) within 3 weeks.

Open-Label Clinical Trials

More formal evidence of SSRI efficacy was reported by O'Reardon, Stunkard, and Allison (2004) in an open-label clinical trial (see Figure 12.1). In their 12-week study 17 adults with body mass index ≥ 27 who met diagnostic research criteria for NES were treated with sertraline (titrated to maximum dose of 200 mg/day—mean dose of 188 mg/day). Sertraline was chosen over other SSRIs such as fluoxetine and paroxetine given its capacity to reduce compulsive eating in binge-eating disorder (McElroy et al., 2000) and because of the negative potential for over-stimulation/insomnia with fluoxetine and weight gain with paroxetine, respectively.

   At the end of the trial significant reduction of sleep interruptions, nocturnal ingestions, and evening caloric intake after the evening meal was observed. A response rate of 67% (with response defined by the standard Clinical Global Impression of Improvement [CGI-I] Scale score of ≤ 2) was reported for those who completed the study (*n* = 12). Remission rate was 29% (CGI-I = 1). Weight loss among remitters was reported to be –4.8 kg (*SD* = 2.6 kg). Of note, sertraline's effects on NES seemed to be independent of its antidepressant effects (O'Reardon, Stunkard, et al., 2004).

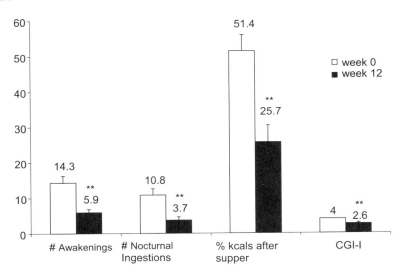

FIGURE 12.1. Intent-to-treat outcome measures from the open-label treatment study of sertraline. # Awakenings, number of times per week that subjects woke up and got out of bed; # Nocturnal Ingestions, nocturnal ingestions per week; % kcals after supper, percentage of total daily caloric intake occurring after the evening meal; CGI-I, overall improvement in study sample. From O'Reardon, Stunkard, and Allison (2004). Copyright 2004 by John Wiley & Sons, Inc. Reprinted by permission.

Additional evidence of benefit from sertraline in the treatment of NES of an open-label nature was reported by Stunkard et al. (2006). They included 50 NES patients (n = 9 normal-weight subjects, n = 41 overweight and obese) in an open-label study using a novel long-distance approach (i.e., sertraline was prescribed by patient's personal physician, who received back-up consultation with an NES specialist from the study staff, as needed). Sertraline again was effective in the treatment of NES as evidenced by statistically significant decreases on the Night Eating Symptom Scale (NESS), evening hyperphagia, nighttime awakenings, and nocturnal ingestions. Furthermore, a significant 3.0 kg reduction in mean body weight in the 41 overweight and obese subjects in the sample was observed (Stunkard et al., 2006).

Placebo-Controlled Trial

The strongest evidence to date to support SSRI efficacy in NES comes from that conducted by O'Reardon et al. (2006) (see Figure 12.2). This

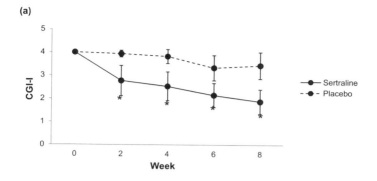

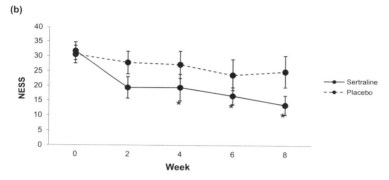

FIGURE 12.2. Results from the 8-week randomized controlled trial of sertraline for NES. (a) CGI-I trends over 8 weeks in the sertraline and placebo groups. p value is significant (< .0125) for weeks 2, 4, 6, and 8. (b) NESS trends over 8 weeks in the sertraline and placebo groups. p value is significant (< 0.0125) for weeks 4, 6, and 8.

(continued on next page)

placebo-controlled trial randomized 34 adult patients with BMI > 18.5 kg/m² and a diagnosis of NES to 8 weeks of either sertraline ($n = 17$) or placebo ($n = 17$). Response rates (defined as CGI-I score of ≤ 2—primary outcome) were 71% and 18% in the medication and placebo groups, respectively, essentially an impressive fourfold better response rate with the active drug. Furthermore, overweight and obese subjects in the sertraline group lost significantly more weight (mean = –2.9 kg, SD = 3.8 kg) after 8 weeks compared to the placebo group (mean = –0.3 kg, SD = 2.7 kg). The largest degree of reduction of symptoms of NES occurred in the first 2 weeks, indicating an early therapeutic effect.

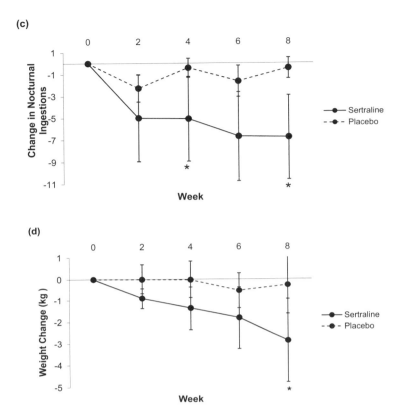

FIGURE 12.2. (*continued*) (c) Change in frequency of nocturnal ingestions per week from the baseline in the sertraline and placebo groups over 8 weeks. *p* value is significant (< .0125) for weeks 4 and 8. (d) Weight change (kg) per week from the baseline in overweight subjects in the sertraline and placebo groups over 8 weeks. *p* value is significant (= .009) at week 8. From O'Reardon et al. (2006). Copyright 2006 by the American Psychiatric Association. Reprinted by permission of the *American Journal of Psychiatry*.

Significant improvements in some secondary measures were also detected: NESS scale score, frequency of nocturnal ingestions, and extent of calorie intake after supper. The dose of sertraline found to be effective in the study ranged between 50 and 200 mg, which is the regular antidepressant dose.

The beneficial role of sertraline in the treatment of NES may extend to other SSRIs and likely also to the dual-acting serotonin and norepinephrine reuptake inhibitors (SNRIs), such as venlafaxine and duloxetine. Unfortunately there are no published data other than case reports with paroxetine and fluvoxamine to support their use currently. There is an obvious need for further pharmacological studies on NES not only to assess the effectiveness of other serotoninergic agents but also to evaluate whether the beneficial effects of sertraline are durable after months or even years of treatment.

Topiramate

Topiramate has also been reported to be helpful in treatment of NES. It is a monosaccharide-type compound with complex pharmacological actions. It inhibits the activity of carbonic anhydrase, blocks voltage-dependent sodium channels, and has a stimulatory effect at the GABA-A receptor.

Anecdotal observation of weight loss in epileptic patients after 6 to 12 months treatment with topiramate suggested a possible role of this pharmacological agent in treating eating-related disorders associated with weight gain (Slater, Reife, & Kamin, 2002). Similar effects were seen in samples of patients treated for migraine and bipolar disorder (McInytre et al., 2002). Furthermore, topiramate induced marked reductions in binge episodes in 69% (9 out of 13) of patients with daytime binge-eating disorder (Shapira, Goldsmith, & McElroy, 2000).

Evidence supporting the use of topiramate in the management of NES is sparse and limited to case reports and case series at this juncture. Winkelman (2003), in a small case series ($n = 4$, two patients with NES and two patients with sleep-related eating disorder), found this agent reduced nocturnal eating and promoted weight loss with a mean reduction of 11.1 kg. The effective dose range appears to fall between 100–400 mg. Tucker, Masters, and Nawar (2004) used topiramate (100 mg/day) to treat a 40-year-old obese patient with NES and comorbid sleepwalking and posttraumatic stress disorder. This patient experienced a 31.7 kg weight loss after 8 months of treatment (Tucker et al., 2004).

Although topiramate is not the only antiepileptic medication with a positive role in the management of eating disorders (i.e., zonisamide has benefit in binge-eating disorder with obesity, phenytoin in some patients with compulsive binge eating, and carbamazepine and valproate in patients with bulimia or anorexia nervosa) (McElroy et al., 2009), it is the only one with evidence of benefit in the treatment of NES. Further research is necessary to confirm a treatment role for topiramate on NES and to assess the usefulness of other antiseizure medications in the management of this specific condition.

Conclusions

Even though there is a plausible theoretical basis for using serotonergic agents in the management of NES, only sertraline is supported by the available evidence. Based on the limited literature a trial of sertraline is the most appropriate first-line treatment approach based on the results from open label studies and a single RCT. Case reports suggest that fluvoxamine or paroxetine are beneficial sometimes with rapid improvement (i.e., within 2 to 3 weeks). An adequate duration trial of 8 weeks, however, should be pursued before judging a trial a failure (O'Reardon et al., 2005). To date there are no guidelines or data on duration of therapeutic benefit of medications on NES, but it has been suggested that an effective medication should be maintained for at least 1 year and then attempt a phased withdrawal over a 2- to 3-month period (O'Reardon et al., 2005).

There has been no systematic study of the potential role of antiepileptic medications. Two case reports support the use of topiramate as an alternative to sertraline to reduce symptoms in these patients. Topiramate may prove to have advantages over sertraline in terms of weight, but this has yet to be demonstrated and sertraline is clearly the better-tolerated agent (O'Reardon et al., 2005).

Dual-acting SNRIs are worthy of future study in particular, given the clinical perception that norepinephrine may have a restraining effect on food intake. Other agents such as melatonin and other hypnotic–sedative agents have not been shown to be beneficial for improving symptoms of NES. In fact, certain sleep medications such as zolpidem and atypical neuroleptics may worsen symptoms of NES (Chiang & Krystal, 2008; Najjar, 2007; Winkelman, 1998).

Clearly, research on pharmacotherapy for NES is still at an early stage. Ultimately, further methodologically sound RCTs will be needed to delineate and improve the pharmacological armamentarium for the management of patients suffering from this unique eating disorder.

References

Allison, K. C., Lundgren, J. D., O'Reardon, J. P., Geliebter, A., Gluck, M. E., Vinai, P., et al. (2010). Proposed diagnostic criteria for night eating syndrome. *International Journal of Eating Disorders, 43*(3), 241–247.

Birketvedt, G. S., Florholmen, J., Sundsfjord, J., Osterud, B., Dinges, D., Bilker, W., et al. (1999). Behavioral and neuroendocrine characteristics of the night eating syndrome. *Journal of the American Medical Association, 282*(7), 657–663.

Chiang, A., & Krystal, A. (2008). Report of two cases where sleep-related eating behavior occurred with the extended-release formulation but not the immediate-release formulation of a sedative–hypnotic agent. *Journal of Clinical Sleep Medicine, 4*(2), 155–156.

Friedman, S., Even, C., Dardennes, R., & Guelfi, J. D. (2002). Light therapy, obesity, and night-eating syndrome. *American Journal of Psychiatry, 159*(5), 875–876.

Lundgren, J. D., Newberg, A. B., Allison, K. C., Wintering, N. A., Ploessl, K., & Stunkard, A. J. (2008). 123I-ADAM SPECT imaging of serotonin transporter binding in patients with night eating syndrome: A preliminary report. *Psychiatry Research: Neuroimaging, 162*(3), 214–220.

McElroy, S. L., Casuto, L. S., Nelson, E. B., Lake, K. A., Soutullo, C. A., Keck, P. E., Jr., et al. (2000). Placebo-controlled trial of sertraline in the treatment of binge-eating disorder. *American Journal of Psychiatry, 157*(6), 1004–1006.

McElroy, S. L., Guerdjikova, A. I., Martens, B., Keck, P. E., Jr., Pope, H. G., & Hudson, J. I. (2009). Role of antiepileptic drugs in the management of eating disorders. *CNS Drugs, 23*(2), 139–156.

McIntyre, R. S., Mancini, D. A., McCann, S., Srinivasan, J., Sagman, D., & Kennedy, S. H. (2002). Topiramate versus bupropion SR when added to mood stabilizer therapy for the depressive phase of bipolar disorder: A preliminary single-blind study. *Bipolar Disorders, 4*(3), 207–213.

Miyaoka, T., Yasukawa, R., Tsubouchi, K., Miura, S., Shimizu, Y., Sukegawa, T., et al. (2003). Successful treatment of nocturnal eating/drinking syndrome with selective serotonin reuptake inhibitors. *International Clinical Psychopharmacology, 18*(3), 175–177.

Najjar, M. (2007). Zolpidem and amnestic sleep-related eating disorder. *Journal of Clinical Sleep Medicine, 3*(6), 637–638.

O'Reardon, J. P., Allison, K. C., Martino, N. S., Lundgren, J. D., Heo, M., & Stunkard, A. J. (2006). A randomized, placebo-controlled trial of sertraline in the treatment of night eating syndrome. *American Journal of Psychiatry, 163*(5), 893–898.

O'Reardon, J. P., Peshek, A., & Allison, K. C. (2005). Night eating syndrome: Diagnosis, epidemiology, and management. *CNS Drugs, 19*(12), 997–1008.

O'Reardon, J. P., Ringel, B. L., Dinges, D. F., Allison, K. C., Rogers, N. L., Martino, N. S., et al. (2004). Circadian eating and sleeping patterns in the night eating syndrome. *Obesity Research, 12*(11), 1789–1796.

O'Reardon, J. P., Stunkard, A. J., & Allison, K. C. (2004). Clinical trial of sertraline in the treatment of the night eating syndrome. *International Journal of Eating Disorders, 35*(1), 16–26.

Shapira, N. A., Goldsmith, T. D., & McElroy, S. L. (2000). Treatment of binge-eating disorder with topiramate: A clinical case series. *Journal of Clinical Psychiatry, 61*(5), 368–372.

Slater, J. D., Reife, R. A., & Kamin, M. (2002). Weight changes in epilepsy patients treated with topiramate. *Neurology, 58*(7, Suppl. 3), A4221.

Spaggiari, M. C., Granella, F., Parrino, L., Marchesi, C., Melli, I., & Terzano, M. G. (1994). Nocturnal eating syndrome in adults. *Sleep, 17*(4), 339–344.

Stunkard, A. J., Allison, K. C., Lundgren, J. D., Martino, N. S., Heo, M., Etemad,

B., et al. (2006). A paradigm for facilitating pharmacotherapy at a distance: Sertraline treatment of the night eating syndrome. *Journal of Clinical Psychiatry, 67*(10), 1568–1572.

Stunkard, A. J., Allison, K. C., Lundgren, J. D., & O'Reardon, J. P. (2009). A biobehavioural model of the night eating syndrome. *Obesity Reviews,10*(Suppl. 2), 69–77.

Stunkard, A. J., Grace, W. J., & Wolff, H. G. (1955). The night-eating syndrome: A pattern of food intake among certain obese patients. *American Journal of Medicine, 19*(1), 78–86.

Tucker, P., Masters, B., & Nawar, O. (2004). Topiramate in the treatment of comorbid night eating syndrome and PTSD: A case study. *Eating Disorders, 12*(1), 75–78.

Winkelman, J. W. (1998). Clinical and polysomnographic features of sleep-related eating disorder. *Journal of Clinical Psychiatry, 59*(1), 14–19.

Winkelman, J. W. (2003). Treatment of nocturnal eating syndrome and sleep-related eating disorder with topiramate. *Sleep Medicine, 4*(3), 243–246.

Chapter 13

Cognitive-Behavioral Therapy and Night Eating Syndrome

Kelly C. Allison

As I have learned over the past decade of working with those who have night eating syndrome (NES), health care providers who are not aware of the literature on NES may attribute the problem to bad habits and may not recognize NES as a condition that requires careful treatment. NES is not simply a vice, nor is it solely an eating disorder, at least as they historically have been conceptualized. NES also shares aspects of sleep and mood disorders at its core. Both biological and psychological factors likely play important roles in the development and persistence of this condition, as detailed in earlier chapters.

Persons with NES have reported to me that their friends, family, and doctors blame night eating on poor self-control, believing that everyone should be able to manage their own eating habits. One woman wrote, "Thank goodness I have discovered that this is a real disorder. I feel like a pig and somehow—like a person with a dirty secret. I am embarrassed about my lack of self-control and angry that I am sabotaging my health and my weight loss goals with this behavior."

In NES the temporal intake of food is delayed, but the sleep period is normal, causing a conflict between the drives to eat and sleep (O'Reardon et al., 2004). Thus many sufferers wake and feel compelled to eat in order to fall back to sleep, and/or they eat before going to sleep in order to prevent initial insomnia.

My colleagues at the University of Pennsylvania and I first focused attention on pharmaceutical targets for treating NES in the early 2000s (see Chapter 12 [Patel, O'Reardon, & Cristancho]), but as we discovered more about patients' thoughts and psychosocial factors, we began turning our attention to conceptualizing a psychotherapy for NES. I outline this process and the preliminary research data below and present the treatment manual in Chapter 14.

Cognitive-Behavioral Therapy

Cognitive-behavioral therapy (CBT) has been well validated for the treatment of many psychiatric disorders, including depression, insomnia, and eating disorders. Depression, which also affects many persons with NES (Allison, Grilo, Masheb, & Stunkard, 2005; Lundgren, Allison, O'Reardon, & Stunkard, 2008; Striegel-Moore et al., 2008), has long been treated with CBT. In fact, the approach was originally formulated for the treatment of depression, based on Aaron T. Beck's cognitive triad: the tendency to regard oneself, one's future, and one's experiences/the world in a negative light (Beck, Rush, Shaw, & Emery, 1979). The dysfunctional thoughts that are generated within this worldview are addressed in the context of CBT, with the goal of generating new, alternative thoughts that are more realistic and positive, which, in turn, improve the patient's mood. A "mega-analysis" has shown that patients with severe depression responded as well to CBT as to antidepressant medication (DeRubeis, Gelfand, Tang, & Simons, 1999).

Beck et al. (1979), in their classic text *Cognitive Therapy of Depression* defined CBT as

> an active, directive, time limited, structured approach used to treat a variety of psychiatric disorders. . . . It is based on an underlying theoretical rationale that an individual's affect and behavior are largely determined by the way in which he structures the world. His cognitions . . . are based on attitudes or assumptions (schemas), developed from previous experiences. (p.3)

Judith Beck (2011) goes on to explain the key elements of CBT. These include (1) an ever-evolving formulation of the patient and his or her problems in cognitive terms; (2) a sound therapeutic alliance; (3)

collaboration and active participation by the patient; (4) a goal-oriented and problem-focused approach; (5) an initial emphasis on the present; (6) education of the patient to be his or her own therapist and emphasis on relapse prevention; (7) time-limited therapy; (8) structured sessions; (9) teaching patients to identify, evaluate, and respond to their dysfunctional thoughts and beliefs; and (10) using a variety of techniques to change thinking, mood, and behavior. These same elements should be included in the application of CBT for any treatment population.

CBT and Eating Disorders

Fairburn (1981) pioneered this approach for eating disorders when he described CBT for bulimia nervosa (BN), which he later adapted for binge-eating disorder (BED; Fairburn, Marcus & Wilson, 1993), and most recently updated into his enhanced CBT for eating disorders (CBT-E; Fairburn, Cooper, & Shafran, 2008). Other groups have also established CBT as an effective treatment for BN and BED (e.g., Peterson & Mitchell, 1996; Wilfley et al., 1993, 2002). When compared to other treatment approaches, including pharmacotherapy, CBT has been proven to be as effective, and in most cases more effective, in treating BN and BED (Hay & Claudino, 2010). In its application to BN and BED, reductions in symptoms have been fairly consistent. Binge and purging episodes are typically eliminated in 30–50% of patients with BN, and binges remit in 60–70% of patients with BED (see Wilson, 2010, for a review).

In treating eating disorders, the "behavioral" aspect of the therapy is particularly important and is more prominently stressed than in the application of CBT to depression. These factors include self-monitoring the timing and amount of food intake, including the setting, and, in the case of binge episodes, the precipitants. Eating at regular intervals throughout the day is also an essential element, and weight is monitored at each appointment. The additive effect of combining behavioral and cognitive techniques was illustrated nicely in an early, seminal study where Fairburn, Jones, Peveler, Hope, and O'Connor (1993) compared behavior therapy alone, CBT, and interpersonal therapy for the treatment of BN. While the use of behavior therapy produced some reductions in binge–purge frequency, these reductions were not statistically significant or clinically meaningful, as compared to those produced after 19 sessions of treatment with CBT, and relapse was quicker over the ensuing year.

Thus the behavioral techniques are an important part of the therapy, but they should be used in combination with the cognitive aspects for long-term, meaningful success. Of note, CBT was more effective than interpersonal therapy at the end of the 20-week treatment, but by 1 year, the effects of interpersonal therapy increased such that the reductions in binge–purge episodes did not differ between treatment groups. Thus CBT remained the treatment of choice with more rapid results, but interpersonal therapy emerged as a viable alternative; this latter approach has yet to be applied to NES.

Elements of the CBT approach for disordered eating is especially relevant for normal-weight night eaters, as this group typically reports higher levels of purposeful daytime food restriction and overexercise (Lundgren et al., 2008) as opposed to overweight night eaters. This difference is also expressed through a higher percentage of daily energy consumed after dinner between these groups; if the normal-weight group is restricting more during the day, then, necessarily, the percentage of intake after dinner would be greater. Patients are often anxious about starting to eat earlier in the day for fear of weight gain. Regular weighing is helpful in reducing this fear while reinforcing the necessity of regular daytime eating.

CBT and Insomnia

CBT for insomnia (CBT-I) is also considered an effective treatment approach for insomnia, an important element of NES. People with insomnia may have predisposing characteristics that increase their risk of sleep disruption, such as proneness to worry, repression of negative emotions, and physiological hyperarousal. As with NES, insomnia may not develop until it is precipitated by a stressful life event. Morin et al. (1999, 2006) have demonstrated that CBT benefits 70 to 80% of patients with primary insomnia. For eating disorders, depression, and insomnia alike, CBT generally provides sustained benefits, while the benefits of drugs often dissipate when they are discontinued (Agras, 1997; Morin et al., 2006). Combined drug and CBT-I treatments show added effect, but providing a maintenance phase with discontinuation of the hypnotic while offering additional CBT-I sessions has proven beneficial (Morin et al., 2009). Nonetheless, hypnotics are often the frontline treatment for insomnia (Simon & VonKorff, 1997; Smith et al., 2002), likely due to their accessibility and immediate results.

The basic tenets of CBT-I (Perlis, Jungquist, Smith, & Posner, 2005) include improving sleep hygiene, restriction of time in bed, sleep education, stimulus control, and disabusing anxiety-related beliefs about one's inability to sleep. *Sleep hygiene* improvements focus on regulating bedtime and morning awakening time, exercising, decreasing alcohol and caffeine use, avoiding napping, not sleeping with the television on, and making the bedroom dark and comfortable. *Restriction of time in bed* limits time in bed to the total amount of sleep time typically experienced per night. This technique helps to consolidate sleep and improve feelings of fatigue. *Sleep education* includes conveying information about the sleep cycle, which typically lasts about 90 minutes, and the normal variances in total sleep time across the population. *Stimulus control* promotes the use of the bed for only sleep and sex, as well as instructs the patient to rise from bed after about 15 minutes of wakefulness. Finally, *lying in bed and worrying* about not being able to fall asleep typically produces more anxiety and arousal, interfering with sleep onset. Cognitive restructuring of these thoughts is helpful, as are relaxation techniques.

In summary, these CBT-I elements are included in the CBT approach for NES to help reduce both nocturnal ingestions and their associated awakenings.

Behavioral Weight Loss

CBT treatment for NES was based in part on CBT for BED in which dieting was prohibited (Fairburn et al., 1993). This rejection of weight control measures in CBT for BED resulted from the hypothesis that restricting food intake would cause binge episodes. The National Task Force on the Prevention and Treatment of Obesity (2000), however, has stated that there is sufficient evidence to indicate that dieting does *not* cause binge-eating problems. Wadden and colleagues (2004) demonstrated this finding. Among obese women seeking behavioral weight loss, no cases of BED developed, and very few objective binge episodes occurred during treatment. Likewise, there is no evidence that would directly link caloric restriction to the occurrence of nocturnal eating episodes. Therefore, the goal of weight loss is included as an important aspect of this treatment for overweight and obese patients. To this end, calorie monitoring is included in food and sleep logs for those who are overweight or obese, and calorie goals between 1,200 and 1,500 kcal for women and between 1,500 and 1,800 kcal for men are recommended. For normal-weight patients, attention is focused on maintaining weight while shifting food intake to regular hours across the day.

CBT for NES

NES Themes

In an earlier research study, Stunkard, O'Reardon, and I asked patients to record thoughts in diaries before and after their night eating episodes. Based on these experiences, we found that there were different themes associated with these nocturnal ingestions (Allison, Stunkard, & Thier, 2004). The most common of these was experiencing specific food cravings, feeling anxious or agitated, needing to eat to fall back to sleep, and experiencing a strong compulsion to eat to feel the satisfaction of having food in one's stomach (sometimes, but not typically accompanied by physical hunger). Other, less common themes were feeling stressed, depressed, or bored.

Most participants reported that, after eating, they were able to resume sleep quickly. These themes were incorporated into an assessment tool, the Night Eating Assessment (included in Chapter 14), which patients complete before each late evening and nocturnal eating episode across the first week or two of treatment (depending on how many episodes they were experiencing per week). Examples of the four most common themes are presented in Table 13.1. These thoughts were extracted from participant logs kept over the course of a week.

CBT Techniques

Specific techniques prescribed in CBT are used. Among these, Dysfunctional Thought Records (DTRs) based on those used for depression at the Beck Institute for Cognitive Behavior Therapy have been developed with examples germane to patients with NES. These records are based on the following premise:

$$Situation \rightarrow Emotion \rightarrow Thought \rightarrow Outcome$$

The patient first identifies the situation, such as sitting down to watch television after dinner. Then he or she works to identify the automatic thought that is relevant, such as, "I really need to eat that bag of chips I bought today." The patient also identifies the emotion that accompanies that thought, such as boredom, stress, or loneliness.

Thus an initial key intervention with NES patients is establishing a link between the evening snacking episodes and nocturnal ingestions with their thoughts and feelings. Behavioral interventions are also important in modifying eating behaviors specific to NES. As Beck et al. (1979) indicate:

TABLE 13.1. Characteristic Thoughts for the Four Themes Most Often Associated with NES

Theme	Thoughts before night eating	Thoughts after night eating
Feel an overwhelming compulsion to eat	"I'm very relaxed. I really am not hungry, but I feel an overwhelming compulsion to eat."	"I'm disgusted that I ate just before going to bed and by my lack of control and willpower."
Anxious/agitated	"I was very tired and just wanted to go to sleep. I was anxious and upset because we are going away on vacation Saturday and my husband has yet to pack. So we had a little argument before bed."	"When I got up and found the chocolate I knew I was in trouble. I started to eat it very fast and my heart was pounding. It is very hard for me to stop once I start, but I only ate a little and then went back to bed."
Cravings	"I woke up at 2:00 A.M. I had just purchased pastry cakes earlier in the day. I knew they were there and wanted them. I knew if I didn't go downstairs and eat a pack I wouldn't get back to sleep."	"I thought, 'Good. Now I can go right back to sleep as soon as I go up to my bed.'"
Need to eat to sleep	"Very tired, can't sleep. If I just eat something I will be able to sleep. My stomach bugs me—if I don't eat, I will just keep getting up."	"Hope I can sleep through to morning. Very tired. Just want to sleep all the way through. Don't want to get up again."

Behavioral methods can be regarded as a series of small experiments designed to test the validity of the patient's hypotheses or ideas about himself. As the negative ideas are contradicted by these "experiments," the patient gradually becomes less certain of their validity, and he is motivated to attempt more difficult assignments. (p.118)

Experiments with stimulus control are encouraged throughout treatment. Another cognitive technique that is used to address beliefs about needing to eat in order to fall asleep is the "downward-arrow" technique. This approach encourages the patient to uncover the underlying meanings that the patient carries about him- or herself and to generate alternative ideas about the meaning of his or her behaviors. Socratic questioning also helps to make these discussions more concrete and meaningful.

Sample CBT Exchange

PATIENT: When I wake up at night, there is no way I will fall asleep without eating something.

THERAPIST: What would happen if you tried to stay in bed without eating?

PATIENT: I would just keep thinking about all I have to do tomorrow and how I won't be rested enough to get through the day.

THERAPIST: Have you tested this before? What's the worst that has happened?

PATIENT: I've tried before, but I always end up giving in and eating, so I don't know what would happen if I didn't go to the kitchen. I feel like a failure.

THERAPIST: So you're afraid to not eat, for fear that you will be up all night, but you feel like a failure if you do eat.

PATIENT: Yes. I feel so torn about it. I think about how hard I've tried to lose weight over the years, only to mess it all up with my night eating. It's gotten to the point that I don't even argue with myself about eating—I just do it because I know it will get me back to sleep.

THERAPIST: Well, it's likely that you have tried different strategies to stop your night eating, but not all of them together at once. Is this right?

PATIENT: Yes. I've tried setting out a specific snack or putting up a sign, but I do it for one night, and then give up.

THERAPIST: We need to give you the best chance at succeeding with not eating during the night. To achieve that, you need to put several tools in place at once. First, we need to help you access the level of distress that you feel during the day and make that felt when you wake up at night. Let's write some of these thoughts down together so you can post them in your home. Second, let's think about where we can put your typical night-time snack foods to limit your access to them. Third, let's plan a reasonable time in the evening for you to declare the kitchen "closed."

At this point, I would work together with the patient to identify relevant places to post signs, such as the back of the bedroom door, in the bathroom, at the top of the stairs, at the entrance to the kitchen, on a cabinet, and/or on the refrigerator. We would also use stimulus control to move favorite snack foods out of easy access, such as to the basement, garage, a roommate's bedroom, or a locked cabinet. We would also plan to place barriers between the bedroom and the kitchen. This could include using painter's tape across the entrance to the kitchen (this tape removes easily without damage to walls and can be used regularly), or placing a rope or chain or piece of furniture across the doorway. The plan could also involve making the typical night eating routine uncomfortable, by piling their favorite snacking chair with objects or keeping the house colder than usual during the winter (and using extra blankets, instead). The more difficult the act of eating becomes, the less comfort it provides, and the higher the likelihood the patient has of accessing the reasons they can so readily list during the day for not eating.

In this example, the continued use of questions uncovers the patient's fear that not eating will lead to a sleepless night, which will lead to impaired functioning during the day. Underneath these possible behavioral consequences lies the fear that this individual is a failure for not being able to control and stop this nighttime eating. Once revealed, cognitive restructuring can help to dismantle this core belief, and behavioral techniques can help challenge the beliefs held about the dire consequences of abstaining from eating. As Beck suggested, this approach turns patients into their own researchers by challenging them to complete these experiments and note the outcomes. These results are then brought to the next therapy session and examined for continued problem solving and strategizing.

Results from the Pilot Study of CBT for NES

My colleagues and I tested this CBT approach for the treatment of NES in an uncontrolled pilot study (Allison, Lundgren, Moore, O'Reardon, & Stunkard, 2010). Participants were recruited from a large, comprehensive assessment study of NES (O'Reardon et al., 2004; Boston, Moate, Allison, Lundgren, & Stunkard, 2008). NES diagnosis was confirmed with a two-stage assessment including screening and interview with the Night Eating Questionnaire (NEQ; Allison et al., 2008) and the Night Eating Syndrome History and Inventory (see Chapter 11 [Lundgren, Allison, Vinai, & Gluck]), and a week-long food and sleep log. Participants were consuming at least 25% of their intake after dinner and/or were waking up at night to eat at least three times per week (this study was completed before the new research criteria [Allison, Lundgren, O'Reardon, et al., 2010] were established). Of the 67 participants who were eligible from the larger trial for this treatment study, 25 were enrolled.

The therapy consisted of 10, 1-hour, individual sessions of CBT for NES, occurring over 12 weeks. Participants were, on average, 47 years old with a mean body mass index (BMI) of 29.5 kg/m²; eight were of normal weight, seven were overweight, and 10 were obese. Sixty-eight percent were Caucasian and 24% were African American. Psychiatric comorbidity was high with current or lifetime rates of: 4% for BN (not current), 24% for BED, 36% for any mood disorder, 48% for any anxiety disorder, and 40% for substance abuse or dependence.

Dropout for the trial was substantial; 14 of the 25 completed at least 8 of the 10 sessions, with seven of these withdrawing by week 2. It seems likely that the work burden of the treatment may have been too much for some of them, whereas comorbid psychopathology was a limiting factor for others. Mixed-models analysis was used to minimize the impact of this large dropout rate on outcome data, but this remains a limitation to external validity.

Despite this limitation, the treatment produced significant reductions in the primary and secondary outcomes (Allison, Lundgren, Moore, et al., 2010). Evening hyperphagia, as measured using food logs, decreased significantly from 35% at baseline to 24.9% at session 10. Awakenings per week decreased from 13.5 per week to 8.5 per week, and nocturnal ingestions dropped from 8.7 per week to 2.6 per week. Total calories per day dropped from 2,356 kcal to 1,759 kcal, with an accompanying change in weight of −3.1 kg.

While all of these outcomes were statistically significant, it is evident that participants were still reporting more than two nocturnal ingestions per week, and their percentage of food intake after dinner barely dipped below the diagnostic cutoff of 25%. Upon further examination, participants decreased the amount they were consuming most significantly during nocturnal ingestions (from 15.1% to 5%), but not during the after-dinner period until bedtime (21.8% to 21.0%). Thus this treatment seemed more effective in reducing nocturnal ingestions than evening hyperphagia.

Normal-Weight versus Overweight Participants: Outcomes

Although the numbers were low, we wanted to get a sense of the efficacy of this treatment for normal-weight as compared to overweight and obese participants. The normal-weight night eaters reported a higher percentage of daily food intake at baseline as compared to the overweight/obese group (46% vs. 31%); the difference in awakenings per week (19.6 normal weight vs. 10.7 overweight) and nocturnal ingestions per week (13.1 normal weight vs. 6.7 overweight) were not statistically different, but they seemed clinically different. Caloric intake also seemed clinically different, with the normal-weight group consuming 2,011 kcal per day as compared to 2,531 kcal per day at baseline. With these small groups standard deviations were large, so bigger trials seem warranted to examine these observations.

Although these groups differed at baseline on core NES symptoms, there was no interaction between weight groups for the primary outcome measures (see Figure 13.1). Both groups significantly decreased the proportion of calories consumed after dinner and the number of nocturnal ingestions per week. However, as the normal-weight group started at baseline with more severe levels, they likewise ended the trial more symptomatic than the overweight/obese group.

This pilot study produced some interesting findings that bear further investigation. Randomized controlled trials with adequately powered sample sizes are needed. Furthermore, attention to indoctrinating patients to the requirements of therapy (e.g., keeping a daily food and sleep log and the active nature of the therapy) and building a strong therapeutic alliance is necessary to reduce the number of dropouts. Likewise, more work is needed to improve strategies for reducing the grazing behavior that occurs between dinner and bedtime; as it stands, this therapy did not improve this behavior. Finally, some modifications were made for normal-weight participants, particularly the exclusion of the behavioral weight loss component. Larger samples across weight classes are needed to determine whether more specific approaches are needed based on weight status or the level of other disordered eating behavior.

Summary

CBT for NES was conceptualized from established approaches for each of its elements: disordered eating, insomnia, and mood. For those who are overweight, behavioral weight loss is included, while attention to purposeful daytime food restriction and overexercise is targeted for normal-weight patients. Overall, the data are promising, but larger, controlled trials are needed to test CBT for NES, and more work is needed to improve outcomes, most specifically for reducing evening hyperphagia.

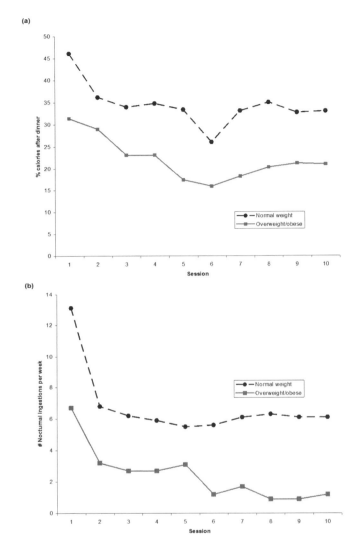

FIGURE 13.1. (a) Change in proportion of calories consumed after the evening meal for normal-weight (n = 8) and overweight/obese (n = 17) participants. The proportion of calories decreased over time, $F(10, 139)$ = 5.23, $p < .0001$, and the levels of caloric intake differed between the weight groups, $F(1, 23)$ = 6.16, p = .02). (b) Change in number of nocturnal ingestions per week for normal-weight (n = 8) and overweight/obese (n = 17) participants. Nocturnal ingestions per week decreased significantly and at similar rates for both weight groups, $F(9, 123)$ = 8.23, $p < .0001$. From Allison, Lundgren, Moore, O'Reardon, and Stunkard (2010). Used by permission of the Association for the Advancement of Psychotherapy.

References

Agras, W. S. (1997). Pharmacotherapy of bulimia nervosa and binge-eating disorder: Longer-term outcomes. *Psychopharmacology Bulletin, 33*, 433–436.

Allison, K. C., Grilo, C. M., Masheb, R. M., & Stunkard, A. J. (2005). Binge-eating disorder and night eating syndrome: A comparative study of disordered eating. *Journal of Consulting and Clinical Psychology, 73*(6), 1107–1115.

Allison, K. C., Lundgren, J. D., Moore, R. H., O'Reardon, J. P., & Stunkard, A. J. (2010) Cognitive behavior therapy for night eating syndrome: A pilot study. *American Journal of Psychotherapy, 64*(1), 91–106.

Allison, K. C., Lundgren, J. D., O'Reardon, J. P., Geliebter, A., Gluck, M. E., Vinai, P., et al. (2010). Proposed diagnostic criteria for night eating syndrome. *International Journal of Eating Disorders, 43*, 241–247.

Allison, K. C., Lundgren, J. D., O'Reardon, J. P, Martino, N. S., Sarwer, D. B., Wadden, T. A., et al. (2008). The Night Eating Questionnaire (NEQ): Psychometric properties of a measure of severity of the night eating syndrome. *Eating Behaviors, 9*, 62–72.

Allison, K. C., Stunkard, A. J., & Thier, S. L. (2004). *Overcoming night eating syndrome*. Oakland, CA: New Harbinger.

Beck, A. T., Rush, A. J., Shaw, B. F., & Emery, G. (1979). *Cognitive therapy of depression*. New York: Guilford Press.

Beck, J. S. (2011). *Cognitive behavior therapy: Basics and beyond* (2nd ed.). New York: Guilford Press.

Boston, R. C., Moate, P. J., Allison, K. C., Lundgren, J. D., & Stunkard, A. J. (2008) Modeling circadian rhythms of food intake by means of parametric deconvolution: Results from studies of the night eating syndrome. *American Journal of Clinical Nutrition, 87*(6), 1672–1677.

DeRubeis, R. J., Gelfand, L. A., Tang, T. Z., & Simons, A. D. (1999). Medications versus cognitive behavior therapy for severely depressed outpatients: Mega-analysis of four randomized comparisons. *American Journal of Psychiatry, 156*, 1007–1013.

Fairburn, C. G. (1981). A cognitive behavioural approach to the treatment of bulimia. *Psychological Medicine, 11*, 707–711.

Fairburn, C. G., Cooper, Z., & Shafran, R. (2008). Enhanced cognitive behavior therapy for eating disorders ("CBT-E"): An overview. In C. G. Fairburn (Ed.), *Cognitive behavior therapy and eating disorders* (pp. 23–34). New York: Guilford Press.

Fairburn, C. G., Jones, R., Peveler, R. C., Hope, R. A., & O'Connor, M. (1993). Psychotherapy and bulimia nervosa: Longer-term effects of interpersonal psychotherapy, behavior therapy, and cognitive behavior therapy. *Archives of General Psychiatry, 50*, 419–428.

Fairburn, C. G., Marcus, M. D., & Wilson, G. T. (1993). Cognitive-behavioral therapy for binge eating and bulimia nervosa: A comprehensive treatment manual. In C. G. Fairburn & G. T. Wilson (Eds.), *Binge eating: Nature, assessment, and treatment* (pp. 361–404). New York: Guilford Press.

Hay, P. J., & Claudino, A. M. (2010). Evidence-based treatments for the eating disorders. In W. S. Agras (Ed.), *The Oxford manual of eating disorders* (pp. 452–479). New York: Oxford University Press.

Lundgren, J. L., Allison, K. C., O'Reardon, J. P., & Stunkard, A. J. (2008). A descriptive study of non-obese persons with night eating syndrome and a weight-matched comparison group. *Eating Behaviors, 9*, 352–359.

Morin, C. M., Bootzin, R. R., Buysse, D. J., Edinger, J. D., Espie, C. A., & Lichstein, K. L. (2006). Psychological and behavioral treatment of insomnia: Update of the recent evidence (1998–2004). *Sleep, 29*(11), 1398–1414.

Morin, C. M., Hauri, P. J., Espie, C. A., Spielman, A. J., Buysse, D. J., & Bootzin, R. R. (1999). Nonpharmacologic treatment of chronic insomnia. *Sleep, 22*, 1134–1156.

Morin, C. M., Vallières, A., Guay, B., Ivers, H., Savard, J., Mérette, C., et al. (2009). Cognitive-behavioral therapy, singly and combined with medication, for persistent insomnia: A randomized controlled trial. *Journal of the American Medical Association, 301*, 2005–2015.

National Task Force on the Prevention and Treatment of Obesity. (2000). Dieting and the development of eating disorders in overweight and obese adults. *Archives of Internal Medicine, 160*, 2581–2589.

O'Reardon, J. P., Ringel, B. L., Dinges, D. F., Allison, K. C., Rogers, N. L., Martino, N. S., et al. (2004). Circadian eating and sleeping patterns in the night eating syndrome. *Obesity Research, 12*, 1789–1796.

Perlis, M. L., Jungquist, C., Smith, M. T., & Posner, D. (2005). *Cognitive-behavioral treatment of insomnia: A session-by-session guide*. Springer: New York.

Peterson, C. B., & Mitchell, J. E. (1996). Treatment of binge-eating disorder in group cognitive-behavioral therapy. In J. Werne (Ed.), *Treating eating disorders* (pp. 143–186). San Francisco: Jossey-Bass.

Simon, G. E., & VonKorff, M. (1997). Prevalence, burden, and treatment of insomnia in primary care. *American Journal of Psychiatry, 154*(10), 1417–1423.

Smith, M. T., Perlis, M. L., Park, A., Smith, M., Pennington, J. M., Giles, D. E., et al. (2002). Comparative meta-analysis of pharmacotherapy and behavior therapy for persistent insomnia. *American Journal of Psychiatry, 159*, 5–11.

Striegel-Moore, R. H., Franko, D. L., Thompson, D., Affenito, S., May, A., & Kraemer, H. C. (2008). Exploring the typology of night eating syndrome. *International Journal of Eating Disorders, 41*, 411–418.

Wadden, T. A., Foster, G. D., Sarwer, D. B., Anderson, D. A., Gladis, M., Sanderson, R. S., et al. (2004). Dieting and the development of eating disorders in obese women: Results of a randomized controlled trial. *American Journal of Clinical Nutrition, 80*, 560–568.

Wilfley, D. E., Agras, W. S., Telch, C. F., Rossiter, E. M., Schneider, J. A., Cole, A. G., et al. (1993). Group cognitive-behavioral therapy and group interpersonal psychotherapy for the nonpurging bulimic individual: A controlled comparison. *Journal of Consulting and Clinical Psychology, 61*, 296–305.

Wilfley, D. E., Welch, R. R., Stein, R. I., Spurrell, E. B., Cohen, L. R., Saelens, B. E., et al. (2002). A randomized comparison of group cognitive-behavioral therapy and group interpersonal psychotherapy for the treatment of overweight individuals with binge-eating disorder. *Archives of General Psychiatry, 59,* 713–721.

Wilson, G. T. (2010). Cognitive-behavioral therapy for eating disorders. In W. S. Agras (Ed.), *The Oxford manual of eating disorders* (pp. 331–347). New York: Oxford University Press.

Chapter 14

Cognitive-Behavioral Therapy Manual for Night Eating Syndrome

Kelly C. Allison

Cognitive-behavioral therapy (CBT) for night eating syndrome (NES) is brief, but intensive. As described in the previous chapter, it is essential to explain the nature and the level of effort associated with this active psychotherapy. Building the therapeutic alliance early on, particularly by showing empathy for the struggles patients may have faced with their NES symptoms, seems essential for full patient engagement and trust.

An initial assessment should take place before starting the therapy. I would suggest using the Night Eating Syndrome History and Inventory (NESHI), as described in Chapter 11 (Lundgren, Allison, Vinai, & Gluck). Once the history and current pattern of the night eating is established, treatment can begin. The treatment has not been studied as a group intervention and is written for application in an individual setting. This approach has not been tested for patients presenting with sleep-related eating disorder (SRED; Chapter 9 [Howell & Crow]), as they are typically sleepwalking or experiencing a clouded state of consciousness that would make application of cognitive-behavioral techniques difficult. In addition, patients who have severe anxiety or panic may have difficulty reducing their night eating without attention to their anxiety disorder. Likewise, therapists should address severe depression or suicidal ideation in treatment before focusing on the night eating. More research is needed to explore the interplay of comorbid disorders and NES (as described in Chapters 7 [Latzer & Tzischinsky] and 8 [Rempfer & Murphy]).

In this chapter, I review the three stages of CBT for NES and the specific approaches used therein.

Three Stages of Therapy

Stage 1

The first stage of CBT for NES focuses on developing the therapeutic alliance, explaining the rationale for CBT, and educating the patient on the basic techniques of CBT, such as monitoring of sleeping, eating, mood, and the automatic thoughts associated with these events (sessions 1–4). Basic exploration of the impetus for NES is explored in the first week using Nighttime Eating Assessment forms (Figure 14.1). These worksheets are paired with the food and sleep log (Figures 14.2 and 14.3).

Through the use of dialogue and food and sleep logs, the circadian pattern of food intake is explored in detail during this initial stage of treatment. The therapist works with the patient to establish scheduled meals and snacks during the waking hours, no more than 4 hours apart, and to keep a detailed food and sleep log. In addition to energy intake information, this log includes assessment of sleep onset and morning awakening, presence of initial insomnia, frequency and duration of awakenings, and presence of morning anorexia to assist in diagnosing NES.

During the early sessions, an official time is chosen for the kitchen to be "closed." Experimentation with behavioral techniques will begin with nighttime awakenings and ingestions, including attention to the energy and nutrient content of the snacks. A behavioral chain describing patients' typical patterns of nighttime eating is completed during session 2 and given to patients for reference at home (Figures 14.4 and 14.5).

For those patients who are overweight or obese, they will start to keep information regarding caloric intake at session 3, with the help of a calorie counter book (e.g., *The Doctor's Pocket Calorie, Fat & Carbohydrate Counter*), website (e.g., *www.sparkpeople.com*), or a smartphone application to inform food choice decisions. If patients have a weight loss goal, they will be encouraged to maintain a calorie goal of 1,200–1,500 calories for women and 1,500–1,800 calories for men. Patients weighing more than 250 pounds keep an intake goal of 1,500–1,800 kcal. Those who are extremely obese, typically those over 350 pounds, should consult a dietician for specific energy requirements. Overall, consultation with a

Directions: Mark an × on the line for how much you are experiencing each feeling before you eat at night.

Day: _____   Time: _____

1. **Physical hunger**—*feeling physical signs of hunger*

   _____

   not at all   **extremely**

2. **Craving food**—*desiring specific foods*

   _____

   not at all   **extremely**

3. **Compelled to eat**—*having a drive to eat, to put something in your stomach, not necessarily for a specific food*

   _____

   not at all   **extremely**

4. **Anxious**—*having anxiety-provoking thoughts, ruminations, racing thoughts, etc.*

   _____

   not at all   **extremely**

5. **Agitated**—*having the physical feeling of not being able to sit still or remain in bed, often linked to anxiety*

   _____

   not at all   **extremely**

6. **Sad**—*feeling depressed or wanting to eat to help improve depressed mood*

   _____

   not at all   **extremely**

7. **Bored**—*looking for an activity to pass the time*

   _____

   not at all   **extremely**

8. **Tired**—*feeling fatigued and just wanting to get to sleep*

   _____

   not at all   **extremely**

FIGURE 14.1. Nighttime Eating Assessment.

Wake-up time: _____7:30 am_____ Bedtime: _____10:30 pm_____

Day: __Saturday__ Date: __August 23__ Desire to eat breakfast? Y N

Time	Food and Beverage	Amount	Calories	Check if NES episode
8 am	Black Coffee	1 cup	5	
12:30 pm	Pizza Hut Pepperoni Pizza (1/8 medium pizza)	2 slices	560	
	Baby carrots	5	20	
	Rice Krispy Treat (3" × 3" × 2")	1 square	90	
	Pepsi 1 can	12 fl oz	150	
	Total:		820	
2 pm	Coffee	2 cups	10	
	Coffee-mate, Hazelnut	1 Tbsp.	25	
	Total:		35	
8 pm	Hamburger Patty (Lean ground beef), broiled	4 oz raw	230	
	Wonder Bread hamburger bun	1 bun	120	
	Tomato	1 slice	5	
	Yellow Mustard	1 Tbsp.	9	
	Ore-Ida french fries, baked	10 med	100	
	Total:		464	
9 pm	Breyers Vanilla ice cream	1 cup	300	
10 pm	Granny Smith apple	1 medium	70	
	Cracker Barrel cheddar cheese	3 oz.	360	
	Total:		430	
1 am	Wonder Bread	2 slices	140	✓
	Skippy peanut butter	2 Tbsp.	210	✓
	Total:		350	
	Day total:		2404	

Time and duration of awakenings:

1. __1-1:30 am__   2. __3-3:30 am__   Did it take > 30 minutes to fall asleep? Y N

3. _____   4. _____

FIGURE 14.2. Example of a completed food and sleep log.

Directions: Complete this daily log to track the timing and amount of your eating and sleeping. Please include details or brands of foods that you have eaten, and measure them, when possible. This can be used to track your progress in treatment.

Wake-up time: _____   Bedtime: _____

Day: _____   Date: _____ Desire to eat breakfast?   Y   N

Time	Food and Beverage	Amount	Calories	Check if NES episode

Time and duration of awakenings:

1. _____   2. _____   Did it take > 30 minutes to fall asleep?   Y   N
3. _____   4. _____

FIGURE 14.3. Blank food and sleep log.

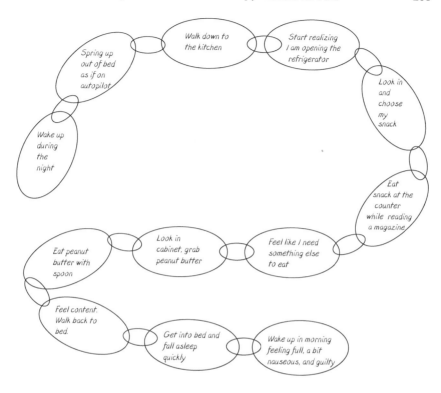

FIGURE 14.4. Example of a completed behavioral chain for NES.

dietician for all patients is encouraged. Clinical experience has suggested that implementing a calorie goal improves motivation for change and compliance among those seeking treatment for NES, as weight management is typically one of the main reasons they are seeking treatment.

Alternative thoughts and behaviors are explored through dysfunctional thought records (DTRs; Figure 14.6), and patients are encouraged to reach out to others for social support. These exercises are practiced in sessions and assigned as homework throughout the course of therapy, with the goal of having the patient challenge first the behaviors and then the dysfunctional thoughts such as "I won't be able to fall back to sleep if I can't have that piece of cake." DTR exercises also help patients identify cognitive errors, such as overgeneralizing, mind reading, or all-or-none-thinking, which will be particularly effective in addressing the depressed mood or anxiety that many persons with NES experience.

Directions: Complete the chain for a typical night eating event. Include the circumstances when you started thinking about wanting to eat and each step that was involved in getting to the food, choosing it, eating it, and then what happened and/or how you felt afterward. Think about where you could change the typical chain of events along the way and write these ideas alongside the chain as an alternative activity or course of action to the usual outcome (i.e., night eating). Display the chain or review it each day/ night to help reinforce the new behaviors you would like to try instead of eating.

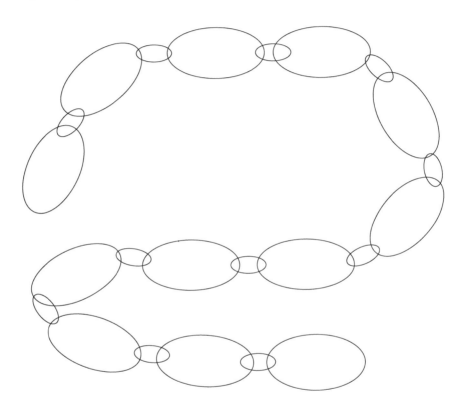

FIGURE 14.5. Blank behavioral chain.

Situation	Emotions	Automatic Thoughts	Alternative Responses	Outcome
Where were you and what was happening when you felt the urge to eat or were in an upsetting situation (include date and time)?	What emotions (sad, angry, anxious, etc.) did you feel at the time? Rate intensity 0–100%	What thoughts and/or images went through your mind? Rate your belief in each (0–100%)	Use the questions and distortions at the bottom to compose responses to the automatic thoughts. Rate your belief in each (0–100%).	Re-rate your belief in your original automatic thoughts (0–100%) and the intensity of your emotions (0–100%).
10:50 pm trying to fall asleep, coughing	Scared (50%) Anxious (70%)	I hate sleeping! I know I will be waking up again to eat. (90%)	Take deep breaths and focus on them. I can fall asleep. If I wake up, I can try the same thing again and hope for the best. (60%) It would feel great to wake up in the morning without eating. (100%)	Scared 30% Anxious 40%

1. What is the **evidence** that the automatic thought is true?
2. Are there **alternative explanations** for that event, or **alternative ways** to view the situation?
3. What are the **implications** if the thought is true? What is most upsetting about it? What's the most realistic view? What can I do about it?
4. What would I tell a good friend to do in the same situation?

Possible Distortions: All-or-nothing thinking, overgeneralization, discounting the positives, jumping to conclusions, mind-reading, fortune-telling, magnifying/minimizing, emotional reasoning, making "should" statements, labeling, inappropriate blaming.

FIGURE 14.6. Example of a completed Night Eating Syndrome Thought Record. Adapted from *Cognitive Therapy: Basics and Beyond*. Copyright 1995 by Judith S. Beck. Adapted by permission of The Guilford Press.

Once the patient increases awareness of these cognitive errors and the situations in which they are most often applied, they are then instructed to start tempering the negative emotional responses. These include the use of food to soothe negative emotions at night that usually occur in response to interpretations of automatic thoughts. See Figure 14.7 for a blank thought record.

Stage 2

Once these initial goals from the first stage of therapy are met, the middle stage ensues (sessions 5–8). During this stage, therapists work with patients to establish the coping skills that have been developed in the first phase, and automatic thoughts are challenged. During this stage the therapist will pay closer attention to the common themes related to night eating episodes that were captured on the Nighttime Eating Assessment forms and to problem solve these situations. Depressed mood and dysfunctional thoughts about eating will continue to be monitored and addressed through the use of DTRs. Behavioral interventions also continue to be emphasized. Behavioral experimentation is essential for decreasing the occurrence of evening and nighttime ingestions and increasing the budding self-efficacy in the patient. While the actual methods to achieve the reductions in nocturnal ingestions may differ, each approach will involve some type of stimulus control of food, including preparing preset portion sizes, locking or hiding away desirable food at night, or engaging in another quiet (nonarousing) activity until sleepiness prevails.

In general, morning anorexia will be addressed by encouraging patients to eat a healthy breakfast as part of their structured meal schedule. The therapist stresses that this process helps retrain the body to expect food during the day and not depend on energy intake at night. It is explained that eating breakfast is not sufficient in reducing evening hyperphagia and nocturnal ingestions, but it is likely necessary. Thoughts regarding fear of weight gain and lack of morning or daytime hunger will be explored. As morning anorexia was the last characteristic to reverse with successful treatment using sertraline, it is expected that in the CBT approach morning hunger will not return until the percentage of caloric intake consumed after the evening meal is decreased.

Mood is also addressed for those many NES patients who struggle with depression. In this middle stage of therapy, not only are automatic thoughts relating to self-worth or loveableness examined, but also the patient's core beliefs or schemata are identified and challenged. The patient will work to generate reasonable alternatives for dealing with

Situation Where were you and what was happening when you felt the urge to eat or were in an upsetting situation (include date and time)?	Emotions What emotions (sad, angry, anxious, etc.) did you feel at the time? Rate intensity 0–100%	Automatic Thoughts What thoughts and/or images went through your mind? Rate your belief in each (0–100%)	Alternative Responses Use the questions and distortions at the bottom to compose responses to the automatic thoughts. Rate your belief in each (0–100%).	Outcome Re-rate your belief in your original automatic thoughts (0–100%) and the intensity of your emotions (0–100%).

1. What is the **evidence** that the automatic thought is true?
2. Are there **alternative explanations** for that event, or **alternative ways** to view the situation?
3. What are the **implications** if the thought is true? What is most upsetting about it? What's the most realistic view? What can I do about it?
4. What would I tell a good friend to do in the same situation?

Possible Distortions: All-or-nothing thinking, overgeneralization, discounting the positives, jumping to conclusions, mind-reading, fortune-telling, magnifying/minimizing, emotional reasoning, making "should" statements, labeling, inappropriate blaming.

FIGURE 14.7. Blank Night Eating Syndrome Thought Record.

these beliefs. Negative beliefs about weight and shape are also addressed throughout the therapeutic process, as these beliefs are often intricately tied to negative affect.

While the treatment is drawn from the experience of experts in the fields of eating disorders, insomnia, and depression, aspects of NES will require unique assessment and problem solving. One of the most unique of these is the varying degree of awareness during the night eating episodes. While patients with NES are aware and are not having parasomnic events (as happens in SRED where persons are eating during episodes of sleepwalking; see Chapter 9 [Howell & Crow]), many report a lowered level of alertness and control over their actions. Clinical experience also suggests that there is variability in the timing and the extent of awareness; many patients report that their first moments of awareness do not occur until they are standing in front of the refrigerator, while others are fully aware from the moment they wake and rise from bed. Many patients are not able to identify automatic thoughts until they are about to eat or are already eating. Treatment of nocturnal ingestions is directed toward increasing awareness progressively earlier in the awakening process so that patients can gradually gain control over each eating episode. Behavioral techniques, such as a bell on the door or some other type of alarm may be used in some cases to raise awareness earlier in the awakening and foraging process.

Stage 3

The final stage of therapy, sessions 9 and 10, transitions the patient to sessions every other week. Progress and successes are reviewed, and ideas regarding how to anticipate future problems will be generated. Patients will be encouraged to practice the strategies and techniques learned in treatment, especially because the patients would now be feeling better and may need encouragement to keep the strategies they learned fresh in their repertoire of coping skills. Therapists also address anxieties or worries about the patients' levels of self-efficacy for facing their challenges alone by becoming more of a consultant than active therapist, thus shifting the responsibility for successes and setbacks on the patient. Overall, this stage helps to reinforce successes and guards against threats to relapse.

CBT Sessions

Following is a summary of the sessions. This description represents a reasonable schedule for what to cover in which session, but some of the content may be introduced earlier within the same phase, as determined by specific patient symptoms or complaints.

Session 1

Introduce the CBT model. Explain the concept of how a cue from a situation evokes a response, which produces a consequence, using examples based on night eating. Explain the concept of NES as a delay or shift in the usual pattern of eating by describing how the human body is "wired" to eat during the day and sleep during the night. In NES, the drive to eat is set at an unusual time, and it disrupts the usual sleeping pattern.

Review symptoms of NES during the past week to establish a baseline. Walk through the example and the format of the food and sleep log (Figures 14.2 and 14.3). Calories are not to be recorded yet, just the amount, types, and timing of food consumed. Exercise/purposeful physical activity should be noted as well. Explain the Nighttime Eating Assessment forms that are to be completed after the kitchen "closing" time, including nocturnal ingestions. The closing of the kitchen is to be established after determining the typical dinner time, cleaning routine, and food preparation for the next day. A portion-controlled evening snack is included in this daily routine. Explain that it is typical for most people to have an evening snack and encourage them to set out a specific portion of the snack, sit down, and fully enjoy it.

Afterward, patients declare the kitchen "closed," and they are recommended only to drink water after that point. They are encouraged to brush their teeth and leave the vicinity of the kitchen. Review the Nighttime Eating Assessment (Figure 14.1) and its purpose, stating that it is used to raise awareness for the reasons he/she is eating at night. Completing this exercise is also used as another barrier by slowing down the typical eating ritual during the night; it serves as a deliberate pause between rising from the couch in the evening or the bed during the night and the act of eating.

Begin to establish regular meal and snack times and sleeping times. If patients are first eating at noon, establish a breakfast time. If patients are not eating until 3:00 P.M. or later, start by establishing lunch and then work toward establishing breakfast the following week. If patients become anxious about gaining weight before their night eating is under control, assure them that weight will be monitored to guard against significant weight gain.

Homework: Complete food and sleep logs and Nighttime Eating

Assessment forms (Figure 14.1) for each late evening snack and nocturnal ingestions.

Session 2

Review homework, food, and sleep logs, and Nighttime Eating Assessment forms from the past week and identify the most common feelings
associated with night eating episodes. Identify a particular night eating
situation. Review automatic thoughts, themes, and decisions and complete a behavioral chain (Figures 14.4 and 14.5) for night eating episodes.
Discuss strategies for decreasing amounts eaten during night through
stimulus-control techniques and portion control. Insert where these
strategies would occur on the behavioral chain. Some strategies include
posting signs, announcing out loud that the kitchen is closed at the desig-
nated time, allowing snacks to occur only in the kitchen, replacing snack
foods with fruits and vegetables, keeping all food out of the bedroom,
and deliberately staying in bed for at least 5 minutes before reassessing
the need to eat. Others have found success with physical barriers, such
as painter's tape (which removes easily from walls and trim) or a small
chain across a doorway, that help remind them to turn back from the
kitchen and go to bed.

Based on the food and sleep log completed by the patient, review
his or her daytime eating schedule and habits. Encourage three regular
meals with small snacks in between. Address concerns about weight gain
by explaining that the body has to be retrained to eat regularly during
the day so it can expect the majority of its food then and not at night.
Explain that his or her body has come to expect to eat at night, and that
it will take some time to retrain it not to expect those calories at night
but to expect them on a regular basis during the day. As his or her eating schedule becomes more regular, the patient will have more control
generally over energy intake, and weight loss efforts (if appropriate) will
be more successful.

Homework: Assign food and sleep log and Nighttime Eating Assessment form (Figure 14.1) (if additional data are needed).

Session 3

Review diary and Nighttime Eating Assessment forms for the past week.
Apply the behavioral chain started in session 2 to specific eating episodes.
Walk through any successful situations to examine what worked well,
then examine nocturnal or late evening eating episodes that the patient

was not able to resist. Problem solve ways to address the difficulties the patient had using any antecedents to night eating and feelings identified on the Nighttime Eating Assessment forms.

Introduce the Calorie Counter book, website, or application to keep track of calories in the food log and set an appropriate calorie goal (as discussed above). Explain that keeping a record of all calories is the best predictor of weight loss. If they do not need to lose weight, they can use their caloric intake to gain perspective on where they need to shift some of their nighttime calories to the day. For all patients, estimate the number of calories they can allot for themselves at night, with the idea of trying to shift energy intake to earlier in the day.

Homework: Assign food and sleep log, including calorie counting for overweight and obese patients wishing to lose weight. Establish regular daytime eating schedule, with breakfast, lunch, dinner, and two to three small snacks. Continue using signs and barriers at night.

Session 4

Review log for past week and recordings of calories. Problem solve any difficulties they had with recording their energy intake, and reiterate that keeping track of their calorie intake is one of the best predictors of weight control and that it raises awareness about the extent of their night eating. Logging also sheds light on the specific food choices they are making during these late-night and early-morning hours.

Introduce DTRs. Work through a night eating situation and identify typical cognitive distortions and alternative responses. Use examples that they have identified in previous sessions or an example from the previous week. Explain that negative feelings that occur from a variety of situations often contribute to night eating. Therefore, it is important to apply the DTRs to any situation, both eating and non-eating-related situations, that causes negative affect. Explain that night eating is often a response to anxiety-provoking or other negative situations and that food is often used during the night to soothe negative feelings. Therefore, working to alleviate negative feelings triggered by situations during the day, as well as the night, should help to alleviate stressors that act as antecedents to night eating episodes.

Use the themes that patients have identified most often in relation to their night eating as part of their examples, and explain the cognitive distortions found at the bottom of the DTR so they can apply them to their own experiences (Figures 14.6 and 14.7).

Homework: Assign food and sleep log and DTRs.

Session 5

Review the food and sleep log, including caloric intake, and DTRs for the past week. Take some time to review the situations described on the DTRs and the effect that these exercises had on their mood and their night eating. Explore any difficulties they had using the forms. Review which night eating themes and cognitive distortions fit the situations described.

Discuss alternatives to eating at night. Introduce deep-breathing exercises and brief progressive muscle relaxation (PMR) exercises to be used when resisting night eating episodes (Figure 14.8). Explain that deep breathing plus PMR can serve two purposes. First, the focus on the body helps to distract thoughts from a food craving or other thoughts that drive the patient to eat. Second, these exercises help to calm and relax them, by slowing down heart rate and central nervous system responses and relaxing major muscle groups so that they can fall asleep easier. Practice the deep breathing and PMR in session and give them the handout to guide their use at home. If the therapist is not familiar with PMR, he or she is encouraged to suggest Internet-based resources or self-help resources.

Directions: Breathe deeply—in through the nose for 5 seconds, out through the mouth for 5 seconds. Repeat several times before starting and before and after each exercise. Tighten each muscle group for 5–10 seconds and release. Repeat each muscle group as needed until you feel all of the tension released in each location.

Clench fists

Bend arm—biceps

Shrug shoulders

Wrinkle forehead

Frown

Clench jaw

Stomach

Arch back

Buttocks and thighs

Point toes

Flex toes

BREATHE DEEPLY THE WHOLE TIME!!!

FIGURE 14.8. Deep breathing and brief PMR exercise.

Homework: Assign food and sleep log, DTRs, and practice breathing plus PMR daily so they can use it when needed before bed and upon nighttime awakenings.

Session 6

Review log, including caloric goals, and DTRs for the past week. Review breathing and PMR exercises and the times they were used during the week. Discuss particular themes and triggers for night eating episodes and precipitants that may occur during the day, and any alternative responses they could generate for automatic thoughts associated with those situations.

Discuss progress with weight and weight loss goals. For normal-weight patients, review any persistence of purposeful daytime restriction and overexercising (the two most common disordered eating activities associated with NES and most commonly seen in normal-weight persons with NES). Review meal patterns and caloric intake. Work together with the patient to identify goals for limiting access to high-calorie foods or foods that they crave, especially in the evening or at night. Encourage them to satisfy cravings for specific foods with portion-controlled servings during the day or with dinner. Explain that this strategy can satisfy the "taste" that they have for a specific food, while helping to prevent them from eating more of the food than they initially desired. This strategy should help prevent dichotomous thinking about foods that may trigger their eating. It helps the patient shift their intake of these foods to the day, as opposed to the evening or night, when their resolve and ability to use portion control is particularly low.

Homework: Assign food and sleep log and DTRs. Continue eating regularly during the day, and continue practicing deep breathing and PMR exercises daily.

Session 7

Review log, including calorie goals, and DTRs for the past week. Examine sleep hygiene behaviors and obstacles for achieving a regular sleep schedule. A sleep hygiene tip sheet to review with patients can be found in Figure 14.9. These often include leaving the television on all night, napping after dinner on the couch, and going to bed well before they are tired enough to sleep. Explain that awakenings will occur less often if they are very tired when they go to bed (sleep restriction). Distractions,

If you have trouble sleeping, either falling asleep initially or waking up during the night, use these tips to help improve your sleep hygiene:

1. Create a dark and quiet bedroom environment. Use room-darkening shades or curtains. Use a sound machine, if needed, to block out noise from others in the home or noise from outside.

2. Use the bed for sleep and intimate moments. Do not spend extra time throughout the day in your bed to do work or watch television.

3. If you have dogs or children who sleep in your bed, you may want to reconsider this arrangement, particularly if you have a small bed. They often move around and can cause more awakenings than you would experience on your own. Your pets may even become conditioned to want food during the night along with you, which may help keep the behavior in place!

4. Go to bed and wake up at the same time every day, including weekends. This will help you to regulate your body's inner clock to expect sleep during those times.

5. Go to bed when you are tired. Do not lie down too early or extend your time in bed in the morning if you had trouble sleeping. Try to confine your time in bed to the hours that you will actually be sleeping.

6. Do not leave the television on all night. Sound and light levels vary from show to show and from shows to commercials. If you are prone to waking up already, these variations in sound and light may increase your risk for waking up during the night.

7. Do not drink caffeine after noon. Do not drink excessive fluids after dinner (to prevent having to use the bathroom during the night).

8. Limit your alcohol intake. As alcohol leaves your system, it can disrupt sleep.

9. Do not smoke.

FIGURE 14.9. Sleep hygiene tips.

---

such as light or volume changes on the TV, can disrupt sleep. Encourage patients to use a fan or white noise machine as background noise during the night (if needed), instead of the TV, and the therapist may even suggest a night light if this eases anxieties about the sleeping environment. Assess the size of the bed and whether any pets or small children share the bed, as these can also serve as an impetus for awakenings. If frequent trips to the bathroom are needed during the night, encourage patients to put up reminder signs to go straight back to bed in order to keep their awareness raised and resolve up not to eat. Patients are also encouraged to keep water by their beds or to drink in the bathroom as a surrogate for eating.

Discuss the role of physical activity in relation to eating, weight loss goals (if appropriate), sleep quality, and overall health. Review the physical activity that they have been doing, and address obstacles to exercising. An example of an exercise log is found in Figure 14.10. Explain that exercise is an excellent tool for weight maintenance and improving health, and that it may help contribute to more restful sleep.

Homework: Assign food and sleep log and DTRs. Continue using deep breathing and PMR, sleep hygiene techniques, and establish a healthy exercise plan.

Directions: Track your physical activity throughout the week. This can be used together with the food and sleep log to track your progress in treatment, as exercise may help reduce night eating and weight, and more generally improve your health.

Day/date	Type of exercise	How many minutes?
	Weekly total:	

FIGURE 14.10. Blank exercise log.

Session 8

Review the food and sleep log, including calorie goals, and DTRs for the past week. Discuss any progress in reducing night eating and positively reinforce any changes. Assess what areas remain most problematic with the help of the logs and DTRs. Review the most effective skills learned that are specific to the problem areas and prepare for a 2-week interval before next session.

Homework: Assign food and sleep log. Use DTRs as needed. Continue using their skills daily, including deep breathing and PMR, sleep hygiene techniques, and exercise.

Session 9

Review the food and sleep log, including calorie goals, and DTRs for the past week. Discuss weight loss, maintenance, or gain across the course of the past 10 weeks. Identify any problems or regression to past behaviors that have occurred with night eating and weight loss efforts. Review skills learned specific to those areas. Discuss anticipating setbacks and how to bolster self-efficacy. Explain that lapses are to be expected, but that it is important not to "throw in the towel" when these lapses occur. Discuss the importance of using the tools that he/she learned so far, including posting visual reminders of individualized goals to help prevent set-backs. Reinforce the progress they have made so far.

Homework: Assign food and sleep logs and DTRs, as needed. Stress the importance of continuing to record food intake, particularly if weight loss is a goal. Next session is in 2 weeks.

Session 10

Review food and sleep log, including calorie and weight loss goals, and DTRs for the past 2 weeks. Discuss reactions to the CBT treatment and again emphasize how to troubleshoot for future setbacks with review of skills learned in program. Highlight the patient's successes and any benefits that the patient can identify related to his/her changes in eating and sleeping patterns.

Arrange for booster sessions as needed. In general, encourage patients to continue to keep their own logs of their food intake, particularly if they have a weight loss goal. They may also wish to keep coming to therapy to continue weight loss and a healthy lifestyle on an ongoing basis, if desired. Discuss goals that patients have regarding night eating and weight that they can continue to achieve.

Maintenance Phase

Booster sessions of CBT will review any lapses in night eating and reinforce the skills learned during the acute therapy. Patients will be reminded of the importance of the maintenance stage, for their long-term well-being.

Chapter 15

Other Approaches
to the Treatment
of Night Eating Syndrome

Laura Pawlow

For a variety of personal, economical, and logistical reasons, clients may prefer to target their night eating syndrome (NES) symptoms with means other than medication or cognitive-behavioral therapy. This chapter provides a review of the promising alternative treatments that have indicated some degree of success in reducing the symptoms of NES. For example, behavior therapy, a system of psychotherapy that relies solely on the application of behavioral principles, has shown promise in reducing night eating in two case study reports. (Also, two studies on predominantly behavioral weight loss strategies suggest that night eaters may be able to lose weight with treatments that do not specifically target the elimination of nocturnal eating.) In addition, progressive muscle relaxation (PMR), a simple technique frequently employed by therapists of many theoretical orientations, led to decreased nighttime consumption, increased morning appetite, and a small degree of weight loss in one randomized controlled study on a NES population. And finally, phototherapy, where clients sit under a specialized source of bright light, was seen to eliminate symptoms of NES in two case reports. Each of these alternate therapies has unique advantages, for example, PMR and phototherapy are very convenient and involve a minimal investment of the client's time and finances. Behavior therapy may be attractive to those wishing to take a less introspective approach to treatment. And behavioral weight loss may appeal to those with NES who wish simultaneously to reduce excess weight and control their problematic night eating. While the findings in this chapter are exciting, the fact that much of this research is case study in nature and has not been independently replicated deserves special attention. Further research, including independent, large-scale, controlled clinical trials, is necessary before broad conclusions may be drawn.

Behavior Therapy and Behavioral Weight Loss

Behavior Therapy and NES

Behavior therapy, or the application of modern learning theory (e.g., classical and operant conditioning) to improve human functioning, became widely popular with the American public in the post-World War II industrial era. At that time, both psychologists and the general population were becoming critical of psychology's almost exclusive emphasis on unobservable phenomena, such as Freud's unconscious. The unobserved, they argued, was also immeasurable and therefore, unscientific. Behaviorist pioneers strove to apply the scientific principle of hypothesis testing to the alleviation of such problems as anxiety and depression by breaking these problems down into discrete, observable, and changeable maladaptive behaviors. Early behavioral clinicians felt that time in the therapy session was much better spent identifying and rectifying problematic behaviors than in spending hours trying to determine the cause of these behaviors.

Currently, a majority of clinicians identify as cognitive-behavioral in approach, meaning that they use techniques from both behavior and cognitive therapy. While cognitive-behavioral therapy (CBT) is widely effective with a range of disorders, pure behavior therapy is also empirically supported for many disorders, including phobias, generalized anxiety, insomnia, obsessive–compulsive disorder, depression, and obesity. Behavior therapy is comparable in price, availability, and length of treatment to CBT. Clients typically commit to weekly, hour-long sessions with a therapist for approximately 16 to 20 weeks and are expected to do homework outside of the treatment session. Because behavior therapy is well established, widely used, and efficacious with many disorders, many insurance plans will cover a set amount of sessions with a licensed provider.

In 1978, Coates reported partial success in the alleviation of night eating in the case of a 30-year-old man with relatively recent-onset NES. As this client had previously been successful at weight loss and smoking cessation by using self-management strategies, he was eager to apply similar principles to control his NES. His therapist engaged successively more limiting response prevention techniques (e.g., posting notes on the refrigerator reminding the client not to eat after bedtime, placing furniture and other obstacles in the client's path to the kitchen, locking kitchen utensils in the trunk of the client's car), with no success. Finally, after several weeks of therapy, a reliable plan emerged. All edibles were stored in the client's refrigerator each night; the refrigerator was then locked with a bicycle chain, and the key given to a roommate. This intervention completely eliminated nighttime eating, restored morning hunger, and resulted in weight loss.

The author suggests that the milder response prevention techniques were ineffective because the client viewed them as challenges which he had the power to overcome. When faced with the increased difficulty of gaining access to his food at night, the client experienced greater levels of anxiety, but was ultimately rewarded with a greater and more reinforcing sense of relief when he was finally able to access the food (e.g., after getting the utensils out of his trunk). Yet when the food was locked up and the key given to the roommate, the author speculated that the client felt that obtaining the food was beyond his control—because the roommate, and not the client himself, controlled access to the food, this was not a challenge the client could overcome, and thus he had no anxiety about it—he simply went back to bed. The client continued to perform this behavior every evening, and at 18-month follow-up reported that this solution was still working for him. Of note, during the course of therapy, the therapist purposefully planned 3 nights of not locking up the food, and the client engaged in night bingeing on all three evenings. While this treatment was successful in that it eliminated night eating and the client was willing to continue locking up the food each night, the clinician considered it only partially successful. Ultimately, the goal would be elimination of night eating through the will of the client, without the elaborate food-locking ritual and the need for a willing roommate to guard the key each night.

Williamson, Lawson, Bennett, and Hinz (1989) used contingency management techniques to eliminate night eating in a 24-year-old woman with bulimia nervosa. Her bingeing occurred primarily at night and was accompanied by rumination (voluntary regurgitation and reswallowing of ingested foods). Although the client considered herself overweight, her body mass index (BMI) was 22. While the client attended group therapy for her bulimia, her nighttime binge episodes were specifically targeted with contingency management. This client highly valued her jewelry and agreed to give it all to her therapist under the condition that she could earn some of it back each week through successful attainment of her treatment goals. Over approximately 20 weeks, the threshold for success was consistently increased. For example, for the first few weeks, "success" was achieved if the client went 2 nights per week without a binge. Over the course of treatment, "success" was eventually defined as making it through the entire week without a nighttime binge. While the client reported some lapses over the course of the program, from week 28 until the end of the 32-week program, she did not engage in any night eating, and this was maintained at both her 3-month and 2-year follow-up visits. Bulimic and rumination symptoms improved during this time period as well; however, since the patient was concurrently undergoing cognitive-behavioral group therapy for her bulimia, care must be taken when drawing any conclusions specifically about contingency management's effects on NES.

Behavioral Weight Loss and NES

Behavior modification has also been applied to weight loss, the prevention of weight gain, and the regulation of eating with a good degree of success (e.g., Wing, 2002). A comprehensive behavioral approach to weight loss incorporates strategies that reduce caloric intake, increase physical activity, and introduce behaviors known to promote weight loss such as regular self-monitoring of weight, keeping food and exercise logs, introducing non-food rewards to encourage weight loss efforts, and practicing simple behavior changes such as eating more slowly and not keeping serving dishes on the table.

Stunkard's original work (Stunkard, Grace, & Wolff, 1955) indicated that those with NES were less successful at losing weight than non-night eaters, and that some with NES even cited adverse effects in response to their weight loss efforts. More recently, Gluck, Geliebter, and Satov (2001) reported that in a weight loss treatment-seeking population, after controlling for body mass index (BMI), those with NES lost significantly less weight than those without over a 1-month period of a medically supervised liquid diet. Similarly, night eaters had significantly higher BMIs than non-night eaters 1 year following bariatric surgery (Powers, Perez, Boyd, & Rosemurgy, 1999). These studies all utilized traditional weight loss methods, suggesting that an intervention that specifically addressees nocturnal eating may be necessary for night eaters wishing to lose weight.

However, recent work by Dalle Grave, Calugi, Ruocco, and Marchesini (2011) suggests that this may not be the case. In their study, 38 weight loss treatment–seeking obese night eaters and 62 matched controls did not significantly differ in mean BMI loss following 21 days of inpatient treatment or at 6-month follow-up. Upon discharge from the inpatient phase of treatment, all participants were encouraged to maintain their newly acquired dietary, physical, and behavioral practices and were given contact information for clinicians specializing in outpatient weight loss. Approximately 62% of the entire sample utilized outpatient obesity specialists while the remainder followed their weight loss plan without professional help. The proportion of night eaters was similar in both groups, and the groups did not differ in BMI loss at 6-month follow-up. See Figure 15.1.

While this is the first study to find that night eaters lost as much weight as those without NES, even more striking is the fact that of the 29 night eaters who participated in the 6-month follow-up assessment

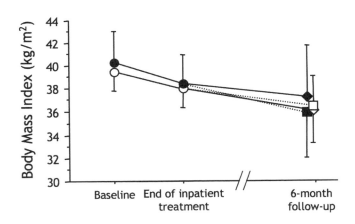

FIGURE 15.1. Body mass index at baseline, at the end of the inpatient program and at 6-month follow-up in obese individuals with NES (closed symbols) and without NES (open symbols). At 6-month follow-up, diamonds identify participants on supervised follow-up; squares and dotted lines are participants managing their weight loss program without professional help, following the initial inpatient treatment (mean ± 95 confidence interval). From Dalle Grave, Calugi, Ruocco, and Marchesini (2011). Copyright 2011 by John Wiley & Sons, Inc. Reprinted by permission.

procedures, only 8 still met criteria for NES, and 18 indicated that they had not engaged in any night eating whatsoever for at least 3 months. As no specific strategies were implemented to specifically target night eating in this intervention, the authors speculate that their unique findings may be attributable to the fact that their weight loss program incorporated a 3-week inpatient stay. During this time, participants were placed on a strict, low-calorie diet (1,200 kcal/day for women and 1,500 kcal/day for men; 55% carbohydrate, 15% protein, 30% fat), engaged in daily 30-minute bicycling and biweekly 45-minute calisthenic exercise sessions, and attended regular psychoeducational group therapy sessions focused on teaching tips and techniques that promote weight loss (e.g., portion control and how to stick to a diet when dining in restaurants). As part of the diet plan, participants had no access to food at night and had a pattern of regular eating (breakfast, lunch, afternoon snack, dinner) imposed on them for the entirety of their inpatient stay. The obligatory daytime intake likely offset nighttime hunger and reset circadian appetite rhythms, while the complete lack of access to nighttime food likely extinguished any anxiety-driven nocturnal eating (similar to the effects found in Coates's [1978] case study). In addition, while this study did not target night eaters per se, Reid et al.'s recent (2010) work indicates that regular aerobic exercise promotes sleep and improves mood in those with sleep disturbances; the nine aerobic exercise sessions per week practiced during the inpatient phase may have bolstered these night eaters' ability to stay asleep at night. While Dalle Grave et al. (2011) suggest that night eaters may not require weight loss programs that specifically target their symptoms, they caution that more studies are needed to examine the effects of traditional weight loss plans that do not include an initial intensive inpatient phase.

Waller et al.'s (2004) study targeted night snacking in an unusual way: by promoting it. The authors suggest that the substitution of a healthful, portion-controlled snack for more traditional, unstructured, high-calorie postdinner fare would attenuate total evening consumption and thereby facilitate long-term weight loss. In their study, overweight adults who self-reported a history of night snacking (but who did not necessarily meet criteria for NES) were randomly assigned to an evening snack or a control group. Over 4 weeks, the evening snack group was instructed to consume one serving (100–135 kcal) of breakfast cereal with two-thirds of a cup of low-fat milk at least 90 minutes after their evening meal. The control group simply followed their typical dietary practices during the same period of time. While there were no differences between the groups at baseline, after 4 weeks, the evening snack participants who had been compliant (cereal consumed on at least 20 of 28 nights) lost more weight than the controls; this difference was marginally significant. Also marginally significant was the correlation between compliance and weight loss: as the number of evenings participants consumed cereal increased, the amount of weight they lost also increased. Compliant snackers also had a significantly lower level of postdinner caloric intake than control participants. These results may generalize to night eaters.

Behavior Therapy and Behavioral Weight Loss: Mechanism of Action

Behavior therapy is grounded in relatively straightforward theory: alter the patient's environment in ways that reduce the likelihood of problematic behaviors and/or increase the likelihood of more adaptive behavior. The practitioner works with the patient to identify troublesome patterns and generate alternate, adaptive means of coping with situations that have traditionally elicited maladaptive behavior. Behavior therapy places limits on the patient by prescribing set behaviors for dealing with challenging situations. Future applications of behavior therapy on NES should focus on other behavioral techniques such as exposure and response prevention, goal setting, and token economies.

Progressive Muscle Relaxation

PMR Therapy and NES

Edmund Jacobsen pioneered the concept of progressive muscle relaxation in his 1938 book *Progressive Relaxation*. He developed a training program targeted at achieving greater muscular relaxation through tensing and subsequently releasing various muscles one by one. His theory was that since muscle tension typically accompanies anxiety, the practice of sitting quietly with focused attention on muscular tension reduction would reduce both the cognitive and physical components of anxiety. Jacobsen's original program consisted of more than 200 different exercises that would take months to complete. His early work was successful at providing relief from a variety of medical conditions, including high blood pressure and ulcerative colitis (Jacobsen, 1938). Jacobsen's success led to a wide array of variations and in 1973 Bernstein and Borkovec developed the abbreviated progressive muscle relaxation technique (APRT) in an attempt to streamline Jacobsen's program while maintaining the integrity of his original efforts. APRT focuses on only 16 muscle groups and can be performed in as little as 20 minutes; its effectiveness coupled with its brevity and ease of use has led it to become a standard fixture in both clinical practice and research (Carlson & Hoyle, 1993). APRT has been found to be effective for a wide variety of issues; King's (1980) review indicated that a single session consistently reduced heart rate, blood pressure, muscle tension, respiration rate, and skin conductance. More recent studies have yielded reductions in anxiety and cortisol levels (Pawlow & Jones, 2002), decreased levels of chronic pain in the elderly (Morone & Greco, 2007), improved quality of life in patients with multiple sclerosis (Ghafari et al., 2009), and improved sleep in breast cancer patients undergoing chemotherapy (Demiralp, Oflaz, & Komurcu, 2010).

PMR is simple, inexpensive, and fast. These factors contribute to its popularity; approximately 3% of the general population indicated using PMR over the past year in both 2002 and 2007 (Barnes, Bloom, & Nahin, 2009). Written scripts and audiotapes can be purchased at a variety of commercial outlets and many versions are available online free of charge. There are no known adverse effects of practicing PMR, but clients should be cautioned that the effects of the technique improve with practice, and early attempts may provide little to no symptom relief.

Pawlow, O'Neil, and Malcolm (2003) conducted the first controlled psychosocial treatment trial for NES. Nightly, 20-minute sessions of APRT were prescribed for 1 week to a group of 10 participants who met criteria for NES; a control group of participants with NES received no such intervention. All participants attended two laboratory sessions, 1 week apart. In the first, participants in the APRT group were seated in a recumbent position in a recliner in a dimly lit room, and the experimenter then led them through a 20-minute scripted session of APRT. Participants in the control group simply sat quietly in the recliner for the same amount of time. After 20 minutes, stress, anxiety, and salivary cortisol were all significantly reduced in the APRT group, but not in the control group. At the end of the first session, all participants were instructed to keep an eating and hunger diary for following week. Participants in the APRT group received an audiotape of the APRT exercise and were instructed to perform it each evening before bedtime. Exactly 1 week later, each participant returned to the laboratory to provide postexperiment data.

As expected, the APRT group experienced significant reductions in stress, anxiety, fatigue, anger, depression, and cortisol levels after performing the APRT exercise for a week; these results replicated those of previous studies on APRT conducted on non-NES samples. Regarding NES symptoms, at the end of the week the APRT group also had a significant reduction in evening appetite and a significant increase in morning appetite. In addition, there were nonsignificant trends of increased breakfast and decreased nighttime consumption as well as weight loss in the PMR group only. These results were promising, especially given the brief duration of the intervention. See Table 15.1.

PMR: Mechanism of Action

NES has been repeatedly linked to stress (e.g., Gluck et al., 2001; Lundgren, Allison, O'Reardon, & Stunkard, 2008), and work by Wichianson, Bughi, Unger, Spruijt-Metz, and Nguyen-Rodriguez (2009) suggests that night eating may be a maladaptive coping response for high levels of stress. NES is also associated with disturbances in the hypothalamic–pituitary–adrenal axis (Birketvedt, Sundsfjord, & Florholmen, 2002). Birketvedt et al.'s (1999) study compared overweight/obese adults with and without NES. The group with NES had significantly higher levels of the stress hormone cortisol for the majority of the day (between 8:00 A.M. and 2:00 A.M.) and also had an attenuated nocturnal increase in melatonin. Melatonin is suppressed by corticotropin-releasing factor (CRF), which is increased by stress. In other words, night eating may be influenced by stress in all the typical ways that stress can lead to eating, but also by stress's disruption of melatonin in the evening. The reductions in CRF that would accompany a decrease in stress could theoretically alleviate melatonin inhibition, resulting in fewer of the sleep disturbances seen in those with NES. Previous research had suggested that a reduction of

TABLE 15.1. Means and Standard Deviations of Hunger and Night Eating Characteristics during Days 1–8 by Group

	Experimental (n = 10)	Control (n = 10)	p
A.M. hunger rating[a]	2.1 (1.3)	1.2 (0.3)	.036
6:00 P.M. hunger rating	6.5 (3.3)	7.8 (2.2)	.309
9:00 P.M. hunger rating	3.8 (1.6)	6.5 (2.4)	.012
No. of nights with postbedtime eating	0.8 (1.3)	2.2 (1.8)	.064
No. of mornings with breakfasts eaten	2.8 (2.7)	0.9 (1.7)	.077
Weight change	–1.8 (3.8)	0.6 (1.0)	.069

Note. From Pawlow, O'Neil, and Malcolm (2003). Reprinted by permission of Nature Publishing Group.

[a] Hunger rating scale ranged from 1 (lowest) to 10 (highest).

stress through psychotherapy alleviated NES (Stunkard et al., 1955). In addition, two studies by Pawlow and Jones (2002, 2005) indicated that brief sessions of APRT significantly reduced stress and cortisol levels in college students. The results of Pawlow et al.'s 2003 study suggest that the same holds true in an NES sample, and that the reduced stress/cortisol levels may have resulted in reductions in some NES symptoms.

If a reduction of stress can relieve NES symptoms, then it follows that similarly proven stress reduction/adaptive coping techniques such as mindfulness meditation, deep breathing, and guided imagery would have similar results. To date, there are no published reports on the use of any of these techniques as a treatment for NES; however, some literature suggests they are successful in reducing binges in both bulimia nervosa and binge-eating disorder (e.g., Kristeller & Hallett, 1999). As these types of relaxation techniques are typically used under the umbrella of cognitive-behavioral therapy, in many studies it is difficult to determine whether the relaxation technique per se produced results. More research is needed to independently replicate the PMR results and to explore the independent effects of similar stress reduction techniques on night eaters.

Phototherapy

Phototherapy and NES

The beneficial effects of phototherapy, or light therapy, on mental illness were first popularized during early descriptions of seasonal affective disorder. In 1984 Rosenthal et al. published a preliminary report describing patients whose depressions followed a seasonal pattern. Hypothesizing that melatonin played an etiological role in this syndrome of seasonal depression, a treatment was sought that would suppress the release of melatonin. Phototherapy was found, for the first time, to provide relief from this form of depression. Encouraged by these results, researchers in subsequent years performed clinical trials on phototherapy for a variety of other psychiatric conditions, including nonseasonal mood disorders (Golden et al., 2005), certain sleep disorders (Fahey & Zee, 2006), Alzheimer's disease (Dowling, Graf, Hubbard, & Luxenberg, 2007), and obsessive–compulsive disorder (Brinkhuijsen, Koenegracht, & Meesters, 2003).

Phototherapy is a relatively inexpensive, convenient, and user-friendly therapy. Light boxes can be readily purchased commercially (typically for between $250 and $500) and are lightweight and portable.

As phototherapy has gained popularity and empirical support, some insurance providers have begun to cover the cost of the light box unit and bulbs; however, many still do not, as phototherapy is not currently approved by the FDA for the treatment of psychiatric illnesses. In 1995, Tam, Lam, and Levitt reported that light therapy at 2,500 lux for 2 hours per day was comparable to 10,000 lux for 30 minutes per day; most clients prefer the shorter treatment period. Clients sit quietly near the lamp (approximately 1 to 2 feet away) and are permitted to do other sedentary activities (e.g., read, sew, watch television) while undergoing treatment. While a 5-year follow-up study indicated no adverse ocular effects due to phototherapy (Gallin et al., 1995), some users have reported headache, nausea, and agitation as side effects (Labbate, Lafer, Thibault, & Sachs, 1994; Terman & Terman, 1999). Phototherapy is contraindicated in patients taking medications that increase photosensitivity, and, similar to other antidepressants, light therapy may be related to an induction of hypomania or mania in some bipolar patients (Chan, Lam, & Perry, 1994).

Recently, Friedman and colleagues reported success in reducing night eating symptoms after the use of phototherapy in two separate case study reports. In the first (Friedman, Even, Dardennes, & Guelfi, 2002), a 51-year-old obese (BMI = 31) woman seeking treatment for her recurrent major depressive disorder (nonseasonal) was also observed to meet criteria for NES. The client's depression had been treated successfully with paroxetine (40 mg/day) for 2 years, but during the previous month had worsened despite continued compliance with her medication. Her treatment team chose to add phototherapy to her current regimen and prescribed 30-minute sessions of 10,000 lux white light therapy each morning. After 14 days, the client no longer met diagnostic criteria for either major depressive disorder or NES. One month after discontinuing her light therapy regimen, her depression was still in remission, but all of her night eating symptoms had returned. Following 12 more mornings of light therapy, those symptoms had completely remitted as well.

In the second case (Friedman, Even, Dardennes, & Guelfi, 2004), a 46-year-old non-obese (BMI = 23) man seeking treatment for fatigue and poor sleep quality was observed to have recurrent major depressive disorder (nonseasonal) as well as NES. Following 14 consecutive mornings of phototherapy (10,000 lux for 30 minutes), the client no longer met criteria for either major depressive disorder or NES. Taken together, these reports suggest that phototherapy may provide relief for comorbid nonseasonal depression and NES in both obese and non-obese patients;

however, large-scale, controlled clinical trials are necessary to independently confirm and expand these findings.

Phototherapy: Mechanism of Action

From the beginning, NES has been conceptualized as involving an abnormal pattern in the typical circadian rhythm of food intake despite a normal sleep–wake cycle, suggesting a dissociation between the internal mechanisms that control the timing of the two. While the behavioral pattern of delayed-onset intake has been reported repeatedly over the decades, recently a clearer picture has emerged regarding neuroendocrine markers of the circadian cycle. Goel et al.'s (2009) study compared 15 female NES subjects to 14 controls; the women participated in a 3-day laboratory-based study where their blood was drawn routinely and their food intake monitored. Only the NES sample had significant deviations in their physiological markers of appetite regulation, suggesting a disruption of their internal clocks.

NES is similar to seasonal affective disorder in that both involve disruptions of mood, sleep patterns, and neurobiological circadian markers, and both respond to SSRI antidepressant medication. These similarities suggest the two disorders may also share a disruption of the suprachiasmatic nucleus (SCN), our body's most prominent biological clock. This cluster of cells in the hypothalamus plays a major role in regulating the release of various hormones in proper amounts according to the time of day; it is located above the optic nerves and normally responds to alterations in natural light over the course of the day. While the SCN typically responds to natural sunlight, it is also responsive to bright light therapy, meaning that appropriately timed phototherapy can help modulate sleep, mood, and appetite-related hormones in a way similar to taking prescription medication would. Beyond these preliminary reports of success with NES, bright light therapy has also been suggested as a treatment for patients with bulimia whose symptoms follow a seasonal pattern (Braun, Sunday, Fornari, & Halmi, 1999; Lam, Lee, Tam, Grewal, & Yatham, 2001) and for weight loss (Bylesjo, Boman, & Wetterberg, 1996).

Clearly, further controlled clinical trials are needed before phototherapy is considered an established treatment for NES. In addition, future work might explore the effects of dawn simulation therapy. This similar form of treatment involves timing lights in one's bedroom to come on gradually (over a period of 30 minutes to 2 hours) before awakening, and was born out of basic research suggesting that animals' circadian rhythms are highly responsive to the gradually escalating dawn signal that accompanies the rising of the sun each morning. Proponents suggest it is more convenient than bright light therapy, as the entire course of treatment is completed before awakening. Dawn simulation therapy has only been studied as a treatment for seasonal affective disorder; in terms of its efficacy compared to phototherapy, the few available data are inconsistent.

Conclusion

Taken together, these data indicate a promising menu of alternative treatments for those suffering from NES. It could be argued that the successful component underlying most of these strategies is an overall reduction of stress and improvement in mood. For example, PMR directly targets psychological and physiological stress though exercises designed to be incompatible with the stress response. Phototherapy directly alters mood through the use of a relaxing procedure (sitting quietly under a bright light) that positively regulates mood, sleep, and appetite-related hormones. While the behavioral and behavioral weight loss techniques discussed in this chapter did not contain a relaxation component per se, they all altered the patients' environments in ways that could be viewed as indirectly stress reducing. As Coates (1978) suggests, the complete elimination of the choice to eat at night that was implemented in his study and during the inpatient phase of Dalle Grave et al.'s (2011) study not only provides a simple barrier to night eating, but could also be viewed stress reducing in that it eliminates the patient's anxiety-ridden *choice* as to whether to engage in night eating. Similarly, the enforced structure of having a preplanned snack in Waller et al.'s (2004) study may provide the night eater with peace of mind because he or she doesn't have to struggle with the decisions of if, what, and how much to eat. NES is clearly associated with stress, and nocturnal eating may be a coping mechanism for those who can't identify healthier methods of dealing with their stress. Perhaps stress reduction through either traditional means or by simplifying the options available to night eaters is the key to managing this disorder. Clinicians dealing with this population would be wise both to monitor and aim to reduce their patients' stress levels throughout the course of treatment.

References

Barnes, P. M., Bloom, B., & Nahin, R. L. (2009). Complementary and alternative medicine use among adults and children: United States, 2007. *National Health Statistics Reports, 12,* 1–23.

Bernstein, D. A., & Borkovec, T. D. (1973). *Progressive relaxation training.* Champaign, IL: Research Press.

Birketvedt, G., Florholmen, J., Sundsfjord, J., Osterud, B., Dinges, D., Bilker, W., et al. (1999). Behavioral and neuroendocrine characteristics of the night eating syndrome. *Journal of the American Medical Association, 282,* 657–663.

Birketvedt, G. S., Sundsfjord, J., & Florholmen, J. R. (2002). Hypothalamic–pituitary–adrenal axis in the night eating syndrome. *American Journal of Physiology, 282,* E366–E369.

Braun, D. L., Sunday, S. R., Fornari, V. M., & Halmi, K. A. (1999). Bright light therapy decreases winter binge frequency in women with bulimia nervosa: A double-blind, placebo-controlled study. *Comprehensive Psychiatry, 40*(6), 442–448.

Brinkhuijsen, M., Koenegracht, F., & Meesters, Y. (2003). Symptoms of seasonal affective disorder and of obsessive–compulsive disorder reduced by light therapy. *Journal of Affective Disorders, 74*(3), 307–308.

Bylesjo, E., Boman, K., & Wetterberg, L. (1996). Obesity treated with phototherapy: Four case studies. *International Journal of Eating Disorders, 20,* 443–446.

Carlson, C. R., & Hoyle, R. H. (1993). Efficacy of abbreviated progressive muscle relaxation training: A quantitative review of behavioral medicine research. *Journal of Consulting and Clinical Psychology, 61,* 1059–1067.

Chan, P. K., Lam, R. W., & Perry, K. F. (1994). Mania precipitated by light therapy for patients with SAD. *Journal of Clinical Psychiatry, 55,* 454.

Coates, T. J. (1978). Successive self-management strategies toward coping with night eating. *Journal of Behavior Therapy and Experimental Psychiatry, 9,* 181–183.

Dalle Grave, R., Calugi, S., Ruocco, A., & Marchesini, G. (2011). Night eating syndrome and weight loss outcome in obese patients. *International Journal of Eating Disorders, 44*(2), 150–156.

Demiralp, M., Oflaz, F., & Komurcu, S. (2010). Effects of relaxation training on sleep quality and fatigue in patients with breast cancer undergoing adjuvant chemotherapy. *Journal of Clinical Nursing, 19*(7–8), 1073–1083.

Dowling, G. A., Graf, C. L., Hubbard, E. M., & Luxenberg, J. S. (2007). Light treatment for neuropsychiatric behaviors in Alzheimer's disease. *Western Journal of Nursing Research, 29*(8), 961–975.

Fahey, C. D., & Zee, P. C. (2006). Circadian rhythm sleep disorders and phototherapy. *Psychiatric Clinics of North America, 29*(4), 989–1007.

Friedman, S., Even, C., Dardennes, R., & Guelfi, J. D. (2002). Light therapy, obesity, and night eating syndrome. *American Journal of Psychiatry, 159,* 875–876.

Friedman, S., Even, C., Dardennes, R., & Guelfi, J. D. (2004). Light therapy, nonseasonal depression and night eating syndrome. *Canadian Journal of Psychiatry, 49*(11), 790.

Gallin, P. F., Terman, M., Reme, C. E., Rafferty, B., Terman, J. S., & Burde, R. M. (1995). Ophthalmologic examination of patients with seasonal affective disorder, before and after bright light therapy. *American Journal of Ophthalmology, 119,* 202–210.

Ghafari, S., Ahmadi, F., Nabavi, M., Anoshirvan, K., Memarian, R., & Rafatbakhsh, M. (2009). Effectiveness of applying progressive muscle relaxation technique on quality of life of patients with multiple sclerosis. *Journal of Clinical Nursing, 18*(15), 2171–2179.

Gluck, M. E., Geliebter, A., & Satov, T. (2001). Night eating syndrome is associated with depression, low self-esteem, reduced daytime hunger, and less weight loss in obese outpatients. *Obesity Research, 9,* 264–267.

Goel, N., Stunkard, A. M., Rogers, N. L., Van Dongen, H. P. A., Allison, K. C., O'Reardon, J. P., et al. (2009). Circadian rhythm profiles in women with night eating syndrome. *Journal of Biological Rhythms, 24*(1), 85–94.

Golden, R. N., Gaynes, B. N., Ekstrom, D., Hamer, R. M., Jacobsen, F. M., Suppes, T., et al. (2005). The efficacy of light therapy in the treatment of mood disorders: A review and meta-analysis of the evidence. *American Journal of Psychiatry, 162,* 656–662.

Jacobson, E. (1938). *Progressive relaxation.* Chicago: University of Chicago Press.

King, N. J. (1980). Abbreviated progressive relaxation. *Progressive Behavior Modification, 3,* 147–182.

Kristeller, J. L., & Hallett, C. B. (1999). An exploratory study of a meditation-based intervention for binge eating disorder. *Journal of Health Psychology, 4*(3), 357–363.

Labbate, L. A., Lafer, B., Thibault, A., & Sachs, G. S. (1994). Side effects induced by bright light treatment for seasonal affective disorder. *Journal of Clinical Psychiatry, 55,* 189–191.

Lam, R. W., Lee, S. K., Tam, E. M., Grewal, A, & Yatham, L. N. (2001). An open trial of light therapy for women with seasonal affective disorder and comorbid bulimia nervosa. *Journal of Clinical Psychiatry, 62*(3), 164–168.

Lundgren, J. D., Allison, K. C., O'Reardon, J. P., & Stunkard, A. J. (2008). A descriptive study of non-obese persons with night eating syndrome and a weight-matched comparison group. *Eating Behaviors, 9*(3), 343–351.

Morone, N. E., & Greco, C. M. (2007). Mind–body interventions for chronic pain in older adults: A structured review. *Pain Medicine, 8*(4), 359–375.

Pawlow, L. A., & Jones, G. E. (2002). The impact of abbreviated progressive muscle relaxation on salivary cortisol. *Biological Psychology, 60,* 1–16.

Pawlow, L. A., & Jones, G. E. (2005). The impact of abbreviated progressive muscle relaxation on salivary cortisol and salivary immunoglobulin A. *Applied Psychophysiology and Biofeedback, 30,* 375–387.

Pawlow, L. A., O'Neil, P. M., & Malcolm, R. J. (2003). Night eating syndrome: Effects of brief relaxation training on stress, mood, hunger, and eating patterns. *International Journal of Obesity, 27,* 970–978.

Powers, P. S., Perez, A., Boyd, F., & Rosemurgy, A. (1999). Eating pathology before and after bariatric surgery: A prospective study. *International Journal of Eating Disorders, 25*, 293–300.

Reid, K. J., Baron, K. G., Lu, B., Naylor, E., Wolfe, L., & Zee, P. C. (2010). Aerobic exercise improves self-reported sleep and quality of life in older adults with insomnia. *Sleep Medicine, 11*(9), 934–940.

Rosenthal, N. E., Sack, D. A., Gillin, J. C., Lewy, A. J., Goodwin, F. K., Davenport, Y., et al. (1984). Seasonal affective disorder: A description of the syndrome and preliminary findings with light therapy. *Archives of General Psychiatry, 41*, 72–80.

Stunkard, A. J., Grace, W. J., & Wolff, H. G. (1955). The night-eating syndrome: A pattern of food intake among certain obese patients. *American Journal of Medicine, 19*, 78–86.

Tam, E. M., Lam, R. W., & Levitt, A. J. (1995). Treatment of seasonal affective disorder: A review. *Canadian Journal of Psychiatry, 40*, 457–466.

Terman, M., & Terman, J. S. (1999). Bright light therapy: Side effects and benefits across the symptom spectrum. *Journal of Clinical Psychiatry, 60*, 799–808.

Waller, S. M., Vander Wal, J. S., Klurfeld, D. M., McBurney, M. I., Cho, S., Bijlani, S., et al. (2004). Evening ready-to-eat cereal consumption contributes to weight management. *Journal of the American College of Nutrition, 23*(4), 316–321.

Wichianson, J. R., Bughi, S. A., Unger, J. B., Spruijt-Metz, D., & Nguyen-Rodriguez, S. T. (2009). Perceived stress, coping, and night eating in college students. *Stress and Health, 25*(3), 235–240.

Williamson, D. A., Lawson, O. D., Bennett, S. M., & Hinz, L. (1989). Behavioral treatment of night bingeing and rumination in an adult case of bulimia nervosa. *Journal of Behavior Therapy and Experimental Psychiatry, 20*(1), 73–77.

Wing, R. R. (2002). Behavioral weight control. In T. A. Wadden & A. J. Stunkard (Eds.), *Handbook of obesity treatment* (pp. 301–316). New York: Guilford Press.

Chapter 16

Epilogue

Jennifer D. Lundgren
Kelly C. Allison
Albert J. Stunkard

After nearly 50 years of neglect in the literature, night eating syndrome (NES) is gaining research and clinical attention, and those suffering from this disorder are beginning to find help. Our main aim in this volume is just that: to help those who suffer from NES by providing health care professionals with the scientific knowledge and clinical tools necessary to research and treat NES more effectively. We hope that the historical account of NES provided in the beginning of this book provides all readers, professional and lay, with a context for better understanding the development and treatment of NES over the past 50 years.

We hoped to begin this volume with the most basic aspects of NES and to conclude with clinically relevant application, so that both research and clinical audiences would find something of value in it. NES research is in its infancy compared to other eating- and weight-related conditions. Important discoveries in the biology of NES, however, have been made. What is known about the biology of NES was presented in three chapters with a particular focus on pathophysiology, circadian rhythm, and genetics. From these chapters we can conclude:

1. Key neuroendocrine and neurotransmitter systems, including cortisol, melatonin, leptin, ghrelin, insulin, and serotonin, likely play a role in the development and/or maintenance of NES.
2. Persons with NES exhibit a circadian delay in food intake, intact circadian sleep cycle (but with evidence of disturbed sleep homeostasis and architecture), and associated circadian dysregulation of neuroendocrine factors.
3. NES aggregates in families and the heritability of NES may be lower than other eating disorders, such as BED. NES and BED appear to share some genetic liability, but there are likely unique genetic factors, as well as shared and nonshared environmental factors that influence the development of NES.

These are exciting discoveries, but as the authors of each chapter have described, more research is necessary to build on this work. Much of what is known about possible pathophysiological and neuroendocrine aspects of NES comes from only a couple of studies. Replication is necessary. Similarly, only one published study has reported the heritability of NES, and these data were based on screening questions, not a comprehensive assessment of NES. As research in the biological factors associated with NES moves forward, three priorities emerge. First, additional neurotransmitter systems and their interaction with serotonin should be explored in relation to the development and maintenance of night eating. This interaction is especially important as the field works to characterize the relationship between NES and sleep-related eating disorder (SRED) more rigorously. Second, NES has been long conceptualized as a disorder of circadian rhythm. This is intuitive and makes "common sense," but very little physiological data are available to test this hypothesis. Behavioral food intake data support this conceptualization, but the few neuroendocrine studies (with notably small sample sizes) comparing persons with NES to weight-matched control participants are contradictory. There are methodological differences between studies, which could explain different findings. Future research should continue to explore alterations in circadian rhythm among night eaters. Finally, behavioral and molecular genetics studies are needed to better understand the biological underpinnings of NES.

Better understanding of the biological causes and consequences of NES is crucial not only because it informs science, but also because it informs the prevention and treatment of NES. For example, exploration of additional neurotransmitter systems might pave the way for alternative pharmacotherapies. Similarly, better understanding of the role of circadian rhythm and genetics could improve efforts at prevention. Thus persons most at risk could be identified earlier.

Not only will improved understanding of the biology of NES promote prevention and treatment efforts, but it will contribute to describing more fully the relationship between NES and other psychiatric and medical conditions. As reviewed in this text, much of the research on NES has focused on its comorbidity with obesity and eating disorders, as well as mood and other psychiatric disorders. As Colles and Dixon point out in their comprehensive review of NES in the context of obesity (Chapter 6), the question "Does NES cause obesity?" remains to be answered. In our view, this question remains unanswered because of a lack of appropriately designed studies to accurately address this question. As important as they are, prevalence and epidemiological studies that assess participants at only one time point cannot address change across time. So although we know that the prevalence of NES is higher among obese persons than among the general population, it is imperative that future studies assess cohorts across time.

Because much of the NES research has included obese samples, and at times specifically excluded persons with other eating disorders, recent studies finding frequent night eating among persons diagnosed with anorexia nervosa (AN) , bulimia nervosa (BN), and binge-eating disorder (BED) suggest that night eating, much like binge eating, co-occurs across a spectrum of disordered eating behavior. At the time of our preparing this book, DSM-5 has not been published. There is evidence, however, that NES is likely to be included in the eating disorder not otherwise specified (EDNOS) diagnostic category. If this happens, we hope that it will prompt researchers to conduct more studies of the frequency, antecedents, and consequences of night eating behavior among persons diagnosed with other eating disorders, especially BN and BED. The few studies, both genetic and behavioral, reviewed in this book that examined the relationship between NES and other eating disorders suggest that there is potentially significant overlap between night eating and binge-eating behavior. Whether this results from methodological artifact (e.g., differentiating evening hyperphagia from evening binge eating) or biological or behavioral shared vulnerability remains to be answered.

Eating disorders, however, are not the only psychiatric disorder showing significant overlap with NES. As Rempfer and Murphy review in Chapter 8, both mood and anxiety disorders are frequently diagnosed in persons with NES. As they point out, there is overlap among major depression, generalized anxiety disorder, and NES in mood, appetite, and sleep features. This could contribute to the high rates of comorbidity, and it is also likely that for some individuals, night eating develops in an attempt to remedy sleep problems that occur in the context of preexisting mood and anxiety disorders. Similar to the question "Does NES cause obesity?", the causal relationship between NES and other psychiatric disorders will remain unanswered until future studies follow cohorts across time. Shorter studies using real-time ecological assessment methods may also improve our understanding of the relationship between night eating, mood, and anxiety (e.g., ecological momentary assessment techniques could be used to study the emotional and behavioral antecedents and consequences of night eating behavior).

Another area in which future research is necessary in order to move the field forward is sleep. The relationship of NES with sleep disorders, in particular SRED, remains understudied. For years, the eating and sleep research communities have conceptualized NES and SRED as distinct disorders. There is evidence to suggest that, in fact, NES and SRED may share similar behavioral features (e.g., ingestion of food at night), but may have distinct etiologies and treatments. It is also possible, however, that much of the distinction between NES and SRED is arbitrary and relatively untested. Take for example, the construct "awareness of eating behavior." Historically, one of the ways in which NES and SRED were differentiated was the individual's level of awareness during nocturnal eating episodes: persons with SRED were described has having little or no awareness (amnestic eating), while persons with NES were described as having much or full awareness. Careful review of studies and anecdotal descriptions from patients would suggest that researcher and clinician conceptualization of awareness is subjective.

In addition, as Howell and Crow point out in Chapter 9, amnestic nocturnal eating is not a criterion for SRED, and they provide evidence to suggest that amnestic eating may be specific to hypnotic medication use, not SRED per se. Because of the association of SRED with amnestic eating, patients diagnosed with SRED, compared to NES, are more likely to eat nonfood substances or engage in dangerous food preparation. There is little evidence to suggest, however, that persons diagnosed with SRED who are aware of their nocturnal eating actually eat dangerous or peculiar foods at night. Finally, although the sleep and eating disorder fields have developed different treatments for NES and SRED, there is some treatment overlap in that both appear to respond to the anticonvulsant topiramate. We hope that this book will encourage eating and sleep researchers, as well as clinicians assessing and treating NES and SRED, to become more curious about their relationship.

The final section of this book focused on assessment and treatment of night eating. Of all of the information included in this text, this sec-tion is the most important for the alleviation of suffering caused by night eating. We are often struck by the number of people who contact us from across the globe requesting treatment for NES. Repeatedly, people have shared frustrated accounts of seeking treatment for their night eat-ing only to be dismissed or misunderstood by their health care provider. In fact, due in part to frequent requests for treatment by individuals who lived a distance from Philadelphia, we initiated a long-distance treatment study using the medication sertraline. As reviewed by Patel, O'Reardon, and Cristancho in Chapter 12, participants were treated with sertraline by their own physician while we assessed them via phone regularly for 8 weeks. Treatment response was quite similar to that found in our ran-domized clinical trial of sertraline for NES, with significant pre- to post-treatment improvements in the Night Eating Symptom Scale, evening hyperphagia, nocturnal awakenings and ingestions, Beck Depression Inventory scores, and body weight.

We hope that this final section of the book provides clinicians with concrete tools for better assessment and treatment of patients who suffer from NES. In particular, we present several assessment tools for NES, including an updated Night Eating Syndrome History and Inventory that corresponds to the new research diagnostic criteria (outlined in the intro-duction). The treatment chapters offer clinicians and patients a range of interventions, and we hope that Allison's cognitive-behavioral treatment manual (Chapter 14) provides guidance for clinicians who want to treat NES through psychotherapy alone or in combination with pharmaco-therapy.

As highlighted in the lone pilot study of CBT for NES, the treatment seems to work well in reducing nocturnal ingestions, but we still have work to do in honing the treatment to induce larger decreases in evening hyperphia. In addition, data suggest that normal-weight and overweight/ obese persons with NES may manifest their symptoms differently, with more inappropriate compensatory strategies, such as excessive exercise and purposeful daytime food restriction. We may need to create different modules to address (1) weight loss in overweight and obese patients and (2) compensatory behaviors in under- or normal-weight patients.

Taken together, our experience, and that of our patients', suggests that much more work is needed to develop, test, and disseminate evi-dence-based assessment and treatment for NES. There are several ways to accomplish this. First, more treatment outcome studies are needed to confirm or disconfirm previous findings. In addition to replication tri-als, studies of novel interventions are necessary to develop the intervention literature further. Also, researchers and clinicians are encouraged to present their treatment outcome work at local, regional, and national/international conferences. Finally, we encourage experienced clinicians to work with health care providers in their communities to teach evidence-based assessment and treatment methods for NES to other providers. We have often consulted with clinicians both in our communities and at a distance to help disseminate these interventions. We hope that, through reading this book, more practitioners will feel confident identifying and treating NES in their practice, and consequently fewer persons will continue suffering from it.

In summary, as we reflect on this book and the state of the literature, we are hopeful that the research and clinical communities have finally gained the momentum necessary to more fully understand and treat NES. As Mitchell stated in the foreword, "The book . . . highlights not only what has been learned but what remains controversial." We agree and encourage readers to take the torch and shed their own light on NES. It is only through continued observation and testing that we as a field will be able to fully understand NES and provide relief to persons who struggle with it.

Index

The letter *f* after an entry indicates figure; the letter *t* indicates table.